Promoting Legal Awareness in Physical and Occupational Therapy

About the Author

Ron Scott is an associate professor in the Department of Physical Therapy, School of Allied Health Sciences, University of Texas Health Science Center at San Antonio. Ron teaches Health Care Systems, Professional Ethics, Patient Care I, Management and Administration, and Differential Diagnosis, and coordinates a Pathology and Pharmacology course in the department's Master of Physical Therapy program.

Ron is also an adjunct assistant professor in the Master of Arts in Health Services Management program at Webster University, where he teaches Organizational Planning, Health Policy Issues, and Law and Health Services courses. He also has a consulting law and risk management practice.

Ron retired from the Army in 1994, where he was a Judge Advocate General (JAG) Corps officer and physical therapist-clinician and manager. He has been married since 1973 to Maria Josefa ("Pepi") Barba Garces. They have two sons, Ron, Jr., an English education major at the University of North Texas, and Paul, a senior at Madison High School.

Ron is the current chair of the American Physical Therapy Association's Judicial Committee, a legal faculty member for APTA's risk management seminar program, and a member of the Editorial Advisory Board for *PT: The Magazine of Physical Therapy*. He has written over 70 articles on orthopedics, quality and risk management, human resources management, and law and ethics. This is Ron's third book, the others being *Legal Aspects of Documenting Patient Care* (Aspen 1994) and *Health Care Malpractice: A Primer on Legal Issues* (Slack 1990).

In his spare time, Ron likes to travel, play guitar, collect Beatles paraphernalia, and write comedy and fiction works.

Promoting Legal Awareness in Physical and Occupational Therapy

RON SCOTT, JD, PT, OCS

Associate Professor

Physical Therapy Department, School of Allied Health Sciences

University of Texas Health Science Center

San Antonio, Texas

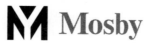 Mosby

St. Louis Baltimore Boston Carlsbad Chicago Naples New York Philadelphia Portland

London Madrid Mexico City Singapore Sydney Tokyo Toronto Wiesbaden

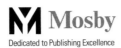

Mosby
Dedicated to Publishing Excellence

A Times Mirror Company

Publisher: Don Ladig
Executive Editor: Martha Sasser
Developmental Editor: Kellie F. White
Project Manager: Mark Spann
Production Editor: Julie Eddy
Designer: TSI Graphics, Inc.
Manufacturing Supervisor: Karen Boehme

Cover photograph by Franz Jantzen, Collection of the Supreme Court of the United States. Pgs. 118–119 Source: Reprinted with permission of the American Hospital Association, copyright 1992. Pgs. 296–297 and 300–302 Source: from *The American Journal of Occupational Therapy*, 48(11). Copyright 1994 by the American Occupational Therapy Association, Inc. Reprinted with permission. Pgs. 291–295 and 298–299 Source: Reprinted with permission of the APTA.

Printed in the United States of America
Composition by TSI Graphics, Inc.
Printing/binding by Maple-Vail

Mosby-Year Book, Inc.
11830 Westline Industrial Drive
St. Louis, MO 63146

Library of Congress Cataloging in Publication Data

Scott, Ronald W.
    Promoting legal awareness in physical and occupational therapy / [Ronald W. Scott].
    p. cm.
    Includes bibliographical references and index.
    ISBN 0-8151-7996-0
    1. Medical care—Law and legislation—United States. 2. Medical laws and legislation—United States. 3. Physical therapists—Legal status, laws, etc.—United States. I. Title.
    KF3821.Z9S367   1996
    344.73'041—dc20
    [347.30441]
                                         96—33589
                                             CIP

96 97 98 99 00 / 9 8 7 6 5 4 3 2 1

I dedicate this book to my life's love, my wife Pepi,
and to our two sons, Ron, Jr. and Paul.

Preface

All licensed health care professionals are justifiably concerned about potential litigation incident to the practice of their professions. This concern stems in part from publicity about the health care "malpractice crisis," in which licensed health care providers from various disciplines have increasingly been named as malpractice defendants in lawsuits brought by patients. This "crisis," although real and of relatively recent vintage, may be somewhat overstated. The greater dilemma involves a general civil "litigation crisis," evidenced by the fact that over 19 million new civil lawsuits of all kinds were filed in the United States during 1992 (the most recent year for which there are statistics). What makes this statistic all the more frightening is the fact that these new cases compound an existing litigation backlog of tens of millions of pending cases awaiting trial, settlement, or other disposition.

While only a small percentage of the new and existing cases in the litigation pipeline are health care malpractice lawsuits, the adverse effects of health care malpractice lawsuits on all parties affected by them can be particularly devastating. Patients who are victims of health care malpractice suffer physical and mental injury. When they are injured by malpractice, these victims incur additional medical expenses to effect a cure for their iatrogenic injuries. They lose wages, salaries, and often future earnings potential. They suffer short- and long-term pain and suffering and even permanent "loss of enjoyment of life" in some cases.

Health care professionals charged with having committed malpractice also suffer adverse consequences from formal and informal allegations of wrongdoing. They suffer emotional and physical injury from stress related to the allegations and loss of business reputation. The stress they feel often has adverse effects on their familial and personal relationships. These health care professionals feel real pain for having possibly breached their sacred duty owed to patients under their care.

In the case of serious bodily injury or death of a patient, often a health care professional will face legal and administrative actions in settings other than just the civil legal system. In cases involving serious injury and allegations of intentional misconduct or reckless disregard for patient welfare, providers may also face legal actions brought by the government in criminal court. Adverse administrative action affecting professional licensure may also result. When cases involve possible ethics violations, disciplinary processes before providers' professional associations may also ensue.

Society, too, is a victim of health care malpractice. The administrative costs associated with adjudicating malpractice claims and litigating lawsuits is enormous. The costs for additional medical and related care for malpractice victims is likewise extremely high, as are malpractice settlement and judgment awards for past, present, and future damages. Additionally, a significant proportion of aggregate health care costs are attributable to "defensive practice" secondary to a fear of malpractice litigation exposure.

While the fear of and actual costs associated with health care malpractice legal actions take a significant toll on providers, patients, and society as a whole, other types of litigation are much more pervasive and costly. Included among these other types of health-related litigation are *business litigation actions* such as breach of contract, tortious interference with an existing contractual relationship, and business disparagement; *employment-setting actions*, such as wrongful discharge from employment, employment discrimination, and sexual harassment; and *criminal and civil actions* brought by governmental entities against health care professionals, such as *antitrust actions* and Medicare and Medicaid *fraud actions*.

This book is intended to provide a basic overview of health care legal issues for clinicians, clinical managers, health care facility administrators, educators, and professional and post-professional students. Although the material presented focuses on two specific disciplines—physical and occupational therapy—the concepts and issues are applicable to all other health care disciplines whose member-providers care for patients and engage in business pursuits.

The book begins in Chapter 1 by presenting an introduction to the American legal system and its principal component parts: the civil and criminal state and federal legal systems and the administrative agencies that operate at the federal and state levels. Next, the text defines and distinguishes the related concepts of *law* and *ethics*, and discusses how the two concepts have come to be blended over time. Chapter 1 ends with frank discussion about the American litigation and malpractice crises and state and federal tort reform efforts.

Chapter 2 presents a capsule overview of concepts and issues related to health care malpractice. Actual reported case scenarios involving physical and occupational therapists (with universal applicability to all other health care disciplines) are presented, along with easy-to-understand boxed highlights of key malpractice concepts. The chapter also defines and differentiates the concepts of *professional* and *ordinary negligence* and points out how both types of allegations commonly arise in clinical health care practice.

Chapter 3 addresses liability for intentional conduct. *Conduct* includes both affirmative actions (*acts*) and failure to act when one should (*omissions*). Liability for intentional acts and omissions in the health care treatment environment can result both from conduct that can be labeled *malicious*, as well as for conduct that is nonmalicious. Malicious liability-generating conduct includes acts such as commission of sexual battery upon a patient, while nonmalicious intentional acts for which malpractice liability might attach include administration of modality treatment on the wrong limb that results in patient injury. This chapter discusses several key specific intentional "wrongs," including assault and battery, false imprisonment, fraud, invasion of privacy, and sexual misconduct.

Chapter 4 presents a thorough overview of the legal and ethical considerations concerning patient informed consent to treatment. Perhaps no principle in health care delivery is as fundamental as respect for patient autonomy and control over treatment decision-making processes. Every health care professional has the legal and ethical duty to involve patients (or their surrogate decision makers) in treatment decisions. This chapter proposes a specific litany of disclosure elements for universal use by health care clinicians in routine practice, which ensure that patients understand the nature of treatments recommended or ordered, any material (decisional) risks of serious harm associated with proposed interventions, reasonable alternatives (if any) to proposed treatments, and the short- and long-term goals of treatment. The chapter concludes with discussion of informed consent requirements and processes applicable in clinical research settings.

Chapter 5 discusses contract law issues. After introductory material addressing the general nature of contracts and contractual legal obligations—including differentiating *bilateral* from *unilateral* contracts and written from oral agreements—the chapter explains how every health care professional-patient interaction is legally (at least) an implied contractual relationship, albeit with special status under law. The chapter ends with discussion about clinical affiliation agreements, contracts between students and employers, restrictive employment contractual provisions, and express and implied continuing education contractual obligations.

Chapter 6 addresses criminal law issues, including the relative incidence of criminal allegations among health professionals and a summary of the types of reported legal actions brought against them. This chapter also discusses state and federal *jurisdiction* (control over cases) and criminal procedure. Specific criminal actions discussed include employment fraud and misrepresentation and reimbursement fraud.

Chapter 7 overviews the educational legal environment. The chapter begins with discussion about the fundamental right of privacy and its applicability in the educational setting. It next overviews educational disciplinary processes and defines *procedural* and *substantive due process*. The chapter concludes with discussion of liability issues in education, including liability of academic faculty, clinical instructors, students, and institutions.

Chapter 8 addresses employment law. It begins by differentiating employment "at will" from employment under contract. An overview of management-labor relations follows, along with a summary of several key federal employment statutes. These include The Age Discrimination in Employment Act, The Americans with Disabilities Act, The Civil Rights Act of 1964 (Title VII), The Civil Rights Act of 1991, The Employee Retirement Income Security Act, The Family and Medical Leave Act, The Freedom of Information Act, The Polygraph Protection Act, The Pregnancy Discrimination Act, The Privacy Act, and The Rehabilitation Act of 1973. The chapter also addresses the sensitive and salient topic of workplace sexual harassment and the obligations incumbent upon employers and employees, including the alleged victims of sexual harassment. The chapter concludes with discussion of several key human resource management issues, namely recruitment, credentialing and privileging actions, and employee discipline.

Chapter 9 summarizes insurance law as it relates to health care professional liability policies. The discussion includes the insurer-insured relationship, duties incumbent upon both parties, and the differences between occurrence and claims-made professional liability policies.

Chapter 10 encompasses several important miscellaneous business law concepts. These include administrative law issues related to licensure and administrative discipline, antitrust law and its application to health care delivery and providers, attorney-health care professional relations, forms of business organization, the business torts of business *disparagement*, or *trade libel*, and tortious (injurious) interference with an existing or prospective business relationship, advertising professional services, Good Samaritan statutes, legal research, and discussion of the Patient Self-Determination Act.

Chapter 11, the final chapter of the book, overviews health care professional ethics. In addition to discussing ethical issues in the clinical and research settings, this chapter discusses professional association codes of ethics and their relation to legal standards.

Each chapter of the book begins with a synopsis of its contents and ends with a summary of key concepts. Annotated references and suggested readings are included for each chapter for the purpose of providing additional sources for further research and study. Hypothetical case examples appear at the end of each chapter, followed by suggested answers to the problems posed in those cases.

Although this book of necessity utilizes legal terminology when describing complex legal principles, every attempt has been made to be sensitive to the fact that lay readers are not attorneys or jurists. In that regard, I have strived to minimize the use of legal jargon, or "legalese." I also thought it important to summarize key legal concepts and relevant laws in the form of a glossary of legal terms at the end of the book.

Finally, to add to the publisher's disclaimer about the nature of the material presented in this book, readers are cautioned that legal principles are not only complex, but subject to change on an ongoing basis. In fact, law students are frequently reminded by their professors that about 25 percent of current law is supplemented or replaced approximately every ten years. Consider what you read in this text as general legal *information*. For specific legal *advice*—both proactive and in response to specific situations raising legal issues—readers are advised to consult with their personal or institutional attorneys.

Through effective clinical risk management, awareness of the legal environment, and sensitivity to the importance of good interpersonal relations with patients, colleagues, and others in the business environment, health care professionals can begin to solve the litigation crisis—one reader at a time.

Ron Scott

Acknowledgments

I first wish to acknowledge my wife for her endless support of my professional endeavors, especially the completion of this project. I also acknowledge all of my professional colleagues in physical and occupational therapy for their dedication to excellence in patient care and the advancement of the professions. Recognition also is extended to my legal colleagues for their professionalism and perserverence in the pursuit of excellence. Finally, my thanks are extended to my editorial staff at Mosby for their superb work on my manuscript: Martha Sasser, Kellie White, and Amy Dubin.

Contents

Chapter 7 Education Law

Chapter 8 Employment Law

Chapter 9 Insurance Law

Chapter 10 Business Law

Chapter 11 Health Care Ethics

APPENDICES

Promoting Legal Awareness in Physical and Occupational Therapy

Chapter 1

Introduction to Health Care Law and Ethics

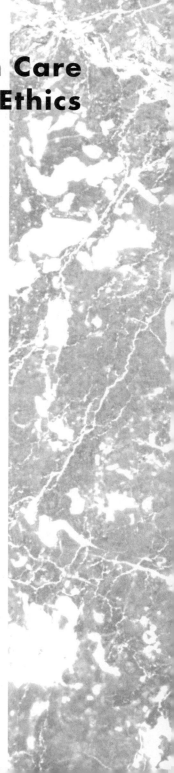

*H*ealth care professionals, like other professionals and citizens, are subject to compliance with legal obligations and personal moral beliefs. Health care professionals are also bound to comply with ethical obligations incident to practice, as reflected in professional association codes of ethics. Sources of legal obligations include: federal and state constitutions, legislatively-created statutory laws, judge-made common (case) law, and administrative rules and regulations promulgated by state and federal administrative agencies.

Legal actions against health care professionals can take place in either criminal or civil courts. Criminal actions brought by the state, incident to health care delivery, are normally limited to situations where there are material issues concerning possible intentional misconduct. Civil legal actions for malpractice are brought by patients against health care providers, where the burden of proof—preponderance, or greater weight of evidence—is lower than in the criminal justice system, where the state must prove a defendant's culpability by the standard "beyond a reasonable doubt."

While there is an obvious civil litigation crisis in the United States, the magnitude of a specific health care malpractice crisis is less certain. Still, tort reform efforts designed to limit health care malpractice plaintiffs' access to court continue to proliferate.

Nature of the American Legal System

The American legal system is divided into two broad subsystems: the criminal legal system and the civil legal system. Every state has its own criminal and civil trial-level and appellate courts, as does the federal government. American criminal and civil law are grounded in British common (judge-made) law and in the legal codes of France, Spain, and other "code" nations. Foundational British common law, the Napoleonic code, and other codes have been substantially replaced or augmented over time with American case (common) law, state and federal statutes, and laws from other sources.

Jurisdiction

State or federal courts in either the criminal or civil legal system exercise jurisdiction, or power, over *litigants* (jurisdiction over parties, or *in personam jurisdiction*), over property that is the subject of litigation (*in rem jurisdiction*), and over specific types of cases (*subject-matter jurisdiction*). The federal courts have (or at least were expected by the founders of the United States to have) limited jurisdiction over issues involving specific federal interests, while state courts are courts of broad, general jurisdiction. State courts have *exclusive* (or at least primary) *jurisdiction* over purely state governmental matters, such as crimes occurring within the state (but not on federal property), domestic and family relations, establishment of private businesses (including incorporation of businesses), insurance, traffic offenses, and health care malpractice and related issues, among many other areas of interest. Federal courts have *concurrent* (shared) *jurisdiction* with states over areas such as the interpretation of state and (most) federal laws.

Federal courts also share jurisdiction with states over what would seem to be exclusively state business, including health care malpractice cases, under a concept known as *diversity of citizenship jurisdiction*. Diversity jurisdiction applies when all parties on one side of a civil case are citizens of different states than the parties on the opposing side of the case. Diversity jurisdiction was originally intended to prevent inequity, or unfairness, to an out-of-state party in a civil case that might occur in a state court. Because of the growing case burden on federal judges, however, diversity jurisdiction has been limited in recent times to cases involving a monetary amount in controversy of greater than $50,000.[1]

The federal courts exercise *exclusive jurisdiction* over limited types of cases for which the Constitution grants the federal courts such power. These types of cases include antitrust actions; bankruptcy proceedings; federal crimes; military law and policy cases; patent, copyright, and trademark actions; and lawsuits brought against the United States.

Sources of Law

Constitutional Law

There are four main sources of law. The preeminent source of legal authority is the federal Constitution, which is universally recognized as the "supreme law of the land." All other laws, regulations, and rules are subordinate in authority to the express provisions of the Constitution and to interpretations of federal constitutional law made by courts. Although there is an historical, ongoing controversy over authority to interpret the Constitution (because of the separation of powers doctrine involving the relative power of the President, Congress, and the Supreme Court), the U.S. Supreme Court is (usually) the final arbiter in interpreting and enforcing the Constitution.

Many cases interpreting the Constitution over the history of U.S. law have directly or indirectly impacted health care delivery, including cases interpreting the meaning and scope of *due process* of law (fundamental fairness) and creating the fundamental *right of* (individual) *privacy*. In fact, the first case in which the Supreme Court established a fundamental right of privacy, *Griswold* v. *Connecticut*,[2] turned on whether a conjugate adult couple could legally purchase pharmaceutical contraceptives for birth control. The *Griswold* case is also the first and only instance where a court created an implied federal constitutional right, and in the majority Supreme Court decision, written by Justice Douglas, one sees how this implied constitutional right of privacy was fashioned from express rights enunciated in the Bill of Rights.

> *Specific guarantees in the Bill of Rights have penumbras [fringe areas], formed by emanations from those guarantees that helped give them life and substance. Various guarantees create zones of privacy. The rights of association contained in the penumbra of the first amendment is one, . . . the third amendment in its prohibition against the quartering of soldiers 'in any house- 'in time of peace without the consent of the owner is another. . . . The fourth amendment explicitly affirms the right of the people to be secure in their persons, houses, papers, and effects against unreasonable searches and seizures. The fifth amendment in its self-incrimination clause enables the citizen to create a zone of privacy which government may not force him to surrender to his detriment. The ninth amendment provides 'the enumeration in the Constitution of certain rights will not be construed to deny or disparage others retained by the people.'*
>
> *The present case [Griswold] concerns a relationship lying within the zone of privacy created by several fundamental constitutional guarantees. . . .*
>
> *We deal with a right of privacy older than the Bill of Rights—older than our political parties, older than our school system. Marriage is a coming together for better or worse, hopefully enduring and intimate to the degree of being sacred. It is an association that promotes a way of life, not causes; a harmony in living, not political faith; a bilateral loyalty, not commercial or social projects. Yet it is an association for as noble a purpose as any involved in our prior decisions.*[3]

Virtually all of the express provisions related to personal rights and liberties in the federal Constitution are found, not in the body of the document, but in the amendments to the Constitution. Personal rights and liberties of citizens were not written into the main Constitution by the founding fathers during the Constitutional Convention of 1787. The personal rights enunciated in the Bill of Rights—added in 1791, were, in large part, fashioned after the Virginia state bill of rights. The first ten of these amendments, originally intended to protect citizens from undue interference with activities of daily living by the federal government (but most later applied also to state governmental intrusion), are collectively known as the "Bill of Rights." These rights are as follows. (Take note of how many of these protections relate directly to the operation of physical and occupational therapy practices.)

Amendment I: Congress shall make no law respecting an establishment of religion, or prohibiting the free exercise thereof; or abridging the freedom of speech, or of the press; or the right of the people peaceably to assemble, and to petition the Government for a redress of grievances.

Amendment II: A well regulated Militia, being necessary to the security of a free State, the right of the people to keep and bear Arms, shall not be infringed.

Amendment III: No quartering of soldiers in private homes during peacetime. [Obsolete.]

Amendment IV: The right of the people to be secure in their persons, houses, papers, and effects, against unreasonable searches and seizures, shall not be violated, and no Warrants shall issue, but upon probable cause, supported by Oath or affirmation and particularly describing the place to be searched, and the persons or things to be seized.

Amendment V: No person shall be held to answer for a capital, or otherwise infamous crime, unless on a presentment or indictment of a Grand Jury, except in cases arising in the land or naval forces, or in the Militia, when in actual service in time of War or public danger; nor shall any person be subject for the same offense to be twice put in jeopardy of life or limb; nor shall be compelled in any criminal case to be a witness against himself, nor be deprived of life, liberty, or property, without due process of law; nor shall private property be taken for public use, without just compensation.

Amendment VI: In all criminal prosecutions, the accused shall enjoy the right to a speedy and public trial, by an impartial jury of the State and district wherein the crime shall have been committed, which district shall have been previously ascertained by law, and to be informed of the nature and cause of the accusation; to be confronted with the witnesses against him; to have compulsory process for obtaining witnesses in his favor, and to have the Assistance of Counsel for his defense.

Amendment VII: In Suits at common law, where the value in controversy shall exceed twenty dollars, the right of trial by jury shall be preserved, and no fact tried by jury, shall be otherwise reexamined in any Court of the United States, than according to the rules of the common law.

Amendment VIII: Excessive bail shall not be required, nor excessive fines imposed, nor cruel and unusual punishments inflicted.

Amendment IX: The enumeration in the Constitution, of certain rights, shall not be construed to deny or disparage others retained by the people.

Amendment X: The powers not delegated to the United States by the Constitution, nor prohibited by it to the States, are reserved to the States respectively, or to the people.[4]

Law derived from state constitutions also is "supreme" vis-a-vis other forms of state law. However, state constitutional law must conform with the federal Constitution. States are free to grant their citizens greater rights than are allowed by the federal Constitution, but cannot take away rights, privileges, and immunities granted to citizens of the United States by the federal Constitution.

Statutory Law

The second source of law is statutory law. Congress and state legislatures enact *statutes* within their scope of authority. Federal statutes, published in the United States Code (U.S.C.), are divided by subject into "Titles." Examples of important federal statutes affecting health care delivery include The Americans with Disabilities Act, The Civil Rights Acts of 1964 and 1991, The Family and Medical Leave Act, The Federal Torts Claims Act, The Patient Self-Determination Act, The Privacy Act, and The Rehabilitation Act of 1973. State statutes enacted by state legislatures are controlling laws in areas where the federal government does not have jurisdiction. Examples of state statutes include those creating health care professional practice acts and insurance statutes.

Common Law

The third source of law is judge-made case law. These court decisions are also referred to as *common law* and encompass all judicial decisions creating legal precedent in areas where legislatures have not enacted statutes. The earliest common law affecting the United States was English common law. Many common law legal precedents are still based on the earliest English common law. Most American civil legal authority comes from common law, including laws related to health care malpractice and business relationships involving health care professionals and others.

Although the common law is considered more flexible and quicker to adapt to societal change than the relatively rigid statutory law, common law is still characterized by relative stability. The concept of *stare decisis*, or "the decision stands", requires all lower courts in a jurisdiction to conform to prior decisions made by a higher level court within the jurisdiction. Standing court decisions, then, are called precedents, and changes in existing precedents take place at the highest level courts—not at the lowest, trial-level courts.

Administrative Law

The final source of law derives from administrative agencies at the federal and state levels. Administrative agencies exercise delegated authority from the executive and legislative branches of government. They are empowered to exercise legislative (rule-making), executive (management), and judicial (enforcement) functions. In their legislative role, administrative agencies promulgate everyday rules and regulations to supplement statutes and executive orders. Such administrative rules and regulations are usually previewed for public comment and debate (such as in the Code of Federal Regulations, or CFR) before attaining the force of law. Once final, though, these rules and regulations govern business conduct in great detail. It is widely accepted as fact that health care professional business people have more interface with administrative agencies than with any other legal entity.

Examples of federal administrative agencies having broad power over the business affairs of health care professionals include The Center for Disease Control (CDC), The Equal Employment Opportunity Commission (EEOC), The Health Care Financing Administration (HCFA), The Occupational Safety and Health Administration (OSHA), The National Labor Relations Board (NLRB), and The Social Security Administration (SSA). Examples of administrative agencies at the state level include health care professional licensure agencies and workers' compensation authorities.

Secondary Sources of Legal Authority

Additional (secondary) sources of law (which legislative, judicial, and executive decision-makers rely on as "authorities") include professional association and institutional practice standards, protocols, and guidelines. Other secondary law sources include accreditation standards and guidelines promulgated by private accreditation agencies, such as the Joint Commission on Accreditation of Healthcare Organizations (JCAHO), the Commission on Accreditation of Rehabilitation Facilities (CARF), and the National Committee on Quality Assurance (NCQA), among others.

Due Process of Law

The Fifth and Fourteenth Amendments to the Constitution require that no person be deprived of the rights to "life, liberty, and property without due process of law." Due process equates to fundamental fairness. It implies that all people will be treated the same under law, and will be given the opportunity to challenge legal actions against them which affect important aspects of their lives.

Substantive Due Process

There are two components of due process—*substantive due process* and *procedural due process*. Substantive due process focuses on whether legal actions—particularly legislation—are substantively fair. For most actions, they must be shown to be rationally or reasonably related to a legitimate governmental purpose. For example, a state statute requiring licensure for physical and occupational therapists is reasonably related to the legitimate governmental purpose of protecting the health and welfare of patients served by these professionals in the state. When legal actions will adversely affect fundamental rights, such as privacy, free speech, voting, and the right to travel, substantive due process requires that such laws be narrowly written to promote a compelling or overriding governmental interest. For example, states may legally prohibit elective abortion in the third trimester, based on the state's compelling interests in protecting developing, viable fetal life.[5]

Procedural Due Process

Procedural due process focuses on administrative requirements for fairness in legal actions. Anyone whose life, liberty, or property interests—including educational degrees, employment rights and professional licensure—would be adversely affected by such action, must: (1) be apprised of the nature of the action proposed, and (2) be given the opportunity to respond on his or her behalf before final action is taken. An example of procedural due process is the legal requirement that, before administrative discipline of a physical or occupational therapist by a licensure board can take place, the *respondent* must be given adequate notice of the charge(s) against him or her and the range of potential adverse actions, and the opportunity to present his or her case to the decision-maker.

Criminal and Civil Law Defined and Distinguished

Criminal law involves legal actions brought on behalf of society for violations of its criminal laws against a defendant or multiple defendants. Criminal legal actions are labeled "public" law, and their case *captions* (titles) reflect this fact. Cases may be titled "*People* v. *Defendant*," "*State* v. *Defendant*," or "*United States* v. *Defendant*."

Civil law, on the other hand, encompasses private legal actions brought by one or more private *plaintiffs* against one or more private *defendants* (including individuals, businesses, and government agencies). All types of private actions are civil law actions, including administrative law cases; cases involving the liability of agents employed by principals; contract law cases; corporate legal actions; domestic relations cases; employment law cases; health care malpractice cases; personal and real property law cases; personal injury cases other than health care malpractice cases; and cases concerning wills, trusts, and estates. (Most private wrongs are termed *torts*, except for cases involving allegations of breach of contract. *Tort* is French for "wrong.")

Parties Bringing Actions in Civil and Criminal Cases

The party bringing criminal and civil charges against defendants differs, too. In civil cases involving private wrongs, the plaintiff is always the victim of the wrong committed (or the victim's legal representative). In criminal legal actions, cases are initiated by prosecutors, who are agents of the state. Because a criminal prosecution is discretionary, the actual victim of a crime does not have an absolute right to compel the government to prosecute the offender.

Standards of Proof

Criminal cases The standards of proof differ greatly between criminal and civil legal actions. In criminal cases—where the stakes for the defendant are much higher than in civil cases and include the sanction of death as a punishment—the government's burden of proof is great. The government prosecutor in a criminal case must prove every element of a criminal charge by the standard of *beyond a reasonable doubt*. This standard requires that the *factfinder* (jury, or the judge, if the criminal defendant does not elect to have a jury trial), be convinced of the defendant's culpability to a moral certainty, so that there can be no lingering question in the mind of ordinary, reasonable persons as to the defendant's guilt.

This is why in the criminal case brought by the State of California against O. J. Simpson in 1994–1995, the jury elected acquittal over a guilty verdict. Jury members were not free of reasonable doubt as to Simpson's guilt for the murders of Nicole Brown Simpson and Ronald Goldman, in part because of the perjury (or poor memory on the witness stand) of Los Angeles Police Detective Mark Fuhrman.

Civil cases: Preponderance of the evidence   In a civil case, the plaintiff's burden of proof is much lower than in a criminal case. In civil cases, plaintiffs normally need only prove their cases by a *preponderance* (or greater weight) *of evidence*. The preponderance standard means that the plaintiff's rendition of facts is at least slightly more credible than the defendant's case presentation.

Clear and convincing evidence   Rarely, a civil plaintiff will be required by a court (or by legal precedent) to prove his or her case by a standard slightly higher than the preponderance standard. This intermediate standard of proof is known as proof by *clear and convincing evidence*. Clear and convincing evidence equates to "much more probable than not" that the plaintiff's version of the case is correct. *Cruzan* v. *Director, Missouri Department of Health*[6] was a case concerning whether the parents of a comatose woman in a persistive vegetative state could compel health care providers to withhold nutrition and hydration from a patient. In upholding the judgment of the Missouri (state) Supreme Court, Chief Justice Rehnquist of the U.S. Supreme Court found that the parents failed to present *clear and convincing proof* that their daughter would have desired withdrawal of such care. (Such proof was later made when the case was returned to state court, and Nancy Cruzan's food and water were taken away. She died December 26, 1990.)

Terminology for Culpability

Another difference between civil and criminal law cases is the terminology used to describe a defendant's culpability. In civil cases, defendants are found to be *liable* when the plaintiff's burden of proof is satisfied. In criminal cases, they are found *guilty*.

Comparative Remedies in Civil and Criminal Cases

The remedies afforded to plaintiffs in civil and criminal cases are also different. In tort civil cases, remedies are designed to make an injured plaintiff "whole." That is the sole purpose of tort law. In breach of contract civil cases, remedies are designed either to put the parties back in the same position they would have been in had the contract never been made (*restitution*), or to award the plaintiff the "benefit of the bargain" (*expectancy*). In other types of civil legal actions, successful plaintiffs may also win awards of *monetary damages*, or they may merely be vindicated in their positions through judicial *declarations of rights and duties*.

In tort cases, successful plaintiffs may win monetary damages of two types: *special* and *general damages*. Special damages replace past, present, and future out-of-pocket monetary losses incurred by the plaintiff as a result of the defendant's wrong-doing, or *tortious conduct*. Included under special damages are lost wages, medical expenses incurred because of the defendant's tortious conduct, and lost future earnings capacity. General damages include monetary awards for pain and suffering and the loss of enjoyment of life resulting from the defendant's culpable conduct. Infrequently, a court will award *punitive* (punishment) *damages* against a civil defendant. Punitive damages are similar to a criminal law monetary *fine*, designed to punish a wrongdoer for egregious misconduct and to deter the offender and others from repeating the offense.

The remedies awarded against defendants in criminal cases are more limited in type, but are also more severe in effect. Criminal defendants—including health care professionals, when charged with criminal misconduct—are *sentenced* when found guilty to *incarceration* or the threat of incarceration (probation). There is a permanent *public record* made of every criminal trial in which a conviction results. When criminal defendants have unjustly profited monetarily from their misconduct (such as with Medicare fraud), a criminal court judge may impose a monetary fine on the defendant in addition to incarceration.

Box 1-1 summarizes the major distinctions between civil and criminal law.

Law and Ethics Defined and Distinguished

Although both legal and ethical obligations are rules of conduct that are grounded in moral theory, they are different in many respects. Ethical rules are formal rules that govern or influence the official conduct of members of a select group, such as a profession. Ethics rules delineate the propriety of official conduct of members of professions, especially concerning business dealings with clients. Aspects of professional conduct commonly regulated by health care professional codes of ethics include (1) the nature of professional-client relations, including (among other considerations) the requirement to maintain information gained about clients in confidence and to

1-1 Civil and Criminal Law Distinguished

Civil Law	Criminal Law
1. Private actions	1. Governmental actions
2. *"Plaintiff"* v. *Defendant*	2. *"State"* v. *Defendant*
3. Proof: Preponderance of evidence	3. Proof: Beyond a reasonable doubt
4. Liability	4. Guilt
5. Monetary damages	5. Incarceration

obtain informed consent to treatment, and (2) the scope of business relationships, including permissible types of business relationships, restrictions on advertising professional services, and other considerations.

Rules governing professional conduct found in codes of ethics are labeled as prescriptive, or *directive*, and use action verbs such as "shall" or "must" in describing acceptable conduct. Those ethics provisions, on the other hand, intended merely to influence official behavior (such as aspirational statements requesting that members of a profession render gratuitous public service), are considered advisory in nature and use action verbs such as "should" or "may." Sanctions may be appropriate for violating ethics provisions that are directives, but not for failing to comply with advisory provisions.

Sanctions for violating ethical rules of conduct typically are levied exclusively by the professional association administering the ethics code in issue. As such, sanctions for pure ethics violations are normally limited in scope, as to who may be sanctioned, as to the range of sanctions that may be imposed, and as to their adverse effect on offenders.

In contrast to ethical rules, rules of law are formal rules of conduct that govern most or all activities of all members of society—citizens and non-citizens alike. No one (except those persons possessing diplomatic immunity, for most offenses) are "above the law." Even legislators, judicial officials, and the chief executive may be sanctioned for violations of law.

The range and effect of sanctions for violations of law are much broader and potentially more severe than for pure ethics violations. Under civil law, sanctions include forfeiture of monetary resources; while under criminal law, the ultimate sanction is death. Under both civil and criminal law, a person adjudged as culpable may lose his or her property interest in practicing a profession under license from the state, after due process of law has been afforded to that person.

Standards of Professional Conduct: The Modern Blending of Law and Ethics

As professions become more complex and sophisticated and as their ethics codes develop and are refined, conduct that is deemed unethical, more often than not, is also conduct that constitutes a violation of criminal law. For example, under the American Physical Therapy Association's Guide for Professional Conduct[7] (governing member-physical therapists), many, but not all, of the express ethical provisions exactly mirror existing legal obligations. Section 1.1C, for example, declares discrimination and harassment in interpersonal relations unethical. Section 1.2 delineates the ethical mandates of confidentiality of information. Section 1.4 requires informed consent before treatment. Section 3.2B7 requires supervision of support personnel. Section 4.3 addresses consent, confidentiality, fraud, and animal rights issues in research settings. Section 4.4B deals with student rights and confidentiality of student information. Section 5.2 spells out permissible and prohibited business arrangements, and Section 7.1B specifically proscribes patient referral for profit.

There are similar references to legal standards within the Occupational Therapy Code of Ethics.[8] Principle 1B prohibits sexual exploitation of, and the exercise of undue influence over, patients. Principle 2B enunciates specific requirements for patient informed consent. Principle 2E addresses confidentiality of patient information. Principle 3F spells out the requirement that support personnel be adequately supervised. Principle 5 deals with misrepresentation and conflict of interest issues. Principle 6 addresses the privacy of staff (employee) information and reporting requirements.

All of the professional ethics code provisions highlighted above reflect legal standards found in federal and state statutes, state licensure regulations, and common (case) law. The American Physical Therapy Association's Code of Ethics and its two supplementary codes, the Guide for Professional Conduct and the Guide for Conduct of the Affiliate Member (physical therapist assistants), and the American Occupational Therapy Association's Occupational Therapy Code of Ethics, are reprinted (with permission) in the Appendices.

Potential Forums for Adjudicating Alleged Violations of Law and Ethics

Whenever a licensed health care professional is charged with negligence or misconduct—whether related to patient care activities or to private pursuits, adverse legal, administrative, and association action may ensue. Take, as a hypothetical example, the case in which a physical therapist is charged with professional negligence related to the death of a patient who drowned in a clinic's therapeutic pool. In this case, the physical therapist left the facility for lunch, while the patient who drowned was left in the care of a physical therapist assistant.

The patient's family or other legal representative representing the *decedent's* estate might bring a civil malpractice action against the therapist for *wrongful death*. (In a wrongful death action, the heirs or legal representative sue to recover the present economic value of reasonably anticipated future contributions lost as a result of the defendant's tortious conduct.[9]) In the ensuing civil malpractice case, the quality of the defendant-therapist's care of the decedent would be challenged as substandard, and, if the decedent's heirs or estate convinced a judge or jury of that characterization by a preponderance of evidence, then they would win a monetary judgment against the therapist.

Because a patient death during treatment was involved, it is likely that coroner's and district attorney's office investigations would be undertaken, which might result in criminal negligence charges being filed against the responsible therapist. If the public prosecutor convinced a judge or criminal jury that the therapist was culpable beyond a reasonable doubt for the patient's death, then a felony or misdemeanor criminal conviction would result.

Similarly, a state licensure board adverse administrative action might take place, particularly because the incident involved a patient death, and because of the possibility of gross negligence or reckless conduct on the part of the respondent-therapist.

Such an administrative action, if substantiated by a preponderance of the evidence, might result in adverse licensure action affecting the therapist's right to practice his or her profession. Such actions might include (temporary) suspension or (permanent or semi-permanent) revocation of the professional license to practice.

Serious adverse action affecting professional licensure (suspension or revocation) can also take place independent of any treatment-related wrongdoing. For example, effective November 1, 1995, Texas physical and occupational therapists, among other professional licensees, face licensure suspension for substantiated nonpayment of child support.[10] The new law, modeled in part on similar laws in effect in Maine and in other states, requires a non-custodial parent to be delinquent in payment of child support for more than 90 days and not be the subject of pending litigation by the state attorney general. As a preliminary step before adverse licensure action, the delinquent parent will be notified of the delinquency and afforded the opportunity for voluntary compliance with payment requirements. If voluntary compliance does not occur, then an attorney from the state attorney general's office will seek licensure suspension before an administrative hearing judge. The professional licensee has the due process rights of notice of the hearing and the opportunity to respond and fight licensure suspension. Once suspended, reinstatement of professional license will occur only after a repayment agreement has been perfected.

In addition to the three types of adverse actions mentioned above, physical and occupational therapist-members of the American Physical Therapy Association and the American Occupational Therapy Association may face private association disciplinary action for ethics violations. In the hypothetical example above, a respondent-physical therapist-APTA member might be charged with a violation of Section 3.2B7, which reads:

> The primary responsibility for physical therapy care rendered by supportive personnel rests with the supervising physical therapist. Adequate supervision requires, at a minimum, that a supervising physical therapist perform the following activities: Direct and supervise supportive personnel in delegated tasks.

One of two possible actions can result. A formal investigation and possible hearings, modeled on state licensure board administrative procedures, can take place with substantive and procedural due process protections afforded to the respondent. Or, if documented proof of a felony conviction or licensure revocation is initially received by the association, immediate interim suspension of membership automatically takes effect, and the respondent's case is adjudicated in an expedited fashion by the American Physical Therapy Association's Judicial Committee.

More detailed information on professional association disciplinary processes appears in Chapter 11.

The Litigation Crisis

The Civil Litigation Explosion

As was mentioned in the Preface, western nations (the United States in particular) are experiencing a civil litigation crisis that seems to be ever-expanding. In 1992, the latest year for which statistics are available, there were 19,707,374 civil lawsuits filed in the United States.[11] If one postulates that there are already an equal number of civil legal cases in existence in the system, then, even if each case had only two litigants—one plaintiff and one defendant—there would be one in seven Americans embroiled in civil litigation at any given point in time.

Which of the states is the most litigious? If you answered either California or New York, you are wrong. The four most litigious states, ranked behind Washington, D.C., are Rhode Island, Massachusetts, New Mexico, and Nevada, respectively. (California ranks thirteenth.)[12]

Why does a litigation crisis exist? There are many sociological reasons for a litigation crisis that are beyond the intended scope of this book. Some of the reasons relate to the nature of our legal system. The United States has five percent of the world's population, yet three-fourths of the world's attorneys. One-third of all legal bills generated in the United States emanate from New York City. With such a large number of attorneys, formal redress of grievances is more easily facilitated, resulting in a disproportionately high volume of litigation.[13]

In addition, the United States is the only western nation that allows attorneys to undertake representation of personal injury clients for a *contingent fee*, where the client contractually agrees to pay a percentage of any recovery to the attorney, but is bound to pay no fee if the plaintiff does not prevail at trial. The client is still liable for the payment of fees and expenses incurred by the attorney in the case, including the filing of court papers, payments to consultants and expert witnesses, and telephone and photocopying expenses.

Some authorities are very critical of the role of lawyers and the law in fueling the litigation crisis. John Leo said in a recent editorial that "[a]ll too often, litigation in America is a lucrative, lawyer-driven enterprise in which the client is not in control and is almost incidental."[14] Philip Howard recently published a highly acclaimed book entitled "The Death of Common Sense: How Law Is Suffocating America," in which he asserts that we have become a nation of enemies in which the rule of law is too often abused.[15]

In cosmopolitan America, citizens may feel nameless, faceless, and relatively powerless. Litigation gives them recognition and a false sense of control. The media, schools, parents, and politicians all contribute to the fervor of litigation, for everywhere one hears "I'll sue you!"

The Health Care Malpractice Crisis—Fact or Myth?

Like the litigation crisis generally, the health care malpractice problem is of recent vintage. While there has been litigation over health care delivery for many centuries, including the 1375 British case of *Stratton* v. *Cavendish* (involving failed hand surgery),[16] the floodgates of health care malpractice litigation did not open until the advent of the consumerism movement post-World War II.

One of the reasons for the health care malpractice litigation crisis is related to changes in benefits for civilian workers after World War II. Employee health benefits became commonplace during and after World War II, making access to health care easy and affordable for millions of families. The benefits grew during the war, in large part, as a means of circumventing mandatory wage and price controls.[17] With enhanced access to care and increased utilization came greater liability risk exposure. Also, as medical and surgical technologies advanced and new drugs were discovered, the risks of patient injury, and of litigation, grew.

Media technology—especially television—became more sophisticated and widely disseminated post-World War II. After troops returned from overseas in the mid and late 1940s, baccalaureate and graduate educational opportunities were seized upon, making veterans and their families into sophisticated, demanding consumers. The consumerism movement helped spark the litigation crisis generally, and the health care malpractice crisis in particular.

Other factors feed the health care malpractice crisis on an ongoing basis. Increasing governmental regulation of health care services, skyrocketing health care costs, and managed care initiatives designed to curb those costs have all contributed to a health care environment that is ever more business-like. When patients perceive that their health care professionals are treating them in a more business-like fashion, they resent it, and tend to respond in kind. So when a patient in the modern health care environment is injured by *iatrogenesis*—i.e., injury or disease caused by health care interventions, that patient is more inclined to claim against or sue his or her health care providers and the institutions vicariously responsible for them.

Tort Reform Efforts

The fundamental purpose of tort law is to award fair and reasonable compensation to persons wrongfully injured at the hands of others. The tort system strives to make victims of wrongdoing "whole" again (or as close to whole as possible through the award of monetary damages). When an imbalance is perceived in the tort system's equitable administration of justice, adjustments are made by legislatures and/or courts to restore balance. Major adjustments to the system are labeled *tort reform*.

The First Wave of Tort Reform: Expanding Litigants' Right of Access

There have actually been two eras of tort reform. The first era of tort reform paralleled the development of the consumerism movement post-World War II. Before and during that time, courts and legislatures began to reverse or at least relax restrictive legal rules that impeded patient-plaintiff access to the legal system and legal redress of grievances. Sweeping legislative and judicial reform took place because of the perception that injured parties were systematically impeded from receiving redress for civil wrongs. Plaintiff-oriented reforms ensued, including the relaxation of restrictive evidentiary rules, the introduction of new theories of recovery in tort, and an expansion of the classifications and amounts of monetary damages awarded to plaintiffs who prevailed in court.

Comparative Fault

One of the first important patient-oriented tort reform measures was the abolition in most states of the harsh evidentiary rule of *contributory negligence*, a rule that, with few exceptions, bars an injured party from any compensation when the injured person is at all partially responsible for his or her own injuries—even if a tortfeasor was substantially at fault. In its place, a system of *comparative fault* was established, under which a patient's tort compensation is subject to being reduced by the degree to which the patient is at fault in contributing to his or her injuries. Although the overwhelming majority of states preclude compensation altogether when a patient is found to be more than 50 percent responsible for his or her injuries, a few states allow a patient to receive tort compensation regardless of the degree of culpability attributable to the patient under a concept called *pure comparative fault*.

Res Ipsa Loquitur

Another first-wave expansive tort reform measure was the easing of an injured party's burden of proof at trial, employing a legal concept known as *res ipsa loquitur* (Latin for "the thing speaks for itself"). Under res ipsa loquitur, whenever a patient is injured as a result of the use of a treatment or modality under the exclusive control of a health care provider, and the injury sustained is of the kind that normally should not occur unless the health care provider is probably negligent (e.g., a burn from a hot pack or heat-molded orthosis), the trial judge in a case may permit the jury to *infer*, or in some cases order the jury to *presume*, negligence against the defendant-provider. For the health care provider to escape liability for the patient's injury once res ipsa loquitur has been invoked, his or her attorney must dispel or rebut the inference or presumption of negligence through the introduction of contrary evidence.

Res ipsa loquitur is not a new concept in law. The doctrine first appeared in 1863 in an English legal case, *Byrne v. Boadle*,[18] in which a beer barrel "mysteriously" rolled out of a second floor window of a factory owned by the defendant. The plaintiff, a passerby below, was injured by the flying barrel. The English court held that because the victim could not prove negligence on the part of the defendant, it was sufficient to show that the incident was of a type that, in the normal course of life events, should not happen absent someone's carelessness, and that the barrel belonged to and was controlled by the defendant.

In the 1940s, courts in the United States began to allow res ipsa loquitur to be invoked by plaintiffs in health care malpractice lawsuits in part as a judicially-imposed penalty for a perceived or factual conspiracy of silence on the part of health care professionals who refused to testify on patients' behalf against professional colleagues in court. The doctrine, however, is relatively rarely allowed in health care malpractice cases, because of the shifting of the burden of persuasion to malpractice defendants in these cases.

There is one reported physical therapy malpractice case in which res ipsa loquitur was petitioned and allowed by the court. The case was *Greater Southeast Community Hospital Foundation* v. *Walker*.[19] In that case, a patient in physical therapy allegedly sustained a shoulder burn from a hot pack left on the skin too long. The trial-level jury found in favor of the plaintiff-patient and awarded her $2,000 in monetary damages. On appeal, the verdict was overturned, and the case was remanded to the trial court for a new trial. The appellate court found that the trial judge improperly allowed the jury to infer negligence against the defendant-physical therapist under res ipsa loquitur, because one of the required elements for its use—exclusive control of the hot pack—was in dispute. At trial, there was conflicting evidence concerning whether the patient had moved the hot pack or protective toweling during treatment. The case never reappeared in the legal literature after its remand, meaning that it probably was settled without resort to retrial.

In the health care setting, the three required elements for allowing a patient-plaintiff to invoke res ipsa loquitur are shown in Box 1-2.

Other patient-oriented tort reform measures include the development and expansion of *strict products liability*, that is, liability for injuries from dangerously defective products without regard to culpability on the part of the person held liable. In addition, there has been an increase in the frequency and amount of punitive damages imposed on health care professionals in malpractice cases, particularly where the court finds that the defendant's egregious conduct was malicious or reckless.

Punitive damages are not awarded in order to compensate an injured plaintiff. They are imposed against tortfeasors as punishment. In addition to their purpose of deterring the wrongdoer from engaging in the same or similar misconduct again,

1-2 Res Ipsa Loquitur: Inference or Presumption of Negligence in a Health Care Malpractice Case

Critical Elements
1. The incident that led to patient injury does not commonly occur absent negligence on someone's part.
2. Because the health care provider exclusively controlled the instrumentality that led to patient injury, the party who was probably negligent is the health care provider.
3. The patient was not contributorily negligent in causing his or her own injury.

they also serve to deter others from following in the footsteps of the tortfeasor. These purposes are labeled *specific* and *general deterrence*, respectively.

In the case where a judge believes that a jury awarded punitive damages in a civil case improperly, the judge has the power to reduce or eliminate the punitive damages award, under a legal concept called *remittitur*. This occurred recently in a premises negligence case involving McDonald's restaurant in which a customer was burned by coffee supplied by the defendant which was allegedly excessively hot.[20] An award of punitive damages can also be modified or overturned on appeal.

Although the concept of punitive damages has received significant attention by federal and state legislatures under more recent, restrictive tort reform initiatives, the courts have upheld it as a legitimate element of monetary damages in malpractice and other civil cases. Recently, the U.S. Supreme Court ruled that the imposition of punitive damages in a civil case is not unconstitutional as an "excessive penalty" under the Eighth Amendment to the Constitution.[21] A summary of first-wave tort reform initiatives appears in Box 1-3.

Prelude to the Second Wave of Tort Reform

The most significant catalyst for a second wave of tort (malpractice) reform, designed to limit the numbers of tort claims and lawsuits and reduce damages awards, was the professional liability insurance crisis of the 1970s and 1980s. During that timeframe, the cost to providers and institutions for professional liability insurance increased dramatically, and the availability of insurance became less certain. In particular, underwriters of professional liability insurance began to issue claims-made vs. occurrence

---

1-3 Summary of First-Wave (Patient Advocacy) Tort Reform Initiatives

- Comparative fault: reducing tort compensation by the degree to which a patient is at fault in contributing to his or her own injuries.
- *Res ipsa loquitur* ("the thing speaks for itself"): an inference or presumption of negligence against a defendant-health care professional arising from unexplained patient injuries.
- Punitive damages: monetary damages awarded against malpractice defendants whose conduct toward injured patients was egregious and malicious. (Insurers do not normally indemnify against punitive damages, so that the responsible health care provider may be personally responsible for their payment.)
- Strict products liability: liability for patient injury from dangerously defective commercial products, without consideration of culpability on the part of the commercial entity supplying the product.

policies to clients, and many health care organizations and physician and non-physician providers and groups began to self-insure against liability exposure. (The topic of professional liability insurance is addressed in greater detail in Chapter 9.)

While the exact number of health care malpractice legal cases in the system at any given time is uncertain, there are a significant number of cases. There are several reasons why malpractice lawsuit frequency rates are not universally publicized. For cases handled by professional liability underwriters, the data on *frequency* (numbers) and *severity* (cost) of litigation are proprietary and not widely disseminated, sometimes not even to professionals insured by these entities. Also, most health care malpractice cases that do go to trial are either settled during trial or not appealed beyond the trial-level, so that case reports are nonexistent, or at least difficult to trace.

Several authors have reported on the number of malpractice claims and lawsuits in the literature. Bovbjerg and Petronis reported a total of 20,016 health care malpractice claims in Florida (92 percent involving physicians) filed by patients from 1975 through August, 1988.[22] The Texas Medical Association reported a steady rise in the number of legal claims brought by patients against Texas physicians from 1,116 in 1983 to 3,496 in 1992.[23] The Department of Veterans Affairs (VA) reported in 1993 that its Tort Claims Information System (TCIS) database held 3,796 health care malpractice claims that had been filed with the agency since the database was established in 1988.[24] Thirty percent of the total number of VA claims in TCIS were still unresolved at the time of the writing of the report. Seventeen of the VA health care malpractice claims reportedly involved allegations of physical therapy negligence.[25] (The VA report cited no occupational therapy malpractice allegations.) The VA reportedly has received approximately 700 claims per year since 1989; the Department of Defense, which operates 168 medical facilities worldwide, receives approximately 900 health care malpractice claims yearly.[26]

A 1984 report by the congressional General Accounting Office (GAO) estimated that, in that year, 73,472 health care malpractice cases were closed.[27] Stewart reported that, between 1985 and 1990, the overall health care malpractice claims rate declined at an average annual rate of 8.9 percent.[28]

Which health care professional disciplines are claimed against and sued most often? The St. Paul Fire and Marine Insurance Company, one of the largest private carriers of medical professional liability insurance, reported that the claims rate against its insured physicians increased slightly from 1993 to 1994, from 14.3 to 14.4 claims per 100 physicians. Average settlements by St. Paul reportedly averaged $36,900 in 1993 and $34,800 in 1994.[29]

Obstetrician-gynecologists (OBGs) reported having a much higher malpractice claims rate than most other physicians, according to the Opinion Research Corporation of Washington, D.C. Nearly 78 percent of OBGs reported being sued one or more times by patients, patient representatives, or estates, with three being the average number of claims or lawsuits against OBGs. In 40 percent of cases, claims were abandoned by patients or settled without a monetary outlay.[30]

Claims frequency and severity data are not widely reported for most other health disciplines. The American Nurses Association reports that registered nurses had a claims frequency rate of 5 claims per 10,000 nurses.[31] The claims frequency rate for physical therapists is approximately 0.51 claims per 100 treatment exposures (averaged over four years, from 1983–1987), according to one (anonymous) large professional liability insurance underwriter.[32] In 1991, another insurance underwriter of physical therapists processed 144 claims[33] based on the following allegations:

- negligent treatment involving exercise (53 claims)
- negligent administration of therapeutic modalities (32 claims)
- negligent evaluative procedures (26 claims)
- negligent monitoring of patient activities (23 claims)
- negligent monitoring of patients receiving modalities (10 claims)

Health care providers are not the only professionals facing significant liability risk exposure in the practice of their professions. Attorneys know this fact all too well. Over recent decades, the attorney-client relationship has devolved from a fiduciary relationship built on absolute trust to a run-of-the-mill, arms-length business arrangement resulting in growing legal malpractice litigation. This situation has resulted in legal malpractice insurance premiums increasing by 63 percent from 1986 to 1994, currently averaging $4,601 per attorney annually. Just as health care professionals are doing, attorneys are reportedly utilizing risk management measures to dampen professional liability exposure, including improving communications between an attorney and client and obtaining informed consent for legal actions undertaken on the client's behalf.[34]

The Second Wave of Tort Reform: Restricting Litigants' Right of Access to the System

As the incidence of health care malpractice claims and lawsuits increased during the 1970s and 1980s and reactive defensive health care practice became commonplace, intensive pressure from medical and insurance lobbyists pressured state legislators to support restrictive malpractice reforms to limit patient-plaintiffs' access to the legal system. This counter swing of the tort reform pendulum began just as the movement toward patient-oriented tort reform was waning. By 1988, 41 of the 50 states had enacted legislative restrictive tort reform measures.[35]

Some of the second-wave tort reform measures enacted by state legislatures include:

- *Requiring plaintiffs in health care malpractice legal actions to undergo administrative hearings addressing the merits of their cases before being allowed to proceed to trial.*

  By 1989, 30 states had enacted statutes concerning administrative scrutiny by medical review panels for health care malpractice cases. New Hampshire, in 1972, became the first state to use health care malpractice review panels, where the procedure is voluntary, and the findings are not admissible as evidence in a subsequent trial.

This administrative procedure is mandatory in 18 states, elective in six, and at a judge's discretion in two other states. In the 13 states where the procedure was challenged as unconstitutional (e.g., violative of *due process* of or *equal protection* under law), it was upheld in nine states and invalidated in four.[36]

In most states, these malpractice review panels consist of attorneys, physicians, and lay members. A panel may reach one of several conclusions: (1) that the defendant-health care professional breached the applicable standard of care (i.e., committed professional negligence), (2) that the defendant-health care professional complied with the applicable standard of care (i.e., did not commit professional negligence), (3) that there appears to be a material issue of fact not requiring medical expert opinion for consideration in a trial on the merits, or (4) that the conduct of the defendant-health care professional was not a causative factor in the patient-plaintiff's alleged injury. Panels may also be required to opine on the existence and degree of patient permanent impairment and disability associated with a finding of professional negligence.

In a study of Louisiana health care malpractice administrative review panels, it was reported that during 1977 and 1978, 40 panels reached decisions on the merits of health care malpractice claims. These panels ruled in favor of defendant-providers 85 percent of the time.[37]

• *Mandating caps on noneconomic monetary damages awarded to plaintiffs for "pain and suffering," or "loss of enjoyment of life."*

California, in 1975, was the first state to limit noneconomic damage awards for health care malpractice plaintiffs to a maximum of $250,000. Since that time, at least 16 states have followed suit.[38] Such caps range in amount from $100,000 to $1,000,000 per individual defendant-provider adjudged culpable. Of the legislatively-established limits challenged, about half were invalidated. Tort law scholars now argue that limits on noneconomic damages are unfair because they are based on median awards from a quarter century ago. The current median noneconomic damages award is about $300,000.[39] These scholars recommend that juries be permitted to award noneconomic damages (under guidelines given by judges) as they believe are warranted, with no restrictive caps on the amounts awarded.

• *Placing monetary limits on plaintiff attorney contingent fees.*

In some jurisdictions, tort reform legislation mandates limits on attorney fees for all classes of personal injury cases (including health care malpractice actions, automobile accident actions, "slip and fall" cases, etc.). In other states, attorney fee limitations apply only to health care malpractice cases. California's Medical Injury Compensation Act (MICRA) is an excellent example of the latter type of statute. Under MICRA, an attorney representing a California patient who is suing a health care professional for malpractice may not receive as a contingent fee more than 40 percent of the first $50,000 recovered, 33 ⅓ percent of the next $50,000 recovered, 25 percent of the next $500,000 awarded, and 15 percent of any recovery that exceeds $600,000.[40]

• *Reforming joint and several liability.*

Under the tort concept of *joint and several liability*, if more than one defendant is responsible for injuries caused to a plaintiff, then each defendant is individually liable to a plaintiff for all monetary damages if the plaintiff prevails at trial. Some states have legislatively reformed joint and several liability so that defendants are only financially responsible for their proportional degree of fault in causing plaintiff injuries.

• *Modifications to statutes of limitations and establishment of statutes of repose.*

Statutes of limitations are laws that set time limits for commencing legal actions after injury, or discovery of injury, at the hands of another person. These "time clocks" for bringing lawsuits require that legal action commence within the time frame provided, or else it is forever barred. There are different time limits for different types of legal actions, such as torts, contractual actions, and criminal actions. Some states have shortened the tort statute of limitations for health care malpractice actions.

Statutes of limitations often have exceptions that permit certain potential plaintiffs to delay filing formal legal actions beyond the normal time limit. If the plaintiff is a minor or is adjudicated mentally incompetent, the statute of limitations may be suspended, or *tolled*, during the period of minority or incompetence. Other exceptions include non-discoverability of the source of an injury (such as when a surgical sponge is inadvertently left within a patient after an operation) or *continuous* (ongoing) *treatment* of the plaintiff by the tortfeasor after injury.

Some states have established strict time limitations for product liability (and other types of) lawsuits, called statutes of repose. The purpose of a statute of repose is to preclude litigation after a specified number of years, irrespective of any *legal disability* affecting the plaintiff, such as minority or incompetence. This is deemed fair because of the possibility that necessary evidence will be lost or destroyed after a period of years, and the likelihood that crucial witnesses will die or otherwise become unavailable to the parties.

• *Relaxing the collateral source rule.*

Under the traditional collateral source rule, a plaintiff's right to receive payments for injuries from sources other than the defendant, such as from the plaintiff's insurance company, without having such payments deducted from damages awarded at trial, is protected. Defendants have long argued that the operation of the collateral source rule unfairly permits double recovery for injuries. Many states, under tort reform, have modified or eliminated the collateral source rule, either permitting juries to learn about collateral payments to plaintiffs and use their discretion to deduct them from tort recoveries, or in some jurisdictions, requiring deduction of monies received from collateral sources from final awards.

• *Requiring periodic payment of monetary damages.*

A large majority of states has changed the traditional lump-sum award payment system into one where future monetary damages are paid out in installments, over the life of the injured plaintiff. One key purpose of this reform measure is to prevent the heirs of the plaintiff from reaping a windfall in the event that the plaintiff dies prematurely.

• *Penalizing plaintiff attorneys and plaintiffs for filing frivolous law suits.*

In recent years, as legal caseloads have increased dramatically, courts have become increasingly impatient with plaintiffs and their attorneys who initiate frivolous legal actions, or employ dilatory delaying tactics to prolong litigation. As a result, courts are increasingly imposing sanctions, including not only dismissal of actions and limiting instructions regarding evidence, but also monetary fines against counsel and their clients. In the federal (civil) courts, frivolous lawsuit penalties arise under Federal Rule of Civil Procedure 11, under which a lawyer for a client certifies in legal papers (*pleadings*) that he or she has read the documents, that, to the best of the attorney's knowledge, there are valid grounds to support the pleadings, and that such pleadings are not being submitted for the purpose of delay.[41]

• *Limiting punitive damage awards.*

In product liability lawsuits, at least seven states (Florida, Georgia, Illinois, Iowa, Missouri, Oregon, and Utah) withhold from victorious plaintiffs in litigation a proportion of any punitive damages awarded to them. The money withheld by these state statutes becomes the property of the state. In Georgia, for example, the state treasury takes 75 percent of product liability punitive damages awarded.[42] Box 1-4 summarizes recent restrictive tort reform initiatives.

1-4 Summary of Restrictive Tort Reform Initiatives

1. Administrative medical (merit) review panels.
2. Imposing caps on noneconomic monetary damages.
3. Placing monetary limits on plaintiff attorney contingent fees.
4. Reforming joint and several liability.
5. Modifications to statutes of limitations and creation of statutes of repose.
6. Relaxing the collateral source rule.
7. Requiring periodic payment of monetary damages.
8. Penalizing plaintiff attorneys and plaintiffs for filing frivolous lawsuits.
9. Limiting punitive damage awards.

The federal government, like the states, is considering federal tort reform legislation. The current Republican plan would cap noneconomic damages at $250,000, and make other modifications to existing laws to cut health-related costs. The Congressional Budget Office recently reported that a $250,000 noneconomic damages cap in medical malpractice litigation cases would reduce physicians' professional liability insurance premiums significantly, resulting in a $200,000,000 reduction in federal payments to doctors over seven years.[43]

Tort Reform Outcomes

The evidence is mixed as to whether tort reform efforts have resulted in a fair balance between patients' right of redress for injuries and cost containment in health care. Statistics show that the costs to insurers and employers for health care are down significantly. A study by the National Insurance Consumer Organization (a consumer rights organization) found that insurance companies paid out a total of $2.7 billion for professional liability claims and lawsuits in 1991, down from $3.2 billion in 1985.[44] Yet, insurance companies collected over $4.9 billion in professional liability premiums from health care organizations and providers in 1991, up from $2.7 billion in 1985.[45]

By 1994, the cost savings from tort reform began to trickle down from insurance companies to business owners. In 1994, after rising 23 percent over the previous two years, the average cost of liability insurance fell 22 percent to $2.55 per $1,000 of gross revenue.[46] Still, health care incurred the highest liability costs of any business, while the insurance industry incurred the lowest liability outlays.[47]

Despite the need for some degree of health care malpractice reform on the part of the states and the federal government, there is also a powerful countervailing equitable consideration favoring protection of the patient's right to seek redress within the legal system for injury incident to health care delivery. Patients do incur injury at the hands of health care professionals, and a small, but significant, percent of injuries are the result of malpractice.

Supporting this contention are the findings of the Harvard Medical Practice Study.[48] This interdisciplinary study involved a retrospective review of 31,429 randomly selected medical records of inpatients hospitalized in acute care, nonpsychiatric hospitals in New York State during 1984. The records were reviewed by expert panels, consisting of board-certified internists and surgeons. The panels found an adverse incident (patient iatrogenic injury) rate of 3.7 percent and attributed these injuries to probable malpractice in 27.6 percent of cases. In 15.8 percent of patient injuries, permanent disability or death ensued. The overall health care malpractice rate for iatrogenic patient injury was estimated to be approximately one percent.[49] Over 98 percent of injury cases attributed to malpractice did not result in a health care malpractice claim or lawsuit. Only about one-eighth of all malpractice claims filed by injured patients studied were from patients who were deemed to have been injured as a result of health care malpractice.[50]

Some health scholars urge that a complete restructuring of the American health care system is the only real solution to health care malpractice reform.[51] The Urban Institute, a Washington, D.C. based research center, recommends an alternative insurance system to replace civil litigation altogether for selected medical injuries, such as severe obstetrical patient injury. Under the proposed "no-fault" system, payment for specified injuries would be automatic, without resort to litigation. Such no-fault compensatory events are labeled "accelerated compensation events."[52]

Some states are developing alternative health care malpractice administrative adjudication systems, with limited right of appeal to state courts.[53] Under President Clinton's 1993 federal Health Security Act, a demonstration project would have examined liability transfer from individual health care professionals to health alliances.[54] This proposal would have created a private-sector analogue to the system already in place for federal health care professionals pursuant to the Federal Tort Claims Act,[55] under which the United States is substituted for individual provider-defendants as the party-defendant in federal sector health care malpractice lawsuits. (The Federal Tort Claims Act is discussed in greater detail in Chapter 2.)

In the keynote address before the American Physical Therapy Association's 1991 Annual Conference, Dr. Timothy Johnson[56] aptly reminded the audience that every component part of the American health care delivery system—providers, attorneys, politicians, the medical products and pharmaceuticals industries, insurance carriers and underwriters, and consumers—shares blame for the current dilemma and has the responsibility to help remedy the situation.

Chapter Summary

The American legal system consists of two broad component parts: the criminal justice system and the civil legal system. Cases brought by governments against private defendants are heard in the criminal system, and cases between and among private parties are adjudicated in the civil system. Allegations of health care malpractice, lodged by patients or their representatives, may give rise to both civil and criminal legal actions.

There are a number of important differences between criminal and civil legal actions, most notably the burden of proof required of the plaintiff, the party initiating an action. In criminal cases, the state is required to prove its case against a criminal defendant beyond a reasonable doubt, while in a civil case, a private plaintiff must prove his or her case by a preponderance, or greater weight, of evidence—a much lower burden of proof.

Because of the growing number of civil legal cases, state legislatures and the federal Congress have initiated tort reform measures to limit the number of cases—including health care malpractice cases—heard by courts. While a large number of health care malpractice legal cases may lack substantive merit, studies have shown that a small, but significant, percentage of cases involving iatrogenic injury are the result of substandard care.

Cases and Questions

1. A patient brings a charge of "inappropriate touching of a sexual nature" against her primary care physician. In which settings can the patient initiate action?

2. You are contemplating writing a letter to your congressman, urging reform of the civil legal system in order to afford greater fairness to litigants, the health care delivery system, and the public-at-large. What original reform measures can you think of to suggest to your congressman?

Suggested Answers to Cases and Questions

1. There are at least four potential forums for adjudicating a case involving an allegation of intentional misconduct such as sexual assault or battery arising in the health care delivery system. The alleged victim of the misconduct may bring a civil legal action for malpractice. He or she may file a criminal complaint with the district attorney, which may lead to a felony criminal legal action against the alleged perpetrator brought on behalf of the state. Either the alleged victim or the district attorney may report the allegation to the administrative agency responsible for licensure of the alleged offender. This may result in an adverse administrative action, potentially affecting licensure of the provider. Finally, any one may report the allegation of misconduct to the provider's professional association, possibly resulting in adverse action for violation of the association's professional ethics code, possibly affecting membership in the private organization. All of these potential adverse actions will have a negative impact on the personal and professional reputation of the provider—irrespective of who eventually prevails in the actions.

2. This problem optimally should be addressed by a group of students or clinicians, and suggestions for improvement in the health care litigation system developed through brainstorming. Remember that during a brainstorming exercise, all ideas are considered to be legitimate, because to arbitrarily exclude ideas as insignificant results in a stifling of creative input.

References

1. 28 United States Code Section 1332.
2. *Griswold* v. *Connecticut*, 381 U.S. 479 (1965).
3. *Ibid.* at 484.
4. U.S. Constitution, Amendments I–X.
5. *Roe* v. *Wade*, 410 U.S. 113 (1973).
6. *Cruzan* v. *Director, Missouri Department of Health*, 497 U.S. 261 (1990).
7. *Guide for Professional Conduct*, American Physical Therapy Association, June 1991.
8. *Occupational Therapy Code of Ethics*, American Occupational Therapy Association, July 1994.
9. Prosser, W.L. *Prosser on Torts*, 4th ed. St. Paul, MN: West Publishing Company, 1971, pp. 901–914.
10. "License Suspension for Non-Payment of Child Support." *Communique*, Texas Board of Physical Therapy Examiners, Fall 1995, p. 1.
11. Davis, Natalie, Courts Statistics Project. Personal communication, March 23, 1994.
12. "California Ranks 13th on List of Most Litigious States." *California Bar Journal*, February 1994, p. 20.
13. Rosen, B. "Why Are Lawyers Taking Over the Country?" *New York Times*, July 12, 1995, p. A14.
14. Leo, J. "The World's Most Litigious Nation." *U.S. News & World Report*, May 22, 1995, p. 24.
15. Howard, P.K. *The Death of Common Sense: How Law Is Suffocating America*. New York: Random House, Inc., 1994.
16. Furrow, B.R., Johnson, S.H., Jost, T.S., Schwartz, R.L. *Health Law: Cases, Materials and Problems*, 2nd ed. St. Paul, MN: West Publishing Company, 1991, p. 379.
17. Cherrington, D.J. *The Management of Human Resources*, 4th ed. Englewood Cliffs, NJ: Prentice Hall, 1995, p. 489.
18. *Byrne* v. *Boadle*, 159 Eng. Rep. 299 (1863).
19. *Greater Southeast Community Hospital Foundation* v. *Walker*, 303 A.2d 105 (D.C. App. 1973).
20. Press, A., Carroll, G., Waldman, S. "Are Lawyers Burning America?" *Newsweek*, March 20, 1995, pp. 32–35. In this case, the trial judge reduced the jury's punitive damages award against McDonald's from $2.7 million to $440,000. *Ibid.* at 35.
21. Wermille, S. "Justices Don't Limit Punitive Damages." *Wall Street Journal*, March 5, 1991, p. A-2.

22. Bovbjerg, R.R., Petronis, K.R. "The Relationship Between Physicians' Malpractice Claims History and Later Claims: Does the Past Predict the Future?" *Journal of the American Medical Association*, 1994; 272:1421–1426.

23. *Medical Professional Liability: An Examination of Claims Frequency and Severity in Texas*. Texas Medical Association, February 1994, p. 13.

24. "Department of Veterans Affairs—Analysis of Medical Malpractice Claims—An Initial Report."*Legal Medicine Open File*. Silver Spring, MD: Armed Forces Institute of Pathology, 1993, pp. 1–9.

25. *Ibid.* at 4.

26. *Ibid.* at 5.

27. "Liability Prevention and You." American Nurses Association, 1992, p. 7.

28. Stewart, L. "Damage Caps Add to Pain and Suffering."*Insight on the News*, November 7, 1994, p. 1.

29. Szabo, J. "Liability Market Seen Mostly Stable, With Little Rise in Premiums." *Physicians' Financial News*, 1995; 13:(7):S2.

30. "Lawsuits—Many Frivolous—Are a Way of Life for OBGs."*Medical Economics*, April 22, 1991, p. 18.

31. "Liability Prevention and You." American Nurses Association, 1992, p. 6.

32. Scott, R.W. *Health Care Malpractice: A Primer on Legal Issues*. Thorofare, NJ: Slack, Inc., 1990, p. 3.

33. Confidential source.

34. Geyelin, M. "Many Lawyers Find Malpractice Lawsuits Aren't Fun After All." *Wall Street Journal*, July 11, 1995, pp. A1,6.

35. "Successful Tort Reform Efforts in 1986–88." American Tort Reform Association, 1989.

36. Insler, M.S. "Louisiana's Medical Review Panel." *Survey of Opthamology*, 1989; 34(3):204–208.

37. *Ibid.*

38. Depperschmidt, T.O. "The Legality of State Limitations on Medical Malpractice Tort Damage Awards." *Hospital & Health Services Administration*, 1992; 37(3):417–427.

39. Felsenthal, E. "Why a Medical Awards Cap Remains Stuck at $250,000." *Wall Street Journal,* November 14, 1995, pp. B1,12.

40. California Business and Professions Code, Section 6146a.

41. Federal Rules of Civil Procedure, Rule 11.

42. Geyelin, M. "States Claim Share of Awards in Liability Suits." *Wall Street Journal*, March 3, 1993, pp. B1,11.

43. Felsenthal, note 39, at B1.

44. Moses, J.M. "Malpractice Claims." *Wall Street Journal*, March 25, 1993, p. B14.

45. *Ibid.*

46. Schultz, E.E. "Employers Are Trimming Liability Costs." *Wall Street Journal*, December 12, 1995, p. B5B.

47. *Ibid.*

48. Localio, A.R., Lawthers, A.G., Brennan, T.A., et. al. "Relation Between Malpractice Claims and Adverse Events Due to Negligence: Results of the Harvard Medical Practice Study, Parts I and II." *New England Journal of Medicine*, 1991; 324:370–384.

49. *Ibid.* at 373.

50. Localio, A.R., Lawthers, A.G., Brennan, T.A., et. al. "Relation Between Malpractice Claims and Adverse Events Due to Negligence: Results of the Harvard Medical Practice Study, Part III." *New England Journal of Medicine*, 1991; 325:245–251.

51. Nutter, D., Helms, C., Whitcolm, M., Weston, W. "Restructuring Health Care in the United States: A Proposal for the 1990s." *Journal of the American Medical Association*, 1991; 265:2516–2521.

52. Bovberg, R., Tancredi, L., Gaylan, D. "Obstetrics and Malpractice: Evidence on the Performance of a Selective No-Fault System." *Journal of the American Medical Association*, 1991; 265:2836–2843.

53. Meyer, H. "Alternative Malpractice Plan Moving in States." *American Medical News*, September 23, 1991, p. 3.

54. "Reform to Relieve PTs of Malpractice Worries." *PT Bulletin*, June 2, 1993, p. 6.

55. Federal Tort Claims Act, 28 United States Code Section 2674.

56. Woods, E. "A Look at America's Changing Health Care System." *Progress Report*, 1991; 20(8):1.

Suggested Readings

1. Cherrington, D.J. *The Management of Human Resources*, 4th ed. Englewood Cliffs, NJ: Prentice Hall, 1995.

2. Furrow, B.R., Johnson, S.H., Jost, T.S., Schwartz, R.L. *Health Law: Cases, Materials and Problems*, 2nd ed. St. Paul, MN: West Publishing Company, 1991.

3. *Guide for Professional Conduct*, American Physical Therapy Association, June 1991.

4. Localio, A.R., Lawthers, A.G., Brennan, T.A., et al. "Relation Between Malpractice Claims and Adverse Events Due to Negligence: Results of the Harvard Medical Practice Study, Parts I, II, and III." *New England Journal of Medicine*, 1991; 324:370–384, 325:245–251.

5. *Occupational Therapy Code of Ethics*, American Occupational Therapy Association, July 1994.

6. Prosser, W.L. *Prosser on Torts*, 4th ed. St. Paul, MN: West Publishing Company, 1971.

7. Scott, R.W. *Health Care Malpractice: A Primer on Legal Issues*. Thorofare, NJ: Slack, Inc., 1990.

8. Scott, R.W. *Legal Aspects of Documenting Patient Care*. Gaithersburg, MD: Aspen Publishers, Inc., 1994.

9. Scott, R.W. "Legal Trends: Tort Reform." *Clinical Management*, 1991; 11(6):11–13.

10. U.S. Constitution, Amendments I–X.

11. Wright, C.A. *Handbook of the Law of Federal Courts*, 3rd ed. St. Paul, MN: West Publishing Company, 1976.

Chapter 2

The Law of Health Care Malpractice

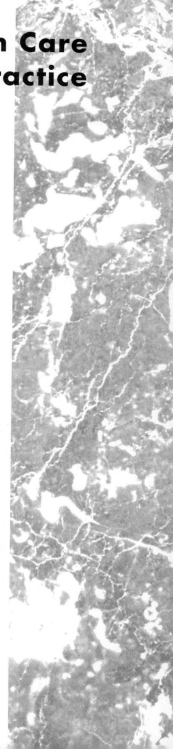

Patient injury incident to treatment can give rise to health care malpractice liability, if, in addition to patient injury, there exists a legal basis for imposing liability. These legal bases for liability include professional negligence, breach of a treatment-related contractual promise, intentional (mis)conduct, and strict liability (without regard for fault) for injury from dangerously defective treatment-related products or abnormally dangerous activities. Defenses to health care malpractice cases include noncompliance with statutes of limitations and procedural requirements for legal pleadings (court documents), and patient contributory negligence or comparative fault. Effective documentation management—including proper creation, use, and filing of incident reports—is critical to effective malpractice risk management.

Introduction

Health care professionals face significant liability risk exposure, primarily because they routinely interact with clients who are injured or ill and often in great physical pain and psychological distress. The concept "malpractice," as used in this chapter, refers to liability on the part of health care providers for patient injury. The traditional term "medical malpractice" only refers to the potential liability of physicians and surgeons for patient injury. In this book, the more inclusive term "health care malpractice" is used, to reflect and emphasize the fact that health care professionals other than physicians and surgeons are also exposed to malpractice liability incident to their professional practice.

> **Health care malpractice:** liability of health care providers for patient injury.

While the vast majority of health care malpractice cases brought by patients are against physicians and surgeons, other health care professionals, including rehabilitation professionals such as physical and occupational therapists, have been claimed against and sued by patients in growing numbers. Since 1969, for example, there have been at least 27 *reported* malpractice cases brought against physical therapists (or hospitals employing them) by patients and one reported case involving alleged malpractice on the part of an occupational thera-pist.[1,2,3,4] Before that time, there had never been a reported physical or occupa-tional therapist malpractice case, except for two New York State criminal cases for the unlicensed practice of medicine.[5,6] One case was brought against a physical therapist-defendant and one against an aide for a physical therapist, in 1933 and 1946, respectively. ·

Approximately one-half of the reported physical and occupational therapy mal-practice cases resulted in court decisions favoring patient-plaintiffs' positions, while slightly less than half were resolved in favor of defendant-physical therapists and their employers. Selected reported physical and occupational therapy malpractice cases will be discussed in later sections of this chapter. Brief descriptions of the two New York State criminal cases involving physical therapist-defendants appear in par-entheticals in the References at the end of this chapter.

Significance of Reported Legal Cases

What is the significance of a "reported" legal case? A reported legal case is one that either was appealed by one or both sides to at least one tier of appellate review or was deemed by legal scholars to be sufficiently significant at the initial trial court-level of adjudication to warrant reporting.

Just because a legal case exists, is appealed, or is reported, does not in any way infer that a finding of liability resulted against a defendant-health care professional. The exclusive burden to prove liability rests with patient-plaintiffs suing defendant-health care professionals. Health care malpractice plaintiffs (i.e., injured patients or their representatives) must prove their cases to the satisfaction of a judge (acting as fact-finder in a *judge-alone* trial) or jury by a preponderance (greater weight) of evi-dence, in order to prevail.

At the end of a trial on the merits of a health care malpractice case, a patient-plaintiff may fail to convince a jury or judge that a defendant-physical or occupation-al therapist committed malpractice. If such is the case, the plaintiff loses his or her case, and the defendant prevails, or wins, and is vindicated in the case.

Even before a formal trial commences, a plaintiff may lose a health care malprac-tice case if the presiding trial judge concludes that there is not any *material* (triable) *issue* in dispute. In such a case, the judge will normally dismiss the case against the defendant-provider through *summary judgment*, that is, a formal finding that the plaintiff's case cannot proceed to trial because of insufficient or defective evidence. Several of the reported physical therapy malpractice cases exemplify judicial exercise of summary judgment.

Factors Increasing Health Care Professionals' Malpractice Liability Exposure

External Factors

Probably the most significant external factor leading to greater health care malpractice liability exposure is the litigious nature of the American public. With nearly 20 million new civil lawsuits filed in the United States in 1992 (with perhaps 30,000 to 50,000 new health care malpractice lawsuits among them), Americans are clearly overly litigious. Another important factor increasing providers' liability risk exposure is the myriad of new and complex governmental and accreditation agency regulations. In a business environment so regulated and so scrutinized by everyone, from administrative agencies to the media, providers can ill afford not to have on retainer, and proactively seek advice regularly from, personal legal counsel.

Another liability-generating factor is the nature of the ever-changing health care delivery system. The health care milieu is moving away from what heretofore has been primarily an altruistic, patient-welfare focused, informal, and friendly system of providing health care for patients, toward an arms-length, business-like, cost-containment-focused, competitive, formal, and defensive system of client management. Fortunately, health management authorities such as Gerald McManis[7] foresee a positive shift in the newly emerging system away from provider- and payer-focused "managed care" to patient-focused "managed health" over the next decade.

Internal Factors

Several factors internal to specific health care disciplines predispose to greater potential malpractice liability exposure. The broadening scope of practice for physical and occupational therapy, for example, allowing for expanded clinical practice procedures may lead to greater liability exposure. For physical therapy, the fact that a majority of states now permit direct access practice, i.e., without physician referral, may lead to greater liability exposure as more physical therapists serve as primary care providers.[8] The trend toward clinical specialty certification may also lead to greater liability exposure—for certified specialists and non-specialists—as the standard of care for specific practice specialties becomes more precisely articulated. Similarly, the trends toward post-baccalaureate professional-level entry to practice and advanced professional degrees and residencies may also alter the legal standard of care, as more prospective expert witnesses who will establish the standard of care in court are educated beyond the baccalaureate level.

Attributes of managed health care delivery, such as creating cross-trained, multi-skilled professionals[9] and the delegation of care (but not legal responsibility) to physical and occupational therapy extenders, will create greater malpractice liability exposure. Also, the recent prominence of rehabilitation professions in the media and on the American health care scene and the trend toward higher professional liability insurance limits carried by physical and occupational therapists, among other disciplines, may lead to greater malpractice liability exposure, as attorneys, patients, and the public-at-large focus greater attention on these disciplines.

Legal Bases for Imposing Liability for Patient Injury

Introduction

Malpractice liability occurs in the health professional-patient relationship whenever a patient is injured during the course of care, and there is a legally recognized basis for imposing malpractice liability. Health care professionals are bound to comply with the foundational ethical principle of *nonmaleficence*,[10] or "do no harm" when caring for patients. However, the myth that malpractice liability occurs any time that a patient is injured in the course of patient care is simply inaccurate. Judges in malpractice cases are required to practice equity, or fairness, and would not allow a jury to award a sympathy verdict in favor of a patient-plaintiff merely because the plaintiff was injured in the course of treatment. One or more of the legally recognized bases for malpractice liability must also be present.

Traditionally, medical (physicians) or health care (all disciplines) malpractice has meant liability for patient injury caused by *professional* (treatment-related) *negligence*. Recently, however, courts, legislatures, and legal scholars have broadened the scope of potential bases for malpractice-related liability to include some or all of the other legal bases for liability associated with patient injury.[11]

Under this broader definition of health care malpractice, a defendant-health care professional may face fault-based malpractice liability for patient injury caused by professional negligence, breach (violation) of a contractual promise made to a patient, and intentional conduct resulting in patient injury. A defendant-health care professional may also face malpractice liability *without regard to fault* for patient injury from dangerously defective treatment-related products and from provider-controlled abnormally dangerous treatment activities (see Box 2-1).

The first three fault-based bases for health care malpractice liability—professional negligence, breach of contract, and intentional conduct—all involve the delivery of care that is adjudged as substandard. *Substandard care* means care that fails to comply with legal and ethical standards and is also defined as care that fails to meet at least minimally acceptable practice standards for the defendant-provider's discipline.

Liability for Professional Negligence

Health care professionals may be liable for malpractice when they fail to care for patients in ways that comply with legal standards of care, including compliance with applicable codes of ethics. Negligent care, for which a physical or occupational therapist may be liable, may be rendered by the physical or occupational therapist (*primary liability*) or by someone under the supervision of the physical or occupational therapist,

2-1 Health Care Malpractice

Traditional definition: liability of health care professionals for patient injury caused by professional negligence.

Expanded definition: liability of health care professionals for patient injury caused by:
- professional negligence
- breach of a contractual promise regarding treatment
- intentional conduct of the defendant-provider incident to care of a patient
- dangerously defective treatment products or modalities
- abnormally dangerous treatment activities

such as a physical therapist assistant or certified occupational therapy assistant or an aide (*vicarious liability*). What the standard of care is, is most often established through expert testimony of health care professionals from the same discipline as a malpractice defendant, by reference to authoritative texts and peer-reviewed publications, or by reference to clinical practice protocols or guidelines.

The Concept of Negligence

Negligence can be considered legally-actionable carelessness. The legal definition of negligence is conduct by a person who owes another a legal duty, which falls below a standard established by law for the protection of others against unreasonable risk of harm.[12] In a health care malpractice scenario, a defendant-health care professional may be negligent in carrying out a duty owed to a patient, and the patient-plaintiff may be contributorily negligent if the patient acts in a manner that falls below a standard that the law imposes on the patient for self-protection against possible harm.[13]

Substandard care: care that fails to comply with legal and ethical standards, i.e., care that fails to meet at least minimally acceptable practice standards for a defendant-provider's specific discipline.

"Conduct" that can form the basis for actionable negligence on the part of a health care provider may involve either an *act* or an *omission*, when the provider had a duty to act. An example of a negligent act might be the act of dislocating the shoulder of a patient with hemiplegia while carrying out passive mobility testing. An example of a negligent omission might be the failure to attach a gait belt to a patient with ataxia during ambulation or activities of daily living (ADL) training.

Contributory negligence: failure, on the part of a plaintiff-patient, to conform to a reasonable standard imposed by law for self-protection against possible harm.

Hint *Conduct constituting negligence can be a positive act, or an omission, or a failure to act, when a defendant had the duty to act.*

Elements of Proof for Professional Negligence

A patient bringing a claim or lawsuit alleging professional negligence on the part of a treating health care professional must fulfill a litany of proof, consisting of four elements: (1) that the defendant-health care provider owed a duty of care to the plaintiff-patient, (2) that the defendant-provider violated the duty owed through conduct that constitutes professional negligence, (3) that, as a direct consequence of the defendant-provider's negligent conduct, the plaintiff-patient sustained injury, and (4) that the type of injuries that the plaintiff-patient sustained warrant the award of monetary damages. The plaintiff has the legal burden to prove each of these elements to a jury or judge (acting as trier of fact) by a preponderance, or greater weight, of evidence. Before an allegation of professional negligence ever becomes a formal claim or lawsuit, the lawyer representing the plaintiff-patient evaluates the merits of the case to satisfy him- or herself that these four elements can be proven in court by a preponderance of the evidence (see Box 2-2).

Duty When does a health care professional owe a special duty of care to a patient? Possible answers include (a) whenever a patient calls for an appointment for evaluation and treatment, (b) when a patient presents him- or herself for care, (c) when a patient signs in at the reception area and is awaiting evaluation and treatment, or (d) when a health care professional accepts a patient for care. Almost always, the special duty of professional care arises only when a health care professional agrees to accept a patient for care.

Occasionally, a health care professional will not know whether a patient's diagnosis or problem falls within the professional's legal scope of practice or ambit of personal competence until after an evaluation is carried out. It is quite proper, and even required by legal and ethical standards, to decline to treat a patient whose problem falls outside a health professional's legal scope of practice or personal competence. In such instances, refusal to treat a patient does not constitute *patient abandonment.*

2-2 Four Required Elements of Proof in a Professional Negligence Lawsuit

1. duty owed by defendant
2. duty violated by defendant
3. causation, i.e., the defendant's negligent conduct caused the patient injury
4. monetary damages are required to be awarded to make the injured patient "whole"

In the United States, unlike in some other countries, there is no general duty to help another person in need of assistance or in peril. Absent some special relationship, such as a pre-established health care provider-patient relationship, an attorney-client relationship, a minister-parishioner relationship, or a parent-child relationship, the general duty to aid another person does not apply. By way of example, consider this hypothetical situation.

> A man is standing on the roof of a tall building. Suddenly, a three-year-old child walks through the door leading to the roof and ambles toward the edge of the roof, which does not have a protective fence. The toddler is walking relatively slowly, and the man has ample time to stop the toddler's movement without any danger to himself. Instead, the man silently observes as the toddler walks off the edge of the building to his death.
>
> Is the man legally responsible for the young child's demise? The answer depends on whether the man owed a legal duty of care to the child. Unless the man was a security guard or another type of employee of the building or somehow enticed the toddler onto the roof, he probably had no legal duty to come to the aid of the child, even though it was a clear, calm day, and he could have easily rescued the child from harm without exposing himself to any danger. Of course, it is beyond debate, under the facts of this scenario, that the man had a moral duty to help the unwitting toddler, but he probably could not be held legally accountable for his failure to act.

Under the same no-duty principle as the one presented in the hypothetical example, health care professionals generally are free to decline to accept patients for care. This commonly properly occurs, for instance, when a provider has a limited-scope practice, such as an exclusive hand therapy practice or spinal manipulation therapy practice. In such circumstances, providers are normally free to reject patients for care who do not fall within the scope of their practice. Health care providers are not free, however, to decline to care for patients for illegal reasons, such as illegal discrimination based on a patient's race, ethnicity, religion, gender, national origin, age, or disability.

Emergency medical treatment and active labor act   In at least one set of circumstances, health care professionals owe an affirmative duty of special care to prospective patients, even if they would not otherwise accept them for care. As part of the 1986 Consolidated Omnibus Budget Reconciliation Act (COBRA), Congress enacted the Emergency Medical Treatment and Active Labor Act (EMTALA),[14] more commonly known as the federal "anti-dumping" law. This federal law was enacted, in part, in response to well-publicized cases of indigent-patient transfers to charity hospitals by for-profit health care facilities not desiring to incur a financial loss by treating indigent patients in labor and other indigent patients with emergencies. The law, applicable to all hospitals receiving federal Medicare funding for patient care, requires such facilities to conduct appropriate medical screening examinations on all patients presenting themselves to emergency rooms and to stabilize bona fide emergency patients, without regard for their ability to pay, before transferring them onto other (e.g., charity) facilities. The anti-dumping law was intended to augment the nebulous common law duty on the part of hospitals to care for indigent emergency patients and to create a uniform standard to replace the few, inconsistent state statutes addressing the problem of patient dumping.

The law, which readers are urged to peruse as an exercise in statutory interpretation, reads in pertinent part:

(b)(1) In general. If any individual (whether or not eligible for [Medicare] benefits comes to a hospital and the hospital determines that the individual has an emergency medical condition, the hospital must provide either—

(A) within the staff and facilities available at the hospital, for such further medical examination and such treatment as may be required to stabilize the medical condition, or

(B) for transfer of the individual to another medical facility in accordance with subsection (c).

(c) Restricting transfers until patient stabilized.

(1) Rule. If an individual at a hospital has an emergency medical condition which has not been stabilized (within the meaning of subsection (e)(3) of this section), the hospital may not transfer the individual unless—

(A)(i) the individual (or a legally responsible person acting on the individual's behalf) after being informed of the hospital's obligation under this section and the risk of transfer, in writing requests transfer to another medical facility;

(ii) a physician . . . has signed a certification that, based upon the reasonable risks and benefits to the patient, and based upon the information available at the time of transfer, the medical benefits reasonably expected from the provision of appropriate medical treatment at another medical facility outweigh the increased risks to the individual and, in the case of labor, to the unborn child from effecting the transfer; or

(B) the transfer is an appropriate transfer (within the meaning of paragraph (2)) to [the receiving] facility.

(2) Appropriate transfer. An appropriate transfer to a medical facility is a transfer—

(A) in which the transferring hospital provides the medical treatment within its capacity which minimizes the risks to the individual's health and, in the case of a woman in labor, the health of the unborn child;

(B) in which the receiving facility—

(i) has available space and qualified personnel for the treatment of the patient, and

(ii) has agreed to accept transfer of the patient and to provide appropriate medical treatment;

(C) in which the transferring hospital provides the receiving facility all medical records . . . related to the emergency condition for which the individual has presented, available at the time of transfer . . . ;

(D) in which the transfer is effected through qualified personnel and transportation equipment, as required, including the use of necessary and medically appropriate life support measures during the transfer. . . .

(d) Enforcement. A hospital or responsible physician that knowingly or negligently violates the Act is subject to termination or suspension of its Medicare provider agreement. A hospital or responsible physician that knowingly violates the Act is subject to a civil monetary penalty of not more than $50,000. . . .

(e) Definitions. In this section:

(1) the term "emergency medical condition" means—

(A) a medical condition manifesting itself by acute symptoms of sufficient severity (including severe pain) such that the absence of immediate medical attention could reasonably be expected to result in—

(i) placing the health of the individual (or, with respect to a pregnant woman, the health of the woman or her unborn child) in serious jeopardy,

(ii) serious impairment to bodily functions, or

(iii) serious dysfunction of any bodily organ or part.

(B) with respect to a pregnant woman who is having contractions—

(i) there is inadequate time to effect safe transfer to another hospital before delivery, or

(ii) a transfer poses a threat to the health and safety of the woman or the unborn child.

(2) the term "participating hospital" means hospital that has entered into a provider agreement under section 1395cc of this title.

(3)(A) the term "to stabilize" means, with respect to an emergency medical condition, to provide such medical treatment of the condition as may be necessary to assure, within reasonable medical probability, that no material deterioration of the condition is likely to result from or occur during the transfer of the individual from a facility or, with respect to an emergency medical condition described in (1)(B), to deliver (including the placenta).

(B) The term "stabilized" means, with respect to an emergency medical condition, that no material deterioration of the condition is likely, within reasonable medical probability, to result from the transfer of the individual from a facility or, with respect to [a pregnant woman having contractions] that the woman has delivered. . . .

(5) The term "transfer" means the movement (including the discharge) of an individual outside a hospital's facilities at the direction of any person employed by (or affiliated or associated, directly or indirectly, with) the hospital, but does not include such a movement of an individual who (A) has been declared dead or (B) leaves the facility without . . . permission.

———

Soon after it became effective on August 1, 1986, EMTALA became the basis for litigation involving allegations of continuing "dumping" of indigent patients.[15,16] Courts continue to wrestle with interpreting what has been labeled as vague statutory EMTALA terms and language.[17]

When does "duty" end? Issues involving patient abandonment   An allegation of improper patient abandonment may arise incident to health care delivery, and may be brought either as a negligent or intentional abandonment charge with different legal consequences. Legally actionable patient abandonment occurs when a treating health care professional improperly unilaterally terminates the professional-patient relationship.

> ***Abandonment:*** **improper unilateral termination by a treating health care professional of a professional-patient relationship.**

The widest imaginable range of variegated clinical treatment activities can give rise to an allegation of patient abandonment, from a clinician momentarily turning his or her back from a patient (with a resultant patient fall) to discharging a patient before the patient reaches the zenith of rehabilitative potential because of inability to continue to pay for care.

In an unreported civil malpractice lawsuit involving a physical therapy student caring for a stroke patient, the patient fell while ambulating with indirect (stand-by) student assistance. The patient's hip fractured as a result of the fall. She claimed negligent abandonment, alleging that her licensed physical therapists always provided direct assistance during ambulation. The case was won by the defendant-hospital on the ground that the plaintiff failed to prove by a preponderance of evidence that indirect assistance was outside the legal standard of care. In addition, the defendant-hospital's attorney called a medical expert witness who opined that the plaintiff's fracture might have been spontaneous, caused by osteoporosis or excessive torsion during sudden turning.[18]

A patient is free to unilaterally and summarily terminate a health professional-patient relationship at any time without legal consequence. The same is not true for a health professional charged with responsibility for caring for a patient. A health care professional may unilaterally terminate a professional-patient relationship when, in the provider's professional judgment, a cure has been effected or maximal recovery or progress has been achieved. Careful documentation of the patient's status upon discharge is always required for the protection of both provider and patient.

It may also be acceptable to discharge a patient for reasons unrelated to goal-achievement, such as failure to pay for services or an irreconcilable personality conflict between provider and patient. In these and in similar circumstances, the freedom to discharge the patient is neither absolute nor without conditions. In the case of discharge for failure to pay for professional services, for example, a health care professional who is a preferred provider in a managed care network may have agreed contractually to treat patients for a fixed price, and may not be free to discharge prematurely nor charge more than the agreed amount, for whatever time period treatment may entail. In the case of discharge because of an irreconcilable personality conflict, the provider must give advance notice of the intent to sever the professional-patient relationship and must also give the patient a sufficient amount of time to locate a suitable substitute, competent care provider. It is highly recommended that a provider discharging a patient under this scenario also actively assist the patient in locating a substitute provider and consult with and transfer the patient's health records expeditiously to the substitute provider to minimize the possibility of legal action by the patient for intentional abandonment.

In the case of negligent abandonment, the same four elements of proof as in any other professional negligence action must be established by the plaintiff-patient. These are (1) that the defendant-health care provider owed a duty of special care to the patient; (2) that, in prematurely and improperly discharging the patient, the defendant-provider breached the legal standard of care; (3) that the breach of duty on the part of the defendant-provider caused injury to the plaintiff-patient; and (4) that the injuries that the plaintiff-patient sustained warrant the award of monetary damages in order to make the patient whole. The language used to present the four professional negligence elements above is similar to language that a defendant-health care provider might see in a formal civil complaint in which the plaintiff-patient details the specifics of his or her lawsuit.

Abandonment and substitute care providers   One of the special circumstances concerning patient abandonment involves whether health care professionals may temporarily transfer the care of patients to substitute health care providers of the same discipline when the primary provider is called away from the facility for additional duties, attends a continuing education course, or goes on vacation. The answer is usually yes. Just as it is legitimate to employ a substitute care provider when a primary health care professional becomes ill, it is normally acceptable to transfer a patient's care to a substitute care professional when duty (or even scheduled vacation) takes the primary provider away from the facility. In the hospital and health maintenance organization (HMO) settings, patients do not normally have a reasonable expectation of receiving professional care from a specific provider. Instead, patients are treated by staff (in the hospital and staff HMO models) or contract (in the group or network HMO models) providers.

In private practice or preferred provider organization settings, however, patients probably do have a reasonable expectation of being treated by specific providers of choice. In such environments, providers are advised to obtain written patient informed consent for substitution of specific primary providers by other professionals. In either situation, providers should always obtain patient consent for substitution and provide a detailed care summary and instructions to the substitute professional. When physical or occupational therapists are involved, referring physicians should also be notified in advance of the substitution of providers. All of these details should be succinctly, but thoroughly, documented in the records of affected patients.

Abandonment and the limited scope practice Another potential problem area involves health care professionals who work only in specific, limited practice settings. For occupational therapists, for example, such settings might include ergonomic work-site analysis and pediatric and hand specialty practices. For physical therapists, limited practice settings might be spine and extremity joint mobilization and manipulation practices. What happens when a current patient asks for treatment for problems unrelated to areas in which the provider offers services? While it would probably still be acceptable to deny care for areas outside of one's specialty practice—even for existing patients—it is recommended that specialty providers clearly delineate their scope of professional practice to patients at the outset of care so that subsequent misunderstandings (and patient dissatisfaction) do not arise.

Duties owed to third parties While a health care professional clearly owes a special duty of care to patients under the professional's care, an additional duty may be owed to third parties associated with patients under care. Specifically, providers may have an affirmative duty to warn third parties, law enforcement, or other authorities of specific danger incident to threats of harm made by patients. Clearly, this duty to warn others about things that patients reveal during confidential evaluation or treatment sessions is in direct contravention of the legal and ethical duties to maintain patient diagnostic and treatment-related information in confidence.[19,20]

The lead case in the area of duty to warn third parties of potential harm from patients is *Tarasoff* v. *Regents of the University of California*.[21] In that California state case, a psychotherapist employed by the University of California was treating a mentally ill patient named Poddar. During therapy sessions, Poddar threatened bodily harm to his former girlfriend. Neither the psychotherapist, nor his supervisors, reported the threats to the potential victim or to law enforcement authorities. Poddar carried out his threat and killed his former girlfriend. Her parents sued the University of California, alleging professional negligence on the part of the psychotherapist and vicarious liability on the part of the University. In ruling in favor of the victim's parents, the California Supreme Court held that a psychotherapist owes an affirmative duty to take reasonable steps to warn identifiable third parties of foreseeable danger of serious bodily

Hint *A psychotherapist owes an affirmative duty to take reasonable steps to warn identifiable third parties of a foreseeable danger of serious bodily harm from patients under their care. This legal duty has been extended to physicians and other providers in many states.*

harm from patients under their care. This legal duty has been extended to physicians and other providers in many states.

Although it is unclear in legal literature as to whether physical and occupational therapists have such a legal duty, there may be an ethical obligation to do so.[22] Physical and occupational therapists, and other non-physician, non-psychotherapist providers are urged to expeditiously consult with personal or facility legal counsel for specific advice should a scenario like that presented in *Tarasoff* arise in clinical practice.

Health care professionals may also have a duty to correct obvious errors made by other providers caring for patients.[23] In *Gassen* v. *East Jefferson General Hospital*,[24] a court held that a contract pharmacy service in a hospital owed a duty to patients to inquire about or correct readily identifiable prescription errors of physicians in the facility. That same kind of duty probably would apply to a physical or occupational therapist who receives a physician referral that requests a contraindicated treatment for a patient.

Breach of duty   The second element that a plaintiff-patient in a professional negligence health care malpractice case must prove is that the defendant-health care professional violated a legal duty owed to the plaintiff by providing substandard care. While every person in society owes a duty to foreseeable others to conduct him- or herself in a reasonable manner (e.g., to drive a car safely), health care professionals, because of their special knowledge, training, and experience, owe an even higher *duty of due care* to patients and others.

In establishing whether a health care professional's conduct met or violated the required professional standard of care, courts do not typically refer to a standard "cookbook" for a list of acceptable vs. unacceptable procedures and interventions. Instead, courts analyze on a case-by-case basis whether what a defendant-provider did in a specific case would have been done or could have been considered acceptable by an ordinary, reasonable professional peer of the defendant, acting under the same or similar circumstances.

There are many sources in which the legal standard of care may be established in court. The most common way to establish what the standard of care is, is to ask experts from the same discipline as a defendant-provider. This usually takes place during pre-trial interviews and (formal) depositions and during trial testimony. It is also common for attorneys and judges to reference official definitions of professional practice and official practice standards published by state licensure administrative agencies, professional associations, or other groups. Institutional and professional practice guidelines and protocols are also relied upon to establish the legal standard of care, as are professional journals, periodicals, and authoritative books.

Parameters of the duty owed   The nature of the duty owed to patients depends, in part, on what is permissible practice under a profession's practice act. When a health care professional carries out treatment that is not permitted under the applicable practice act, the offender is held to the legal standard of the profession whose practice the offender is encroaching upon. For example, in the physical therapy criminal cases cited earlier in this chapter, the physical therapist and masseur who were convicted of the unlicensed practice of medicine would, in civil malpractice cases, have been held to the standard of an ordinary, reasonable *physician* acting under the same or similar circumstances, and not to the standards of physical therapists and masseurs.

The legal definition of a profession is often the first point of research for an attorney attempting to define the legal scope of professional practice. The following detailed definition of physical therapy is from the American Physical Therapy Association's "A Guide to Physical Therapist Practice."[25]

Physical therapy, which is the care and services provided by or under the direction and supervision of a physical therapist, includes:

1) Examining patients with impairments, functional limitations, and disability or other health-related conditions in order to determine a diagnosis, prognosis, and intervention; examinations include, but are not limited to, the following:
   - aerobic capacity or endurance
   - anthropometric characteristics
   - arousal, mentation, and cognition
   - assistive, adaptive, supportive, and protective devices
   - community or work reintegration
   - cranial nerve integrity
   - environmental, home, or work barriers
   - ergonomics or body mechanics
   - gait and balance
   - integumentary integrity
   - joint integrity and mobility
   - motor function
   - muscle performance
   - neuromotor development and sensory integration
   - orthotic requirements
   - pain
   - posture
   - prosthetic requirements
   - range of motion
   - reflex integrity
   - self-care and home management
   - ventilation, respiration, and circulation

2) Alleviating impairments and functional limitations by designing, implementing, and modifying therapeutic interventions that include, but are not limited to, the following:
   - therapeutic exercise (including aerobic conditioning)

- functional training in self-care and home management (including activities of daily living and instrumental activities of daily living)
- manual therapy techniques (including mobilization and manipulation)
- prescription, fabrication, and application of assistive, adaptive, supportive, and protective devices and equipment
- airway clearance techniques
- debridement and wound care
- physical agents and mechanical modalities
- electrotherapeutic modalities
- patient-related instruction

3) Preventing injury, impairments, functional imitations, and disability, including the promotion and maintenance of fitness, health, and quality of life in all age populations.

4) Engaging in consultation, education, and research.

The following is the legal definition of occupational therapy from the Texas Occupational Therapy Practice Act.[26]

Occupational therapy means the evaluation and treatment of individuals whose ability to perform the tasks of living is threatened or impaired by developmental deficits, the aging process, environmental deprivation, sensory impairment, physical injury or illness, or psychological or social dysfunction. Occupational therapy utilizes therapeutic goal-directed activities to evaluate, prevent, or correct physical or emotional dysfunction or to maximize function in the life of the individual. Such activities are applied in treatment of patients on an individual basis, in groups, or through social systems, by means of direct or monitored treatment or consultation.

The occupational and physical therapy professions have both recently published official standards of practice.[27,28] The practice standards for occupational therapy consist of ten standards, addressing the following issues: professional standing, referral of patients, screening examinations, assessments, intervention planning and interventions, transition services, discontinuation of care, continuous quality improvement (CQI), and practice management. The 22 physical therapy practice standards broadly address practice administration, provisions of care (including informed consent, evaluation, planning care, and treatment), professional and student education, research, community service, and compliance with legal and ethical requirements in practice. The occupational and physical therapy practice guidelines are reprinted in Appendix 2, with permission of the American Occupational Therapy Association and the American Physical Therapy Association, respectively.

Certainly, peer-reviewed professional journals, such as the *Journal of the American Medical Association*, *New England Journal of Medicine*, *Journal of the American Physical Therapy Association*, and the *American Journal of Occupational Therapy*, among many others, qualify as *learned works* that health professional witnesses in malpractice cases may rely upon to formulate expert opinions on the professional standard of care. Standard textbooks for the health professional disciplines, such as Trombly's *Occupational Therapy for Physical Dysfunction*[29] and *Muscles: Testing and Function* by Kendall,[30] qualify as *learned treatises*, from which opinions on the professional standard of care may also be based.

Expert witness testimony on the standard of care   Most health care malpractice legal cases are settled well before formal trials occur, through settlement, abandonment of a case, or other disposition. How and whether a case is settled often turns on the strength of expert testimony given at pre-trial depositions. Health care professionals may qualify to serve as experts for a wide range of purposes, from vocational rehabilitation experts to ergonomic experts. In health care malpractice cases, however, they frequently testify as clinician-experts who establish the legal standard of care, and render expert opinions on whether a defendant-provider-peer met or breached the standard of care in treating a plaintiff-patient.

Health care professional experts may serve as expert witnesses for either plaintiff-patients or defendant-health care providers in malpractice cases. They may be asked to testify about patient care evaluation or treatment practices, the use of therapeutic equipment and modalities, informed consent practices, referral and consultation customary practice, and many other practice parameters.

In all cases where expert witnesses are called to testify, experts establish the legal standard of care for the defendant-provider's profession and comment on whether the care rendered by the defendant met or violated legal practice standards, based on one of three geographical frames of reference:

- In the vast majority of states, what fits within acceptable legal standards is care that passes as at least minimally acceptable in the same community or communities similar to the community in which a defendant-health care professional practices (*same or similar community standard*, majority rule).

- In only a very few states, experts are required to compare defendant-providers only to ordinary, reasonable peers practicing in the exact same community (*locality rule*, minority rule).

- In a few states, health care professional-generalists are held to a state- or nationwide standard of comparison, meaning that experts from anywhere within the state, or from across the nation, may testify on the applicable standard of care (*trend*).

The locality rule, which was the rule of law in the majority of jurisdictions earlier in this century, tended to cause unjust results in medical malpractice cases and was gradually supplanted by the same or similar community standard in a majority of states. Under the locality rule, there was often an actual or perceived conspiracy of silence in which professional colleagues in small (or even large) communities refused to come forward to testify as experts for patients against their friends and associates. This conspiracy of silence often resulted in the dismissal of clearly meritorious legal cases, which did not further the primary purpose of the tort legal system: to make whole deserving victims injured by the negligence or misconduct of others (see Box 2-3).

Irrespective of the geographical frame of reference from which an expert testifies, the expert must testify, when commenting on a defendant-provider's care, whether the defendant acted as an ordinary, reasonable professional peer would have acted under the same or similar circumstances. Experts are not allowed to testify about what they themselves would have done under circumstances similar to those at issue in a trial. The legal system is not interested in what an expert would do in practice, but whether what a defendant-provider did constituted at least minimally acceptable clinical practice.

In order to be *legally competent* to testify as an expert, a witness must meet two basic requirements:

- possess in-depth knowledge about the treatment procedure at issue in the trial
- be familiar with the applicable legal standard of care in the place where the alleged professional negligence took place, at the time of alleged patient injury

Since an expert's qualifications are subject to challenge through *impeachment* by opposing legal counsel, an expert must also demonstrate how he or she acquired the special knowledge that makes him or her an expert, i.e., through formal or continuing education, clinical experience, or other training. When, as often is the case, a jury or judge is faced with competing expert testimony on both sides about whether a defendant-provider met or violated the standard of care, the verdict often turns on which expert is most convincing in his or her presentation.

Who may testify as an expert for or against a defendant-provider of a specific health care discipline, on that discipline's legal standard of care? In many states, courts require that expert witnesses be of the same academic discipline as the defendant. This is often referred to as the *same school* doctrine.[31] A number of courts,

2-3 Three Geographical Frames of Reference for Expert Witness Testimony on the Legal Standard of Care

1. **Majority rule:** Expert practices in a similar community (or the same community) as the defendant-health care professional.
2. **Minority rule:** Expert must practice in the exact same community as the defendant-health care professional.
3. **Trend:** Expert practices in any community, state- or nationwide.

however, allow others to qualify and testify as experts in health care malpractice cases based on their personal knowledge about the procedure in issue and of the applicable standard of care for the defendant's profession obtained through formal or informal training or experience.

In the overwhelming majority of physical therapy malpractice cases in the legal literature, physicians and surgeons—not physical therapists—testified as experts, and established the physical therapy standard of care. (One notable exception was the case of *Emig* v. *Physicians' Physical Therapy Services*,[32] in which the state physical therapy association chapter president testified on the physical therapist standard of care.)

In one reported physical therapy malpractice case, *Novey*,[33] in which a post-operative hand surgery patient sustained a tendon rupture during physical therapy care, an occupational therapist was called at trial by the plaintiff-patient as an expert witness to establish the physical therapy standard of care for post-operative hand patients. In the case, the plaintiff, who had severed his middle finger flexor tendons in an industrial accident, underwent surgical repair of the lacerations and was casted. When the cast was removed, the patient was sent to the defendant's physical therapist-employee for rehabilitation. The plaintiff alleged that his tendons were re-torn during physical therapy.

At trial, the patient won his case, and was awarded $12,127.67 in monetary damages. On appeal, the defendant-hospital's attorney successfully argued that the occupational therapist was unqualified to testify as an expert on the physical therapist standard of care, because she was not from the same "school" as the defendant's physical therapist-employee. Because of the appeals court's finding that the occupational therapist-witness was not a proper expert in the case, the case was remanded to the trial court for reconsideration. (The case was not reported again in the legal literature, meaning that it might have been settled upon its remand.)

What is troubling about this case? The Illinois appellate court, like many other courts (and lawyers), apparently had incomplete knowledge about the professions of physical and occupational therapy. There is a common professional standard for hand therapists certified by the American Hand Society, which includes occupational and physical therapists. Physical and occupational therapists also probably share a common standard—based on similar knowledge, training, and experience—in areas such as ergonomics, functional capacity assessments, pediatric practice, and stroke rehabilitation, among many other areas of practice.[34,35,36] Because of incomplete knowledge about these professions on the part of attorneys, physical and occupational therapists are urged to educate their legal counsel about their professions for any type of legal representation.

Fundamental changes in physical and occupational therapy practice made over the past few decades—including autonomous accreditation of professional education programs, postbaccalaureate entry-level professional education, clinical specialty certification, and (for physical therapists and occupational therapists in the military setting[37]), practice without physician referral—have altered and will continue to alter the legal standard of care for these professions to some degree. Health care professionals and facility administrators should be aware of the impact of these changes on the legal standard of care generally and on future therapist-malpractice defendants in particular.

Autonomous accreditation of professional education programs is evidence that the professions of physical and occupational therapy are controlled by practitioners of the same discipline as graduates, clinicians, and academicians. This control of the educational process makes it incumbent upon leaders in these two professions to autonomously establish the professional standard of care in legal proceedings.

The evolution of entry-level professional occupational and physical therapy programs from the baccalaureate level to the master's level affects the legal standard of care, not only for those clinicians possessing advanced degrees, but for all clinicians within the two disciplines. As more and more clinicians obtain master's and doctoral degrees, the overall standard of comparison will change. This likelihood raises a question: Can clinicians with bachelor's degrees testify on the standard of care for professional colleagues who hold higher-level degrees? The answer is yes. Qualification as an expert is not necessarily based on formal education. Rather, it is grounded in familiarity with the treatment procedure in issue in a given case, and firsthand knowledge of the legal standard of care in the geographical area at the time of alleged malpractice.

Clinicians having advanced degrees who are called upon to serve as expert witnesses should bear in mind that the legal standard of care for a given community is not necessarily what advanced-level clinicians would deem appropriate (unless all clinicians in that community have advanced degrees). The standard is what constitutes at least minimally acceptable practice for all practitioners in the community, irrespective of their degrees or years of experience.

Specialty certification also has an impact on the legal standard of care. Although there have been no reported malpractice cases involving board-certified physical and occupational therapists to date, if physician-specialist legal cases serve as precedent, the standard used to assess physical and occupational therapist-clinical specialist conduct will be a national, rather than local or state-wide standard.

Are non-specialists permitted to testify as expert witnesses in legal cases involving defendant-clinical specialists? Yes. Just as with clinicians having different degrees, qualification as an expert witness does not turn on certification, but on demonstrated knowledge about a treatment procedure in issue—whether that knowledge is derived from formal or informal training.

Direct access practice may have a profound effect on the legal standard of care for non-physician health care professionals. For example, consider a physical therapist legally practicing without physician referral in a state where such practice is allowed. If the physical therapist engages in treatment that exceeds the legal scope of practice under the state practice act or if the physical therapist negligently fails to refer a patient to another health care provider, when appropriate, the treating clinicians may be held, in a malpractice action, to the standard of care of the professional to whom the clinician should have referred the patient for consultation. In other words, physical therapists practicing without referral may be held to a physician's legal standard of care if they exceed permissible physical therapy practice limitations.

In such cases, physical therapist-expert witnesses may not be legally competent to testify about the standard of care, since another profession's (medical) standard of care will be involved. The legal ramifications of misdiagnosis and failure to appropriately refer patients to physicians and other appropriate professionals, therefore, make it imperative to practice squarely within the boundaries of state practice acts and individual competency levels, whether clinicians are practicing with or without referral.

Physical and occupational therapists, like other health care professionals, should consider it an honor to be called upon to serve as expert witnesses. Whether sought out because of professional publications, noteworthy clinical practice, or for another reason, it is a civic duty to serve as an expert witness when called upon. It is akin to jury duty, voting, and registering for military service. If physical and occupational therapists do not come forward in future legal cases to establish their own standards of care, other professionals will continue to do so for these professions.

Clinical practice guidelines   Physical and occupational therapists are no doubt familiar with recent clinical practice guidelines for stroke rehabilitation, treatment of pressure ulcers, and low back pain care, published by the Agency for Health Care Policy and Research (AHCPR). AHCPR was created by Congress as part of the Omnibus Budget Reconciliation Act (OBRA) of 1989, and is housed within the U.S. Public Health Service. AHCPR's Medical Treatment Effectiveness Program (MEDTEP) evaluates the efficacy of clinical interventions on desired patient outcomes, through its multidisciplinary Patient Outcomes Research Teams (PORTs).

What are clinical practice guidelines, and how do they mesh into the legal standard of care? Clinical practice guidelines are different from clinical practice protocols. Protocols are relatively rigid decision matrices that call for fairly specific compliance with treatment regimens, such as post-operative tenorrhaphy or anterior cruciate ligament reconstruction rehabilitation instructions.

Clinical practice guidelines, on the other hand, rely more on qualitative clinical reasoning and offer clinicians a number of acceptable treatment options for particular patient presentations. Valid clinical practice guidelines[38] should address all reasonable practice options and potential outcomes of these interventions (and their likelihood of occurrence). Whether or not relative values are assigned to practice options presented, the names of the authors or panels formulating the guidelines and recommendations should be delineated, and the guidelines should clearly state that the process of formulating options and assigning values has been peer-reviewed. Their date of publication should reflect that the guidelines are clinically current.

What, if any, legal precedent do clinical practice guidelines have in establishing the standard of care? To the extent that guidelines are inclusive of all reasonable clinical practice options, they are inclusive of the standard of care, although they are not prescriptive like protocols are. Just as with clinical protocols, however, deviation from acceptable practice standards may shift the legal burden of persuasion to a defendant-health care professional to justify why the clinician deviated from collectively-established practice standards. While the burden of proof remains with a patient-plaintiff in such cases, clearly the defendant who deviates from clinical protocols or guidelines encumbers him- or herself with a trial burden that normally a defendant does not have—the burden to either justify why the clinician disregarded collective wisdom enunciated in standards or to leave it to the jury or judge to guess why.

Advantages of clinical practice guidelines include standardizing treatment processes, memorializing collective professional judgment on the validity and efficacy of treatment options, possibly reducing the number of health care malpractice claims,[39] and providing a framework for clinical decision-making, among others. Disadvantages include limiting available options for clinicians, creating "cookbook" health care, and causing the burden of persuasion to shift to defendant-health care clinicians in malpractice cases to justify deviation from clinical practice guidelines, among others.

Clinicians and administrators should ensure that clinical practice guidelines intended merely to guide clinical decision-making are not misconstrued as representative of *the* standard of care. Facilities and professional associations may wish to include a disclaimer with clinical practice guidelines indicating that the guidelines are not intended to represent the legal standard of care.

Causation   The third element of proof that a plaintiff-patient bears in a health care malpractice professional negligence case is to show, by a preponderance of evidence, that any breach of duty (i.e., violation of the legal standard of care) by a defendant-provider caused injury to the plaintiff-patient. There are two elements of legal causation: *actual cause* and *proximate cause*.

Actual causation means that, "but for" the defendant's substandard care delivery, the plaintiff-patient would not have sustained any injury incident to care. The "but for" designation is also frequently referred to as *sine qua non* (Latin for "without which not").

It is fairly simple in a health care malpractice professional negligence case to establish actual causation. Any direct causal link between a health care professional's conduct (action or failure of action) and a patient's alleged injuries establishes actual causation. This is true even if the defendant-provider's conduct was only a *substantial factor* (along with other possible causes) in the plaintiff-patient's injuries.

Proximate causation poses a more difficult hurdle for plaintiffs in health care malpractice litigation. Under proximate, or *legal*, causation, a court may choose not to hold a defendant-provider liable for professional negligence, even where a breach of duty and actual causation have been established by the plaintiff.

The definition of proximate causation is somewhat elusive, even for legal scholars. In one reported physical therapy malpractice case, *Greening by Greening v. School District of Millard*,[40] the court described proximate causation in detail. In *Greening*, a state-employed physical therapist designed an exercise regime for a student-patient with myelodysplasia. The program was carried out with the patient wearing leg braces, by an aide, under supervision of the physical therapist. During a treatment session, the patient sustained a femoral fracture. The school district (sued by the patient's parents for vicarious liability) prevailed in the case at trial and on appeal. The appellate judge in the case described proximate cause as a natural, direct result of a breach of duty on the defendant-provider's part, with no superseding intervening act breaking the "chain" of causation.

When harm is not reasonably *foreseeable*, courts may limit health care malpractice liability, so as to not unfairly impose liability for unforeseeable results. Note, however, that a patient's pre-existing medical conditions do not necessarily equate to superceding causes of injury that absolve a provider of liability for injuries incident to treatment, if the provider could have learned about the pre-existing conditions through the taking of a thorough history or through other reasonable means. It is only the reasonably unforeseeable consequence for which a court may be willing to cut off liability under proximate causation. Recall the *Piccarillo* case,[41] in which a plaintiff-patient alleged professional negligence because a student physical therapist allegedly failed to provide direct assistance during her late-stage ambulation training. A defense expert witness testified that the plaintiff's fall during therapy and hip fracture might have occurred spontaneously, because of osteoporosis or torsion during turning movements. To the extent that such an event is unforeseeable, it might well constitute a superseding intervening act that would break the chain of (proximate) causation and prevent the imposition of liability.

Damages   The final element of proof in a professional negligence lawsuit is damages. To warrant the award of monetary damages, a plaintiff must show that he or she sustained the kinds of injuries, as a direct result of a defendant-provider's breach of duty, that require the payment of money in order to make the plaintiff "whole" (or as whole as possible).

What kinds of losses warrant the award of monetary damages in a professional negligence health care malpractice case? Monetary outlays for additional medical care to correct or minimize the injury caused by the defendant constitute one element of damages. So do lost wages or salary (from one or more employment sources) resulting from time away from work because of rehabilitation. Economic losses, such as telephone and traveling expenses, are also recoverable, as are (in some states) loss of a reasonable chance of recovery or survival incident to a defendant-health care professional's negligent care. These actual out-of-pocket losses specific to the plaintiff-patient are known as *special damages*.

Finally, damages may be awarded for the monetary value of pain and suffering incident to the defendant-provider's substandard care. Because of the difficulty in quantifying the monetary value of pain and suffering, many states now cap pain and suffering damages at a statutory maximum amount. Pain and suffering damages and damages paid for the loss of enjoyment of life and the fear of contracting a disease related to a defendant's negligence are known as *general damages*.

Immediate family members directly and adversely affected by the plaintiff-patient's injuries may also recover monetary damages for *loss of consortium*. For spouses, loss of consortium damages include the monetary value of lost services, society, and companionship (including sexual relations), incurred over some definite period of time.

For parents, the value of a plaintiff-child's lost economic contribution to the family unit is recoverable in some states.[42]

Other Tort Bases for Malpractice Liability

The two other tort bases for health care malpractice liability are intentional conduct causing patient injury and strict liability without regard for fault. Intentional tort liability is addressed in Chapter 3. A brief description of the two forms of strict liability in tort follows.

Strict, or absolute, liability in tort involves either socially important, but abnormally dangerous, activities that result in patient injury or patient injury from dangerously defective commercial products. The first form of strict liability is called *strict liability for abnormally dangerous activities* (formerly called *strict liability for ultrahazardous activities*); the second is *strict product liability*. An issue of strict liability for abnormally dangerous activity seldom, if ever, should arise in health care clinical practice, because of the emphasis on patient safety and quality management associated with health care delivery. Factors used by courts to assess whether an activity is abnormally dangerous include:

- whether the activity involves a high degree of risk of foreseeable harm
- the severity of the attendant risk of harm
- whether the risk of harm can be eliminated through the stringent safety precautions
- whether the activity constitutes customary common practice
- the social worth or value of the activity to clients and society[43]

Hypothetical examples of activities that could be bases for strict liability for abnormally dangerous activities include high velocity, high amplitude manipulative thrust procedures and extremely high-weight manual cervical traction techniques that result in patient injury. Although in at least one reported medical malpractice case, the court opined that an action for strict liability for abnormally dangerous activity incident to health care delivery might be possible,[44] no reported cases finding such liability were retrieved.

Regarding strict product liability, courts will impose liability upon commercial distributors of unreasonably dangerously defective products that injure buyers or other foreseeable persons. According to the Restatement of Torts (Second) [a model for adoption as law by the states], Section 402A(1):

> One who sells any product in a defective condition unreasonably dangerous to the user or consumer . . . is subject to liability . . . if the seller is engaged in the business of selling such a product.

Strict product liability was first imposed in California in 1944, in *Escola* v. *Coca-Cola Bottling Co.*,[45] a res ipsa loquitur case involving an exploding soda bottle that injured a consumer. All other states soon followed California's lead in establishing strict product liability as a viable cause of action in tort.

The philosophy behind strict product liability is that, between two potentially inno-cent parties—a commercial seller and a consumer of a dangerously defective prod-uct—the seller is the logical party to bear the risk of liability for injuries from the product, since the seller is in the better position to insure against such liability and to monitor product safety. Dangerous product defects can be of three types: design defects, manufacturing defects, and inadequate warnings about potential hazards associated with a possibly dangerous product. Courts may grant immunity from design defect-based strict product liability to sellers of Class III medical devices that are unavoidably unsafe and about which insufficient information is known to ensure product safety (e.g., cardiac pacemakers and penile implants).[46]

Courts traditionally have been reluctant to impose strict product liability on health care professional-defendants, because health care delivery is primarily the delivery (sale) of a professional service and not the sale of a product. This quasi-qualified immunity of health care professionals from strict product liability means that patients injured by defective medical products normally are required to claim against or sue product manufacturers.

Courts will, however, allow patients to sue health care clinicians (also classified under law as "learned intermediaries"[47] for strict product liability when health care clinicians are regularly in the business of selling products to patients, such as TENS devices, home traction units, and exercise equipment. The professions of orthotics and prosthetics also are more vulnerable to strict product liability malpractice lawsuits, since these allied health professions are co-primary service and products-professions.[48]

Ordinary Negligence Incident to Health Care Delivery

Ordinary negligence differs from professional negligence in several key respects. Any person owing a duty of due care to others may face liability for ordinary negligence. Professional negligence, on the other hand, deals with liability of members of learned (licensed or registered) professions. Professionals are rightfully held to a higher standard of care vis-a-vis their clients than are members of the public at large. This is because learned professionals possess superior knowledge and skills gained through advanced formal and informal education, training, and professional development. (Along the same continuum, board-certified professional specialists and their equivalent colleagues, are held to even a higher standard, because of their additional credentials.)

Ordinary negligence allegations formed the bases for legal actions in a significant number of the reported legal cases brought by patients against physical therapists. For example, in *Winona Memorial Foundation v. Lomax*,[49] a patient receiving hydrotherapy in a physical therapy clinic tripped and fell on a protruding floor board midway between the dressing area and the hydrotherapy room. As a result of the fall, she sustained a herniated lumbar disc. She sued the facility for vicarious liability, claiming professional (treatment-related) negligence. The court held (and the appel-late court affirmed) that the case was one involving ordinary (premises) negligence, and not health care malpractice (professional negligence).

Similarly, in *St. Paul Fire and Marine Insurance Company* v. *Prothro*,[50] the court ruled that a fall from a Hubbard tank hoist device constituted a charge of ordinary, not professional, negligence. This case scenario presents a much closer call than that illustrated in *Winona*. In *Prothro*, the patient was post-operative for a total hip arthroplasty. When the Hubbard tank chain broke during transfer of the patient, and the patient fell, the fresh surgical wound re-opened. In the emergency, the patient's bleeding was stopped with a clean, but unsterile, towel. The patient subsequently developed a Staphylococcus aureus infection, requiring removal of the hip prosthesis and leaving the patient with a significant residual leg length discrepancy. On appeal, the Arkansas appellate court affirmed a trial court judgment of $75,000 in favor of the plaintiff-patient.

Finally, in *Emig* v. *Physicians' Physical Therapy Services*,[51] a case in which a patient who was post-operative from hip arthroplasty surgery allegedly fell out of a wheelchair while unattended during physical therapy treatment, the appeals court disallowed expert testimony in the case. This was based on the court's legal conclusion (ruling *as a matter of law*) that the lawsuit was one involving ordinary premises negligence and not health care malpractice.

Premises liability[52] concerns potential liability for monetary damages on the part of owners or occupiers (e.g., lessees ["tenants"]) of land for injuries incurred by patrons and others coming onto the premises. A duty of due care may be owed even to those persons entering or remaining on the premises without authorization, for example, trespassers and burglars.

> ***Premises liability:*** potential liability for monetary damages on the part of owners or occupiers of land for injuries incurred by patrons and others coming onto their premises.

In many states, the law classifies the degree of duty owed to persons entering onto premises based on their status as invitees, licensees, and trespassers. For trespassers, the duty owed under this classification scheme is the lowest, often involving only the duty to post warnings about hidden man-made dangers that pose a substantial risk of serious bodily harm or death. As with most laws, there are exceptions to this bare-bones requirement, particularly for children who might be drawn onto hazardous premises by an "attractive nuisance."

A higher duty is normally owed to business licensees, such as delivery persons and vendors. In addition to the aforementioned duty to warn about hidden hazards, there is usually a duty owed to use all reasonable measures to protect licensees from injuries resulting from operation of the facility. For example, an occupational therapist using work simulation machinery in the clinic would be required to take reasonable steps to prevent a Federal Express delivery person from being injured by that machinery while traversing the clinic on the way to the office to make a delivery.

For states using the "bright-line" duty standard based on victim status, the highest duty owed is toward invitees, including, in the case of physical and occupational therapist-clinic owners, patients and their families and significant others who are allowed into the clinic.[53] Here, the duty owed is to take all reasonable steps to protect the invitees from any foreseeable harm from their exposure to the premises. This includes an affirmative duty to undertake regular inspections of the premises to seek out potential hazards.

A minority of states have abolished the bright-line rules for duty owed to persons coming onto premises based on their status. In these states, the law simply universally requires owners and occupiers of premises to act reasonably under all circumstances to protect all persons coming onto their property from foreseeable harm. The status of the entrant, then, becomes only one factor to be considered in deciding the extent of the duty owed.[54]

What's the significance of the legal distinction between ordinary and professional negligence to health care professionals? The difference is very important to all parties and their attorneys. If a case is filed as an ordinary negligence case, the tort reform measures applicable to health care malpractice legal actions will probably not apply, such as the requirement for administrative panel screening of a malpractice case for merit. There may be a longer statute of limitations (time line for commencing legal action) for ordinary negligence cases than for professional negligence cases because of tort reform. In ordinary negligence cases, the health care professional standard of care is not normally in issue, and often, expensive, contradictory, and confounding expert witness testimony is not needed. In some jurisdictions, it is not even permitted, since juries are perfectly capable of discerning common premises negligence without it. In the event of a finding of liability in an ordinary negligence case—even if it arises in a health care setting—the defendant's name should not be reportable to the National Practitioner Data Bank (which is defined and discussed later in this chapter).

So it appears that a case brought as an ordinary negligence case, rather than as a professional negligence case, can inure to the benefit of all parties. It can also be of great benefit to courts, as trial time may be decreased because less expert witness testimony may be required. Finally, ordinary vs. professional case designation may benefit society as a whole, since cases will probably cost less to bring to trial.

Vicarious Liability for Others' Conduct

The term *vicarious liability* refers to the circumstances under which an employer bears indirect legal and financial responsibility for the conduct of another person, usually of an employee. The concept of vicarious liability dates back to ancient times and in legal circles is often referred to as *respondeat superior* (Latin for "let the master answer").

> **Vicarious liability:** indirect legal and financial responsibility for the conduct of another person, such as an employee or a clinic volunteer.

The basic rule of vicarious liability is that an employer is financially liable for the negligent conduct of an employee when that employee-wrongdoer ("tortfeasor") is acting within the scope of his or her employment at the time the act or omission occurred. Therefore, when a hospital-based physical or occupational therapist, assistant, or aide is alleged to have negligently caused injury to a patient during the course of treatment, the hospital employing the person directly responsible for the patient's injury may be required to pay the monetary judgment, if negligence is proven in court.

An employer's indirect responsibility for an employee's conduct does not in any way excuse from financial responsibility the employee who is directly responsible for negligent patient injury. A tortfeasor is always personally responsible for the consequences of his or her own conduct. Vicarious liability, however, gives a tort victim another party to make a claim against or to sue for monetary damages incident to wrongful injury. If an employer is required to pay a settlement or judgment for the negligence of one of its employees, the employer retains the legal right to seek indemnification from the employee for this outlay.

Is it fair to impose liability on an employer who is innocent of any wrongdoing? In balancing the equities between an innocent victim of negligence and an innocent

> **Hint** *A tortfeasor is always personally responsible for the consequences of his or her own conduct.*

employer of the party directly responsible for negligence, the legal system weighs in favor of the innocent victim of negligence. There are several good reasons for this public policy favoring victims over employers. First, it is the employer, not the patient-victim, who has the exclusive right (and duty) to control the quality of patient care rendered in the facility by all providers. Second, because the employer earns a profit from the activities of its employees, it is only fair that the employer should be held responsible for patient injuries caused by employees. Third, the employer is normally in a much better position than the patient to bear the financial risk of loss—through economic loss allocation (i.e., purchasing liability insurance)—as part of the overall cost of doing business.

An employer may be held vicariously liable for the conduct of non-employees, as well as for employees. In the relatively few reported cases addressing the issue, courts have universally imposed vicarious liability on hospitals for the negligence of their volunteers; in essence, equating unpaid volunteers with employees. For this reason, health care facilities utilizing the services of volunteers should carry liability insurance for volunteers' activities.

Another area of vicarious liability involves general partnership business arrangements, wherein each general partner is considered legally to be the agent of all other general partners. Each general partner, then, is vicariously liable for negligent acts committed by other general partners when those acts are within the scope of activities of the partnership.

There are several important exceptions to vicarious liability. Although an employer may be vicariously liable for employees' negligence, the employer typically is not liable for intentional misconduct committed by employees. An example of intentional misconduct would be commission of battery on a patient by a physical therapist assistant during a treatment session.

Another exception to vicarious liability involves independent contractors—for example, contract physical and occupational therapists and their support personnel working in a health care facility. The legal system generally distinguishes between employees—for whom an employer is vicariously liable, and contract workers—for whom the employer generally is not vicariously liable. This distinction is based primarily on the permissible degree of control the employer may exercise over the physical details of the professional work product of these two classes of workers.

In some jurisdictions, courts hold employers vicariously liable for the negligence of independent contractors under the theory of *apparent agency*, or *ostensible agency* (also called "agency by estoppel"). When a contract professional worker in a clinic setting is indistinguishable from an employee-clinician, for example, a court may hold the employer vicariously liable for contractor negligence. Therefore, it is prudent risk management for employers to take appropriate steps to ensure that patients know when they are being treated by contract workers instead of employees. Methods to accomplish this include requiring contractors to wear name tags identifying them as contractors and posting an informational memorandum about workers' status in the clinic reception or waiting area.

In some cases, an employer may not only be vicariously liable for its employees' negligence, but also primarily, or directly, liable for its workers' conduct under a concept known as *corporate liability*. Until recently, nonprofit hospitals were virtually immune from any liability under a concept known as charitable immunity, granted in large part because of the benevolent character of these institutions. Since then, in at least 22 states,[55] courts have imposed direct liability on hospitals under corporate liability; in essence, courts are treating hospitals like any other ordinary business.

There are at least four theories under which corporate liability may attach. Hospitals have been found liable for the negligent screening and hiring of professional employees, such as physicians, nurses, and allied health professionals. They have also been held liable for the negligent credentialing and privileging of staff professionals. Hospitals have also been held directly liable for negligent failure to adequately monitor safety in their facilities. Finally, hospitals have been held liable under corporate liability for failing to establish effective quality management programs to systematically monitor the quality of health care delivered by all providers within the facility—including employees, contractors, consultants, volunteers, and others.

In a recent Harvard University study, researchers found that systemic problems at the organizational level, rather than individual culpability on the part of specific health care professionals, accounted for many reported iatrogenic patient injuries.[56] They attributed poor information management as a key factor in creating an environment in which medication errors and other mistakes can take place. The authors of the study urge that hospital administrators and clinical managers adopt a systems approach to quality management, similar to that used in the aerospace industry, to minimize the propensity for systemic errors that lead to patient injuries and deaths.

Defenses to Health Care Malpractice Actions

While a defendant in a health care malpractice case normally bears no particular burden of proof in the case, the defendant probably will put forward one or more affirmative defenses in opposition to a plaintiff-patient's *case-in-chief*. Affirmative defenses are ones that normally must be stated in the defendant's *answer*, the first responsive *pleading* to a plaintiff's *complaint*. By its apparent meaning, an affirmative defense is one in which the defendant bears the legal burden of proving the defense to the plaintiff's allegation by a preponderance of evidence.

Two key defenses available to health care malpractice defendants are expiration of the statute of limitations and comparative patient fault in causing injury. Other potential defenses include assumption on the patient's part of the attendant risks associated with a treatment and immunity and release from liability.

Statutes of limitations   For purposes of health care malpractice litigation, the statute of limitations is a time line that begins at a point where a patient knows (or should reasonably know) that he or she was injured at the hands of a health care provider and ends some months or years later at a time fixed by state or federal statute. The alleged victim of malpractice must file a formal civil lawsuit within the confines of that time line or be forever barred from later bringing legal action. The statute of limitations is considered a procedural, rather than a substantive, law.

> **Statute of limitations:** time period after injury during which an injured person must file a civil lawsuit or be forever barred from later initiating legal action.

There are several key purposes to the statute of limitations. First, it affords an injured person sufficient time to investigate the source and nature of an injury, consult with and retain legal counsel (if desired), file a complaint with the responsible party (and/or that party's employer and/or insurer), and attempt to settle the matter short of resorting to trial. Second, the statute of limitations creates a state of certainty (except when its exceptions apply, discussed below) and finality. Under the statute of limitations, legal cases must be commenced and brought to trial within a reasonable timeframe so that witnesses to an event are still alive and available, documents and physical evidence are preserved for inspection, and parties and insurers can anticipate the resolution of pending legal disputes and their likely consequences.

There are a number of exceptions to the statute of limitations that apply in many jurisdictions. If one of these exceptions applies, the statute of limitations is said to be *tolled*, or suspended until the exception is no longer applicable. Some exceptions concern what is termed a *legal disability* involving an alleged victim. For example, in some jurisdictions, the statute of limitations is tolled for minors and mentally incompetent victims for varying time periods. Now, many jurisdictions do not suspend the statute of limitations because of a victim's minority or incompetency. This is the case in the federal civil legal system.[57]

Other exceptions that toll the statute of limitations include the *continuous treatment doctrine* and the *discovery rule*. Under the continuous treatment doctrine, a court may suspend the running of the statute of limitations during the time in which the alleged victim of malpractice and the responsible health care professional maintain an active patient-professional relationship for treatment of the same condition from which injury resulted. The public policy purpose for this exception is that a tort victim should not be expected to interrupt necessary health care intervention for an active condition in order to bring legal action for malpractice.

The principle exception to the statute of limitations is the discovery rule. Under this exception, the statute of limitations may be suspended for the time period during which an injured person cannot reasonably be expected to discover the injury upon which a malpractice claim may be based. The discovery rule has been invoked for conditions such as surgical sponges, needles, or instruments left inside of a surgical patient. Consider the following hypothetical example.

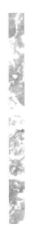

A patient is referred to physical therapy by an orthopedic surgeon with a diagnosis of cervical degenerative joint disease with mild right C5 radiculopathy. The treatment order reads, "Evaluate and treat. Consider traction and/or appropriate mobilization techniques." After taking a thorough history and conducting a comprehensive physical examination, a physical therapist treats the patient using manual cervical distraction and manipulation techniques. The patient does not improve, and after several treatments, appears to have worsened. The physical therapist then ceases treatment, and refers the patient back to the orthopedist for re-evaluation. Nine months later, it is discovered through diagnostic imaging study, that the patient sustained bony injury to the cervical spine, probably from the physical therapist's manipulation treatment. The statute of limitations would probably not begin to run until the date of discovery by the patient of the existence and source of the injury.

Some states, pursuant to tort reform legislation, have placed absolute time limits, called *statutes of repose*, on certain types of civil actions, including strict product liability actions. This means that, regardless of legal disability or plaintiff inability to discover the source of an injury, the outside time limit for initiating affected legal actions covered under statutes of repose is cut off after a set statutory period. Statutes of repose are considered to be an equitable way to solve the problems of perpetual litigation involving products produced long ago and incidents resulting in injury that have become stale because of lost or destroyed evidence or unavailable witnesses.

Several reported physical therapy malpractice cases were lost by plaintiffs because of noncompliance with, or adverse judicial interpretations involving statutes of limitations. In *O'Neal* v. *Throop and Rehab Works*,[58] a patient filed a lawsuit against his orthopedic surgeon and physical therapist for professional negligence, claiming (1) negligent performance by the surgeon of an arthroscopic medial meniscus repair, and (2) negligent failure on the part of the physical therapist to communicate with the surgeon about the plaintiff's alleged slow progress with post-operative rehabilitation. After approximately two weeks of physical therapy treatment, the plaintiff failed, without warning or complaints, to report for further treatment. The plaintiff consulted with another orthopedist, who removed a staple from the patient's knee that purportedly was the source of the patient's problems.

The plaintiff-patient lost the case at trial and on appeal. The appellate court ruled that the plaintiff had failed to comply with the state's two-year tort statute of limitations in initiating legal action. The plaintiff's attorney argued on appeal that the trial judge committed *reversible error* by not ordering the statute of limitations suspended because of the continuous treatment exception. The plaintiff unsuccessfully argued that he had remained under the defendants' care for sufficient time to allow his malpractice action to proceed to trial. He also unsuccessfully urged the appellate court to reverse the trial-level judgment in favor of the defendants on the ground that the defendants committed "fraudulent concealment" of his alleged injuries.

In *Myers* v. *Woodall*,[59] the plaintiff-patient was allegedly injured when an aide transporting the patient from the nursing floor to the physical therapy clinic caused the patient's body to strike a wall while on a gurney. The appellate court affirmed the trial court's summary judgment in favor of the defendant-hospital and physical therapist. However, the appeals court reversed the trial court award of summary judgment in favor of the transport aide directly responsible for the plaintiff-patient's injury, in essence, allowing the lawsuit against the aide to proceed. This ruling reflected the fact that the statutes of limitations for professional negligence (against the defendant-hospital and physical therapist) expired before the plaintiff's lawsuit commenced. A longer statute of limitations was in place in the state for non-professional treatment-related negligence (against the defendant-aide).

Comparative fault   The right of a patient to collect monetary damages for injury incident to health malpractice is not absolute. In many cases, defendant-health care professionals will raise the issue of patient contributory negligence or comparative fault in cases brought against them. Just like health care professionals treating patients have a duty of due care owed to patients under their care, patients themselves have a legal duty incident to care. That duty is to conduct themselves so that their actions do not fall below a standard imposed by (case) law for their own safety and protection. When a patient's conduct falls below the standard imposed by law for the patient's own protection, that careless conduct constitutes *contributory negligence*.

> ***Contributory negligence:*** plaintiff-patient conduct which falls below a standard mandated by law for the patient's own protection from unreasonable harm incident to treatment.

There are two ways that courts assess plaintiff-patient conduct, depending on the state in which a health care malpractice trial takes place. Before the first era of patient-oriented tort reform earlier in this century, most or all jurisdictions used a pure contributory negligence formula for assessing plaintiff-patient conduct. Under this formula, if a patient is at all responsible—even one percent or less—for his or her own injuries incident to treatment, then the patient loses a health care malpractice case brought against a defendant-health care professional or organization. This harsh rule of "all or nothing" was tempered over time with numerous exceptions that permitted meritorious lawsuits brought by plaintiffs to proceed. One of those exceptions (still operational in some jurisdictions) is *last clear chance*. Under the doctrine of last clear chance, application of all-or-nothing contributory negligence is prevented when a defendant has the last clear opportunity to act reasonably to prevent plaintiff injury, but negligently fails to prevent it. Consider the following hypothetical example.

A patient who is recently status-post lumbar laminectomy is undergoing an occupational therapy work capacity evaluation. While preparing to lift a 10-pound weight from one table to another, the patient suddenly moves toward a 75-pound weight which is on the floor and states, "Let's see how much I can lift." Even though it would otherwise be pure contributory negligence for the patient to attempt to lift the heavy weight from the floor without authorization, the patient's harm to himself might not preclude legal action for professional negligence. A legal action might be viable if the occupational therapist failed to take reasonable steps to attempt to halt the patient from attempting to lift the heavy box, under the equitable doctrine of last clear chance.

In most states, a newer method of assessing potential plaintiff fault in a malpractice case applies—*comparative negligence*. Under the doctrine of comparative negligence, plaintiff-patient contributory negligence or wrongdoing does not necessarily eliminate any possibility of a professional negligence malpractice lawsuit against a health care professional. Instead, courts assess proportional patient culpability, and assign a percentage of fault to it. In most states, if the patient's percentage of fault is 50 percent or less, the patient can proceed with a lawsuit and have monetary damages reduced by the patient's proportional degree of fault. In a few jurisdictions, patients can proceed to trial and win a monetary judgment, even if plaintiff comparative fault is greater than 50 percent. This subcategory of comparative negligence is called *pure comparative fault*. Consider the following hypothetical case.

An outpatient being treated in a privately-owned physical therapy clinic for chronic mechanical low back pain is receiving hot pack modality treatment prior to joint mobilization and exercise therapy. Midway through the 20-minute hot pack session, the patient removes five of eight layers of protective toweling without calling for the physical therapist assistant overseeing the modalities area, in order to enhance the heating effect of the hot pack. When the patient's bell sounds ten minutes later, the physical therapist assistant enters the patient's cubicle and removes the hot pack. The assistant notices that the patient has greater-than-normal erythema in the area of treatment and blisters forming over the treated area of skin. Assuming that the state in which the patient files a physical therapy malpractice lawsuit against the physical therapist-clinic owner for professional negligence uses the doctrine of comparative fault to assess damages, at what level would you quantify patient comparative liability? Justify your assessment. Would the patient be permitted to proceed to trial and win any monetary damages under your assessment? Explain.

The defensive comparative fault concepts of contributory negligence and comparative negligence apply in most cases only to health care malpractice cases brought as professional negligence cases. Because, under strict liability cases, culpability on the part of a defendant is not in issue, comparative fault principles are likewise not applied in these types of cases. As always, of course, there are exceptions in the legal literature.[60] Contributory negligence and comparative fault are not valid defenses in cases involving intentional misconduct by defendants, as a matter of equity and public policy.

Assumption of risk   Assumption of the risk is a theoretically possible defense to a health care malpractice lawsuit. A plaintiff is considered to have assumed the risk of an activity under a defendant's control if the plaintiff (1) fully appreciates the nature and extent of the risk of injury associated with the activity, and (2) makes a knowledgeable, intelligent, voluntary, and unequivocal choice to encounter that risk.[61] Assumption of the risk applies, for instance, when a patron having cervical pathology voluntarily elects to ride a tumultuous rollercoaster ride at an amusement park, despite clear, posted warnings of its potential dangers.

As with comparative fault, assumption of the risk is theoretically a defense in health malpractice litigation that should only be available in professional negligence malpractice cases. It is not available in cases involving alleged intentional misconduct by a defendant-provider, nor can it normally be raised as a defense in cases where a plaintiff is a member of a statutorily protected class of persons, such as those persons who are mentally incompetent or minors. Finally, no health care professional may compel a patient to waive liability (indirectly causing a patient to assume the risks of health care interventions) through a contractual *exculpatory release*.

In at least one reported legal case, *Schneider* v. *Revici*,[62] involving a female patient who contractually agreed with her physician to waive any liability on the physician's part for a novel form of breast cancer therapy, the federal court held (in finding that the contract was invalid because it was vague) that assumption of the risk is potentially an available defense to a health care malpractice lawsuit, where the intervention in issue is "unconventional."

The better rule to follow is that patients assume the risk of nothing in the course of health care intervention that would excuse professional negligence on the part of a health care provider owing a duty of special care toward that patient. Therefore, except theoretically, assumption of the risk is inapplicable as a defense in health care delivery.

> **Hint** *Assumption of the risk is inapplicable as a defense to malpractice litigation in conventional health care delivery.*

Immunity   Until very recently, nonprofit religious-based health care institutions enjoyed immunity from legal actions under an equitable legal doctrine called *charitable immunity*. This immunity was granted because of the great public service rendered on behalf of the sick and dying patients who, otherwise, had no place of refuge in society. As health care delivery became equated with ordinary business during this century, however, the charitable immunity exception to tort liability died.

Immunity from legal actions is also a privilege enjoyed by governments under an ancient concept known as *sovereign immunity*. States and the federal government enjoy sovereign immunity from liability (i.e., cannot be sued or compelled to pay out a monetary judgment) unless they expressly waive, or give up, their sovereign immunity. The federal government, in 1946, partially relinquished its sovereign immunity from liability under a statute known as the Federal Tort Claims Act.[63] Under this statute, in the federal-sector health care setting, most patients (except active duty military service members and their family members, when suing the federal government derivatively for wrongdoing against active-duty service members) may bring lawsuits against the federal government for professional and ordinary negligence and for a limited number of intentional wrongs. Many states have adopted waiver-of-sovereign-immunity-statutes similar to the Federal Tort Claims Act.

Under litigation brought pursuant to the Federal Tort Claims Act, individual federal health care employees are personally immune from suit under the Federal Liability Reform and Tort Compensation Act,[64] provided that their conduct falls within official scope of duty. State-employed health care professionals may enjoy similar personal immunity from liability under state statutes.

In some states, selected licensed health care professionals engaging in *pro bono publico* (Latin for "for the public good") health care services may enjoy limited tort immunity from liability.[65] The American Physical Therapy Association's Code of Ethics, *Guide for Professional Conduct*[66] and the American Occupational Therapy Association's *Occupational Therapy Code of Ethics*[67] contain provisions making it an ethical responsibility on the part of professional members to attempt to meet the health needs of socioeconomically disadvantaged patients. (For more detailed information on the history of *pro bono publico* service in the legal profession and in the health services professions, please see Scott, R.W. "For the Public Good." *PT: Magazine of Physical Therapy*, 1993; 1(1):82–85.)

Releases from liability   The release from liability is a standard legal instrument in civil law. For instance, when an insurance company settles a claim with a claimant, release from liability is used to absolve the insurance company forever of further liability resulting from the incident in question. It is also utilized in health care malpractice litigation to absolve a defendant or defendants of further liability exposure in exchange for a monetary settlement made to a plaintiff. These uses of a release are well-established and not generally subject to nullification, except in cases of fraud, duress, undue influence, or other overreaching by a party or by the party's agent.

It is the attempted prospective use of releases in the health care setting that is legally problematic. As a general rule, an attempted exculpatory release that is made a *condition precedent* (pre-condition) of receiving treatment is invalid as violative of public policy. The lead reported legal case involving exculpatory releases from liability is *Tunkl* v. *Regents of the University of California*.[68] In that seminal case, a terminally ill patient was admitted to a state-run charity research hospital for treatment. As a condition of admission, the hospital required the patient to sign a release from liability, which was purportedly justified because the facility was a charity hospital. The patient died and his wife, as *executrix* (personally-appointed legal representative) of his estate, brought suit challenging the exculpatory release and claiming professional negligence regarding her late husband's care. In invalidating the exculpatory release, Justice Tobriner of the California Supreme Court held that California statutory law stated that "all contracts which have for their object, to exempt anyone from responsibility for his own fraud, or willful injury to the person or property of another, . . . whether willful or negligent, are against the policy of the law."[69] The court ruled that there could be no exception for hospitals, even charity or research hospitals, and allowed the executrix's legal action for malpractice to proceed.

In two reported physical therapy negligence cases, courts struck down exculpatory health care releases as unenforceable. *Leidy* v. *Deseret Enterprises*[70] involved a health care malpractice action brought by a post-operative lumbar laminectomy patient against a health spa and a physical therapist-employee. The appeals court reversed a trial-level summary judgment in favor of the spa and therapist and remanded the case for trial, in part based on an attempted exculpatory release from liability that the patient had signed. *Meiman* v. *Rehabilitation Center, Inc.*[71] was a case involving a claim of professional negligence against a physical therapist secondary to the plaintiff-patient sustaining a femoral neck fracture during stretching of a limb which was status-post above-knee amputation. The appeals court reversed a trial-level judgment for the defendants, in part, because of an exculpatory release agreement.

There may be instances where a waiver of liability may be appropriate and enforceable. Consider the case where a competent, hospitalized inpatient voluntarily elects to leave the facility midway through care "against medical advice" ("AMA") Before such a patient leaves the facility, a physician, nurse, or administrative official will discuss the adverse consequences of leaving AMA, and attempt to have the patient sign a release from further liability. Such a risk management measure is appropriate. Similarly, when a patient declines what health care professionals deem to be necessary care because of religious or personal beliefs, it is appropriate to seek a limitation of liability agreement from the patient. What is repugnant to the courts are exculpatory health care releases from liability that are general in nature. Consider the following hypothetical example.

> A post-operative finger flexor tendon surgical patient is receiving outpatient rehabilitation by an occupational therapist. Suddenly one day, the patient states that she is going to quit attending rehab and exercise her hand on her own. Objectively, she is still in need of professional care. As

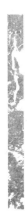

the treating therapist, explain how you would protect the patient's interests and your own interests in this situation. Answer: (1) Fully explain to the patient the consequences of discontinuing therapy prematurely. Ensure that the patient's decision to discontinue treatment is knowing, intelligent, voluntary, and unequivocal. Make sure that there is no point of dissatisfaction regarding your care that can be remedied to the patient's reasonable satisfaction. (2) Notify the referring physician of the patient's action, and carefully document the patient's statements, your counseling of the patient, and your communication with the referring physician. (3) Consult with your legal advisor, and consider asking the patient to sign a release from further liability. Be careful that the release does not attempt to absolve you of any liability incident to care, because such a release would probably be unenforceable as a violation of public policy.

National Practitioner Data Bank

The National Practitioner Data Bank was established pursuant to a federal statute, the Health Care Quality Improvement Act of 1986.[72] Congress enacted this law with several purposes in mind:

- to promote effective professional peer review by the health professions by providing "qualified immunity" from defamation or other bases of liability for statements made during these processes[73]

- to require reporting by hospitals and other health care organizations having peer review of adverse credentialing actions affecting clinical privileges involving physicians, dentists, and other licensed health care professionals

- to require the reporting of adverse licensure action against a licensed health care professional by a state licensure board

- to require the reporting of health care malpractice payments made on behalf of health care professionals to patients or their representatives, either by settlement or judgment[74]

Before the advent of the National Practitioner Data Bank, unscrupulous and incompetent health care providers were often able to "skip" from state to state to avoid adverse licensure disciplinary action with impunity.[75] The Data Bank was intended to prevent these kinds of injustices by making available to employers and licensure agencies critical information about adverse actions taken against licensed health care professionals.

The implementation of the Data Bank was delayed for several years after the effective date of the Health Care Quality Improvement Act, in part because of strong opposition by health care professional associations. The Data Bank was debated in Congress, with substantial lobbyist intervention, until its implementation on September 1, 1990. Regarding health care malpractice payments, any amount, even a nominal, so-called "nuisance" settlement amount, must be reported by payers to the Data Bank.

In its first year of operation (September 1, 1990 through August 31, 1991), the Data Bank recorded 15,782 malpractice payments made by insurers and health care organizations on behalf of licensed health care professionals. Of that number, 11,721 involved physician malpractice payments, 2,360 involved payments made on behalf of dentists, and 1,701 payments were made on behalf of other licensed health care professionals, including physical and occupational therapists. There were 2,779 adverse administrative action reports for the first-year period: 2,285 involving physicians, 470 involving dentists, and 24 involving other licensed health care professionals. The total number of reports made to the Data Bank in the first year was 18,561.[76]

Who has access to the Data Bank? Hospitals and other health care organizations required to query the Data Bank about newly licensed health care professional-employees, state licensing entities, and licensed health care professionals themselves. In limited circumstances (such as when employers fail to query the Data Bank, as required, about new health care professional-employees), plaintiff attorneys have access to information in the National Practitioner Data Bank.[77] Note that employers are also required to query the Data Bank for information about employed or otherwise privileged licensed health care professionals on a regularly recurring basis—every two years.[78]

There are currently no provisions under the Health Care Quality Improvement Act for public access to information about health care professional adverse administrative actions or malpractice payments. Some legislators and consumer advocacy groups are lobbying for changes in the statute to allow for such public disclosure.[79] Meanwhile, one consumer advocacy group, Public Citizen, has published a 13,000-page, two-volume text listing what the group labels as 10,289 "questionable " physicians. The group bases its labeling on publicly-available reports of serious disciplinary action by state or federal administrative agencies.[80]

Patient Care Documentation Management

Patient care documentation has malpractice implications, just as affirmative care delivery does. Physical and occupational therapists have fared relatively well thus far in the health care malpractice litigation crisis, in large part because of the uniqueness of the relationship these professionals have with their patients. Because physical and occupational therapists and their assistants devote so much time to patient care, these professionals become privy to many details about patients' medical histories and personal lives that other health care professionals simply do not have the time to hear. In this capacity, they have a unique opportunity to communicate vital information about patients (consistent with privacy considerations) to other health professionals having a need to know. The information conveyed then becomes assimilated into interdisciplinary care plans to speed recovery, enhance patient functioning, and alleviate pain.

Communication of pertinent information about the patient to other providers who are simultaneously treating that patient, therefore, is the principal purpose of patient care documentation. Concise, objective, timely documentation of a provider's evaluation, diagnosis, and treatment of a patient conveys to other health professionals who treat that patient—now or in the future—insight into the patient's specific needs. Standards for formats and frequency of patient care documentation are established by statutes; licensure regulations; institution, group, or network standards; accreditation and third-party payer mandates; and professional association guidelines.

The American Occupational Therapy Association and the American Physical Therapy Association have established documentation guidelines for their respective professions.[81,82,83] The association documentation guidelines contain a disclaimer that the guidelines are intended to be foundational material used to develop more specific guidelines for individual and group practices, as appropriate. The association documentation guidelines are not intended to create a legal standard of care for purposes of malpractice litigation.

Because communication through patient care documentation is so critically important to a patient's well-being, the failure to document vital care information in the patient's record accurately, clearly, objectively, and in a timely manner constitutes professional negligence, which may be legally actionable, depending on the consequences of an omission. This type of professional negligence action for the negligent failure to communicate vital patient information to others having a need to know exists independently of any other legal action based on the quality of care rendered.

There are many other legitimate purposes for patient care documentation, including the risk management purpose of memorializing important facts about an event for possible use in subsequent litigation. Patient care documentation is also used as a basis for planning and continuity of care, as a primary source of information for quality measurement and evaluation of patient care activities, to provide information necessary for reimbursement decisions and utilization review, to identify training needs, as a resource for patient care research and education, and to memorialize informed consent to treatment and patient wishes concerning advance directives, among other purposes (see Box 2-4).

Hint *Documentation of patient care is as important as the rendition of patient care itself.*

The patient treatment record is a legal document, referred to as a business document, which is admissible in court as evidence in health care malpractice and other civil and criminal legal proceedings. As part of the legal duty owed to a patient, a treating physical or occupational therapist is responsible and accountable for accurate, clear, objective, and timely documentation of the patient's chief complaint(s), relevant history, evaluative findings, informed consent to intervention, treatment, discharge, and, if appropriate, follow-up care.

Information documented about a patient serves simultaneously to protect both the patient and the treating clinician. If a patient brings a malpractice lawsuit against the clinician—often years after care is rendered—what is documented in the treatment record about the patient's care may well be the best or even only objective evi-

2-4 Purposes of Patient Care Documentation

- communicate critical information about a patient to other health care professionals concurrently treating the patient and having a need to know
- basis for patient care (post-discharge) planning and continuity of care
- primary source of information for the measurement and evaluation of patient care activities, as part of a systematic quality management (improvement) program
- justification for reimbursement
- source document for utilization review activities
- identification of deficiencies in documentation and patient care performance and formulation of training needs
- resource for patient care research and education
- business document
- legal document
- provide substantive evidence on whether patient care rendered meets or breaches the legal standard of care
- memorialize disclosure elements and patient informed consent to treatment
- memorialize patient choices concerning life-sustaining interventions to be taken in the event of the patient's subsequent incompetence, in the form of advance directives

dence of what transpired between the patient and the health care professional at the time of treatment. This is especially important in busy clinical practices, where, because clinicians evaluate and treat hundreds or thousands of patients in a given year, memories naturally tend to fade over time.

When expert witnesses take the stand for or against defendant-physical or occupational therapists to testify about whether care rendered to plaintiff-patients met or violated the legal standard of care, they rely primarily on what is documented in treatment records to formulate their professional opinions. From the standpoint of health care malpractice, documentation of patient care serves as the primary basis for expert testimony about whether the standard of care was breached or met in a given case, the standard of care being the benchmark that delineates negligent and non-negligent care.

When a treating physical or occupational therapist (or other health care clinician) is required to testify as a defendant or witness in a legal proceeding, how can the clinician recall a given patient's relevant history, evaluative findings, treatment plan, disposition, and follow-up care, when the event occurred months or years earlier?

While attorneys often try to jog the memories of *percipient* (fact) or expert witnesses through leading questions (where not objected to, or where allowed by judges), more often than not, reference to treatment records is often indispensable in order to refresh lapsed memories regarding past events.

When a treating health care clinician's memory (as a witness) is incomplete, patient care documentation in the treatment record can be relied upon in one of two ways during direct testimony in a legal proceeding. The preferred way is for the clinician to first review the treatment record while on the witness stand, as a stimulus to jog the witness's present memory. After reviewing the documentation, the treatment record is taken away from the witness, and the witness testifies. This form of recall is called *present recollection refreshed*.

If a clinician's present recollection cannot be refreshed by reviewing the treatment record, then the treatment record itself may have to be admitted into evidence as substantive evidence of the care rendered to the patient under an exception to the hearsay rule.[84] This exception is called *past recollection recorded*. In order to substitute the treatment record for live testimony, however, the clinician must swear or affirm that the treatment record was accurate at the time it was written.

A health care professional should always document in a patient's treatment record as if the entry were being prepared for court, because this may in fact occur. A health care professional will be more inclined to document more carefully if he or she imagines the documentation being blown up to giant size in a courtroom. The following simple, common-sense documentation tips will help physical and occupational therapists and assistants to avoid legal dilemmas concerning patient care documentation:

- Always write on every line in the record (to avoid the temptation to correct an entry after-the-fact).

- Write with one pen, using black (or blue) ink. In the rare case in which a pen runs out of ink midway through documenting an entry, indicate in a brief parenthetical that the first pen ran out of ink, and continue with a second pen.

- Correct mistaken entries by drawing a single, straight line through the error and initialing (and dating, if this is customary practice) the correction. (Do not add words such as "error" or "mistaken entry," because such words may give rise to an inference in the eyes of a jury of negligent care delivery.)

- Except when correcting contemporaneous mistakes, do not edit prior documentation entries.

- Do not back-date an omission in a patient treatment record. Once an omission is noted, document critical omitted information in a new entry with today's date.

- Write legibly. Print, type, or dictate as required to help you to communicate clearly. Remember that the failure to communicate vital patient information clearly and in a timely manner constitutes professional negligence.

- Do not express negative personal feelings about a patient in the treatment record, such as, "Patient is an obvious malingerer." Lack of objectivity in documenting patient evaluation and treatment can give rise to an inference of noncompliance with the legal standard of care.

- Do not argue with or disparage other health care professionals in the treatment record. Again, such behavior gives rise to an inference of negligent care.

- Avoid including in patient care documentation extraneous verbiage not related to diagnosis or treatment of patients. Such information as, "Patient is a pleasant, 43-year-old Beatles record collector," probably has no place in a general patient treatment record.

- Avoid using terms and abbreviations not universally understood by all health care professionals caring for the patient. Use of cryptic, esoteric terminology constitutes a negligent failure to communicate patient information.

- Avoid documenting patient status using ambiguous terminology, such as, "tolerated treatment well," without specifying the parameters of the meaning of the phrase. Health care malpractice insurers caution that such ambiguous phraseology is too vague to be useful in defending a health care malpractice charge.[85]

Even innocent corrections of prior treatment entries may be construed by courts as intentional alteration of treatment records, which can have profound adverse legal consequences for health care professionals who become defendants in malpractice cases. A court may rule that altered treatment records are inadmissible, or that a jury may infer or must presume negligence against a defendant-health care provider. Intentional alteration of treatment records may also give rise to the awarding of punitive damages against a defendant-provider should be plaintiff prevail in the case. Punitive damages are not normally payable by a provider's malpractice liability insurer. The legal term for intentional treatment record loss or alteration is *spoliation*.

Although specific rules concerning the use of adverse incident reports vary from facility to facility, certain universal rules apply when documenting adverse, potentially-compensable events involving patients. Potentially-compensable events that warrant the generation of incident reports include patient injury or expression by a patient of serious dissatisfaction with care.

An incident report serves two purposes: (1) to alert management to possible safety hazards requiring investigation and possible correction, and (2) to memorialize important facts about an adverse event for the purpose of preventing liability on the part of the organization.

Always document adverse patient incidents concisely and objectively. Do not assign blame or speculate as to the cause of injury in the incident report.

> ***Spoliation:*** the intentional loss or destruction of patient treatment records.

Document as fact only those things that you personally perceive. What others related to you, as recorder, constitute hearsay, and should be bracketed in quotation marks to clearly identify the hearsay statements as emanating from someone other than the recorder.

Normally, information documented in an incident report is immune from discovery by a plaintiff-patient and his or her attorney. This qualified immunity normally requires that incident reports be clearly labeled as "quality assurance/improvement documents" or a "report prepared at the direction of the organization's attorney for possible use in litigation."

Do not file a copy of a incident report or mention its creation in the treatment record. The information contained in its does not relate to patient evaluation or treatment. Do create a concurrent treatment entry in the record detailing patient injury and provider interventions on the patient's behalf. Consider the following hypothetical example.

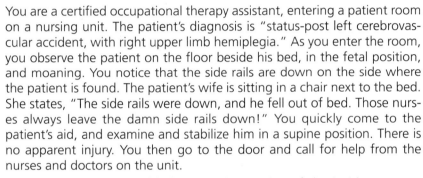

You are a certified occupational therapy assistant, entering a patient room on a nursing unit. The patient's diagnosis is "status-post left cerebrovascular accident, with right upper limb hemiplegia." As you enter the room, you observe the patient on the floor beside his bed, in the fetal position, and moaning. You notice that the side rails are down on the side where the patient is found. The patient's wife is sitting in a chair next to the bed. She states, "The side rails were down, and he fell out of bed. Those nurses always leave the damn side rails down!" You quickly come to the patient's aid, and examine and stabilize him in a supine position. There is no apparent injury. You then go to the door and call for help from the nurses and doctors on the unit.

How do you document (a) the narrative portion of the incident report, and (b) the progress note in the patient's treatment record?

(a) The narrative portion of the incident report might read: "Upon entering the patient's room, I observed the patient on the floor next to his bed. The patient was in the fetal position and was moaning. The side rails were down. The patient's wife, who was seated in a chair next to the patient's bed, stated, 'The side rails were down, and he fell out of bed. Those nurses always leave the damn side rails down!' I examined and stabilized the patient in the supine position, after noting no apparent injury. Nursing and physician notified."

(b) The progress note might read: "Upon entering the patient's room, I observed the patient on the floor next to his bed. The patient was in the fetal position and was moaning. Patient examined and stabilized in the supine position, after noting no apparent injury. Nursing and physician notified."

For an in-depth discussion about comprehensive patient treatment records management, including storage, retention, and destruction, see Guarino, K.S.

"Developing a Comprehensive Records Management Plan." *Health Lawyer*, 1994; 7(3):15–16. This legal article presents a frightening example of how broad a litigation discovery request for "records" or "documents" may be phrased in a pleading.[86]

Selected Recently Reported Physical Therapy Malpractice Cases Involving Allegations of Negligence

Case 1: Incident reports   A patient filed a strict product liability civil lawsuit against a medical device manufacturer.[87] The patient allegedly was shocked during physical therapy treatment by a neuromuscular stimulation device. The treating physical therapist, who was not named as a defendant in the patient's lawsuit, had generated an adverse incident report at the time of patient injury. The stated purpose for the creation of the incident report was to alert management to a potential patient safety problem, so that it could be rectified as part of the hospital's interdisciplinary quality improvement and safety program.

As part of pre-trial discovery, the defendant-device manufacturer sought to compel the release of the physical therapist's incident report, after the hospital denied the defendant's request for voluntary release. The trial judge ordered the incident report released to the defendant, however, the hospital sought interim, or *interlocutory*, appeal of the judge's decision.

On appeal, the higher-level appeals court ruled that the incident report, which was generated for the legitimate purpose of promoting quality care and patient safety as part of a systematic quality management program, was immune from involuntary release to anyone outside of the organization's peer review and quality assurance committees. Protection from release of incident reports made pursuant to quality assurance program requirements is guaranteed by statute.

Cases 2 and 3: Ordinary vs. professional negligence   A patient undergoing hydrotherapy treatment in physical therapy filed, as an ordinary negligence malpractice lawsuit, a case alleging injury from a laceration resulting from contact with a sharp object in the whirlpool tub.[88] The trial court judge ruled that the plaintiff's allegation constituted a professional, not an ordinary, negligence lawsuit, and granted summary judgment in favor of the defendant-hospital on the grounds that the plaintiff failed to follow statutory procedural requirements concerning professional negligence health care malpractice cases. Specifically, the plaintiff did not notify the defendant of a claim before filing suit as required by statute. The appeals court agreed with the trial judge's decision and affirmed the trial-level summary judgment in favor of the defendant-hospital.

A patient who had just undergone an amputation (making her a double lower-limb amputee secondary to diabetes mellitus) was referred by her physician for prosthetic gait training in physical therapy.[89] During the physical therapy initial evaluation, the patient fell while executing a turning maneuver in the parallel bars. The patient sued the hospital for vicarious liability for the alleged (ordinary) negligence of the evaluating physical therapist, demanding monetary damages for physical injury and pain and suffering.

The trial court ruled that the patient's case involved an allegation of professional, not ordinary premises, negligence. The court declared a judgment in favor of the defendant-hospital, since the plaintiff had not complied with the state statutory requirement to include an expert opinion on the theory of professional negligence with the pre-trial pleadings in the case.

On appeal, the patient-plaintiff argued that her case should be considered as an ordinary premises liability case, which would obviated the need for an expert opinion on professional negligence. The appeals court rejected the patient's plea.

While her case against the hospital for vicarious liability was on appeal, the plaintiff filed a separate lawsuit against the physical therapist responsible for her post-amputation evaluation, this time alleging professional negligence. The trial court in this second case dismissed the plaintiff-patient's action on the grounds of *res judicata* (Latin for "the matter has been settled"). The appeals court hearing this second appeal affirmed the lower court's dismissal of the case, declaring that once a judgment against the hospital for vicarious liability had been rendered, a case against the physical therapist individually for direct liability was barred.

Cases 4 and 5: Summary judgment   A patient filed a professional negligence health care malpractice lawsuit against a treating physical therapist, alleging substandard care in the administration of electrical stimulation therapy.[90] The patient was status-post arm fracture, and had Kirschner wires holding the open reduction, internal fixation in place. The patient claimed that the muscle re-education treatment, performed by a physical therapy aide, was negligently done. The patient allegedly was shocked by a surge in current, purportedly causing the Kirschner wires to bend, and some even to rupture.

The trial court judge granted summary judgment in favor of the defendant-physical therapist, on the technical grounds that the plaintiff's expert witness's *affidavit* (sworn statement) did not have appended to it the documents upon which the plaintiff's expert had relied in formulating the expert opinion. This deficiency rendered the plaintiff's expert opinion "legally defective." The only documentation that the court had to rely on to rule on summary judgment, then, was the defendant-physical therapist's sworn statement, in which the therapist declared that the care given comported with the legal standard of care. With no admissible conflicting evidence to refute the therapist's affidavit, the court ruled in the defendant's favor. The appellate court affirmed the trial-level decision.

A patient, who was a worker's compensation client secondary to shoulder injury, underwent occupational and physical therapy treatment at the defendant-rehabilitation center.[91] During the patient's discharge evaluation, he allegedly sustained a back strain. On physician follow-up, the patient was sent back to the rehabilitation center for further therapy.

The patient continued to complain of back symptoms with activities of daily living training. In order to establish a precise diagnosis, the center's director referred the patient to a psychologist for a mental evaluation. Based in part on the psychologist's assessment, the center discharged the patient from the clinic.

The patient consulted with a second physician, who diagnosed the patient as having preexisting, multilevel lumbar spondylolysis. The second orthopedist carried out a lumbar discectomy and fusion on the patient. The patient subsequently initiated a professional negligence lawsuit against the rehabilitation center.

Based on available affidavits and other evidence, the trial court granted summary judgment in favor of the defendant-rehabilitation center, concluding as a matter of law that the plaintiff-patient's evidence was insufficient to proceed on to trial. On appeal, the plaintiff-patient alleged that the record before the trial judge during the defense motion for summary judgment did demonstrate material issues of fact in dispute, warranting a full trial on the merits. Allegedly, the evidence creating material issues consisted of the defendant's physical therapist's affidavit and pre-trial *deposition*.

The appeals court disagreed with the plaintiff's position and affirmed the summary judgment granted by the trial judge in favor of the defense. The appeals court specifically stated that the physical therapists employed by the defendant-center and their assistants did not breach the legal standard of care in this case.

One additional point was noteworthy in this case. In *dicta* (judicial remarks not directly related to the court's decision), the appellate judge authoring the court's opinion stated that there was a relative dearth of case law concerning physical therapy malpractice issues. The judge went on to state that physical therapy (and presumably, occupational therapy) malpractice actions were to be treated exactly like physician malpractice cases, thus equating the status of the allied health professions with medicine.

Chapter Summary

The term *health care malpractice* encompasses civil legal actions initiated by patients or their representatives against health care providers and/or health care organizations for patient injury incident to the delivery of professional care services. However, patient injury alone is insufficient to allow a patient to prevail against a health care professional or organization. The injury must be coupled with a recognized legal basis for imposing health care malpractice liability.

The legal bases for imposing health care malpractice liability consist of professional negligence; intentional, treatment-related conduct resulting in patient injury; breach of a treatment-related contractual promise made by a health care provider; and strict liability (without regard to fault) for injuries from abnormally dangerous clinical procedures or from dangerously defective treatment-related products.

The overwhelming majority of health care malpractice legal cases are based on allegations of professional negligence. A plaintiff-patient alleging professional negligence by a defendant-health care professional must prove a litany of four elements, each by a preponderance, or greater weight, of evidence at trial. These elements are (1) that the defendant-provider owed a legal duty of special care toward the plaintiff-patient, (2) that the provider breached the duty owed by delivering care that was objectively substandard, (3) that the breach of duty directly caused the patient injury, and (4) that the award of monetary damages is appropriate and necessary to make the patient "whole."

Defenses available to defendant-health care professionals and organizations in malpractice cases are of two general types: technical (procedural) and substantive. Technical defenses, demonstrated in many of the reported malpractice cases lodged against physical and occupational therapists, include plaintiff-patient noncompliance with the applicable statute of limitations, failure to comply with procedural requirements for affidavits and other pleadings and documents submitted to courts, and personal immunity from liability (as when the federal government is responsible for official conduct of federal workers under the Federal Tort Claims Act). Substantive defenses include plaintiff-patient contributory negligence or comparative fault and proof by the defendant of compliance with the legal standard of care, making a plaintiff-patient's injuries merely a non-actionable adverse event.

Health care professionals—individually and collectively, and health care organizations and networks, can and must develop and implement effective risk management strategies to minimize malpractice exposure and liability. Such measures include documentation skills and management, effective communications with patients and professional colleagues,[92] empathy[93] and respect[94] for patients, systematic quality and risk management,[95] continuing and continuous professional education and training,[96] and perhaps, the development of valid clinical practice guidelines.[97]

Cases and Questions

1. Patient *A* is undergoing outpatient stroke rehabilitation in occupational therapist *B*'s section of an interdisciplinary privately-owned rehabilitation center. *A* ambulates using a four-legged cane. On his way from the reception area to the treatment area, *A* trips on a frayed edge of carpeting and falls and breaks a tooth. *A* expresses an intention to file a claim against the clinic for malpractice. Is *A*'s claim for malpractice valid? If so, under what theory of liability? What steps should the therapist take immediately after injury?

2. Patient *C*, an outpatient in a sports physical therapy clinic, is being treated for an anterior cruciate ligament deficiency with closed-chain functionally-focused exercise. *Z*, the clinic owner and treating physical therapist, promised *C* that her involved (dominant) knee strength would be equal to the uninvolved leg after six to eight weeks of rehabilitation. During a session, *C* falls, twisting and injuring her involved knee. The incident was clearly no one's fault. Does *C* have a valid claim for physical therapy malpractice? Under which theory or theories might she proceed?

3. *D*, a physical therapist, is a certified orthopaedic clinical specialist. She operates a private practice. *D* treats patient *E*, an outpatient with a diagnosis of mechanical low back pain, with back extension exercises under an "evaluate and treat" order from Dr. *F*, a neurosurgeon. At the end of the first session, *E* suddenly complains of increased left lower limb radicular symptoms and severe low back pain. A subsequent MRI study reveals an intervertebral disc herniation at L4-5. *E* undergoes a surgical discectomy the next day. On these facts alone, is *D* liable for malpractice? From which disciplines might health care professionals testify as experts in a subsequent physical therapy malpractice trial?

Suggested Answers to Cases and Questions

1. Patient *A*'s case is probably an ordinary premises negligence case and not a professional treatment-related negligence case. This is so because the source of injury was a frayed rug, causing the same kind of fall that could occur in a retail store, a private home, or anywhere else.

The main advantage for the plaintiff of the case being labeled as ordinary negligence is that the plaintiff avoids the many administrative hurdles that attach to professional negligence legal actions, such as submission of the case to an administrative merit panel and submission of expert opinions along with court pleadings. In an ordinary premises negligence case, expert testimony on the occupational therapy standard of care is inapplicable. Experts are unnecessary, since the nature of an ordinary fall is within the common knowledge of lay jurors, without the need for clarification by experts.

For the defendant, the main advantage of the case being labeled as ordinary negligence is that a finding of liability does not result in the health care professional's name being reported for inclusion in the National Practitioner Data Bank. For both parties, an ordinary negligence case should be less time-consuming, less intense, and less expensive than a health care malpractice case.

The first step that the occupational therapist should take after injury is to ensure that the patient is safe and stable. After injuries are ascertained, emergency consultation with a physician or dentist should be accomplished and the patient transferred for care by these professionals. Express empathy with the patient's situation, and show that you care.

Complete an incident report. In addition to accurate documentation of administrative data, such as time, place, lighting, and other relevant details about the incident, carefully complete the narrative part of the report objectively and completely. Attribute any hearsay statements made by others to their source. Do not file or mention the incident report in the patient's treatment record.

Complete an entry in the patient's treatment record regarding injuries incurred by the patient and actions taken by you and your staff on the patient's behalf. Be sure to send a copy of the patient's record with the patient for emergency medical treatment.

2. It is given in the problem that patient *C*'s knee injury was no one's fault. This, however, does not prevent the filing of a health care malpractice claim or lawsuit. Some people erroneously believe that malpractice liability automatically attaches anytime a patient is injured during treatment. Such is not the case. Malpractice liability requires patient injury, plus the presence of one of the recognized legal bases for imposing liability. Here, one of these bases for liability—breach of contract—may seem to be present, since a therapeutic promise was made to the patient by the physical therapist. However, the accidental fall that caused the patient injury probably would excuse the physical therapist from the contractual promise to achieve a therapeutic result, under the contractual defense of "impossibility of performance."

3. As was explained in the answer to problem 2 above, patient injury during treatment alone does not create health care malpractice liability. The patient must also prove, by a preponderance of evidence, the existence of one of the legal bases for imposing liability. If such a connection can be established, a malpractice case may proceed to trial.

If the case proceeds to pre-trial depositions and to trial, expert witnesses for the plaintiff and defendant may be physical therapists (under the "same school" [discipline] doctrine) or other health care professionals from related disciplines having similar knowledge, training, and experience about orthopaedic physical therapy as the defendant and knowledge of the applicable standard of care in effect in the community in which the defendant practices.

References

1. Scott, R.W. *Health Care Malpractice: A Primer on Legal Issues for Professionals.* Thorofare, NJ: Slack, Inc., 1990.

2. Scott, R.W. "Malpractice Update." *PT: Magazine of Physical Therapy*, 1993; 1(12):62–64.

3. Scott, R.W. "Lessons From Court." *Aon Direct Group Risk Advisor*, 1995; 1(1):5.

4. *Oslund* v. *United States*, 701 F. Supp. 710 (D. Minn. 1989).

5. *People* v. *Mari*, 183 N.E. 858 (N.Y. 1933). (Conviction of physical therapist for the unlicensed practice of medicine in treating rheumatism patient *affirmed.*)

6. *People* v. *Dennis*, 271 N.Y.S. 2d 912 (App. Div. 1946). (Conviction of masseur employed by physical therapist for the unlicensed practice of medicine *affirmed.*)

7. Coile, R. *The New Governance: Strategies for an Era of Health Care Reform.* Ann Arbor, MI: Health Administration Press, 1994, p. 231.

8. *1993 APTA State Licensure Reference Guide.* Alexandria, VA: American Physical Therapy Association, pp. 29–30.

9. Hamby, E.F. "The Use of the Multiskilled Practitioner to Manage Care."

Orthopaedic Physical Therapy Clinics of North America, 1995; 4(3):335–350.

10. Beauchamp, T.L., Childress, J.F. *Principles of Biomedical Ethics*, 4th ed. New York: Oxford University Press, 1994, pp. 189–258.

11. Peterson, R.G. "Malpractice Liability of Allied Health Professionals: Developments in an Area of Critical Concern." *Journal of Allied Health*, 1985; 14:363–372.

12. Prosser, W.L. *Handbook of the Law of Torts*, 4th ed. St. Paul, MN: West Publishing Company, 1971, p. 143.

13. *Ibid.* pp. 416–417.

14. Emergency Medical Treatment and Active Labor Act, 42 United States Code Section 1395dd.

15. *Owens* v. *Nacogdoches County Hospital District*, 741 F. Supp. 1269 (E. Dist. Texas 1990). (16-year old indigent pregnant patient allegedly denied care during active labor; judgment in favor of plaintiff.)

16. *Thornton* v. *Southwest Detroit Hospital*, 895 F. 2d 1131 (6th Cir. 1990). (Female stroke patient, discharged from hospital to home because of inability to pay for intensive rehabilitation; summary judgment in favor of the hospital affirmed, based on the fact that the patient's condition had stabilized.)

17. *Cleland* v. *Bronson Health Care Group*, 917 F. 2d 266 (6th Cir. 1990). (terms "appropriate" and "stabilize")

18. *Piccirillo* v. *Staten Island University Hospital*, 1993 WL 725742 (Supreme Court, Richmond County, New York).

19. *Occupational Therapy Code of Ethics*, Principle 2.E, reads:
    Occupational therapy personnel shall protect the confidential nature of information gained from educational, practice, research, and investigational activities.

    American Occupational Therapy Association, Commission on Standard and Ethics, 1994.

20. *Guide for Professional Conduct*, Principle 1, Section 1.2A (Confidential Information) reads:

    Information relating to the physical therapist-patient relationship is confidential and may not be communicated to a third party not involved in that patient's care without the prior *written* [emphasis added] consent of the patient, subject to applicable law.

    American Physical Therapy Association, Judicial Committee, 1995.

21. *Tarasoff* v. *Regents of the University of California*, 17 Cal. 3d 425 (1976).

22. *Guide for Professional Conduct*, Principle 1, Section 1.2D reads:

    Information may be disclosed to appropriate authorities when it is necessary to protect the welfare of an individual or the community. Such disclosure shall be in accordance with applicable law.

    American Physical Therapy Association, Judicial Committee, 1995.

23. Brushwood, D.B. "Hospital Pharmacist's Duty to Question Clear Errors in Prescriptions." *American Journal of Hospital Pharmacy*, 1994; 51:2031–2033.

24. *Gassen* v. *East Jefferson General Hospital*, 1993 Westlaw 514862 (La. App. Dec. 15, 1993).

25. "A Guide for Physical Therapist Practice," Volume I: A Description of Patient

Management. Chapter 1: Management of Physical Therapy Services, Definition of Physical Therapy. *Journal of the American Physical Therapy Association*, 1995; 75:711–712.

26. Texas Occupational Therapy Practice Act, Article 4512e-1, Tex. Rev. Stat. Ann.

27. "Standards of Practice for Occupational Therapy." *American Journal of Occupational Therapy*, 1994; 48:1039–1043.

28. Standards of Practice for Physical Therapists. HOD 06-91-25, 1991.

29. Trombly, C.A. *Occupational Therapy for Physical Dysfunction*, 4th ed. Baltimore, MD: Williams and Wilkins, Publishers, 1995.

30. Kendall, F.P., McCreary, E.K., Provance, P.G. *Muscles: Testing and Function*, 4th ed. Baltimore, MD: Williams and Wilkins, Publishers, 1993.

31. *Novey* v. *Kishwaukee Community Health Services*, 531 N.E. 2d 427 (Ill. App. 1988).

32. *Emig* v. *Physicians' Physical Therapy Services, Inc.*, 432 N.E. 2d 52 (Ind. App. 1982). (This case involved an elderly plaintiff-patient who fell from a wheelchair, allegedly while unattended. At the appellate level of disposition, the trial-level judgment in favor of the defendant was reversed and the case remanded for reconsideration.)

33. *Novey*, note 31.

34. *Commonalities and Differences Between the Professions of Physical Therapy and Occupational Therapy*. Alexandria, VA: American Physical Therapy Association, 1994.

35. Mehn, J.H., Dennis, S.W., Rybski, D.A. "PT/OT Role Delineation in a Combined Department." *Clinical Management*, 1986; 6(3):30–33.

36. Breske, S. "Turf Wars in the Clinic: PTs and OTs Struggle to Find Common Ground." *Advance for Physical Therapists*, October 30, 1995, pp. 10–11.

37. *Army Regulation 40-48: Non-Physician Health Care Providers (AR)*. Washington, DC: Department of the Army, 1986, Chapter 5, Paragraph 5-1, Credentialing, reads:

    a. The credentials committee will recommend to the military treatment facility (MTF) commander those clinical privileges of assigned occupational therapists who perform the *primary* [emphasis added] evaluation, diagnosis, and treatment of patients seeking care for neuromusculoskeletal disorders of the upper extremity. The MTF commander will—

      (1) Determine in writing the scope and limits of clinical privileges of the assigned occupational therapists, and

      (2) Designate in writing the supervisory physician.

    b. Clinical privileges will be determined upon initial assignment, change of assignment, and annually unless more frequent evaluation is necessary. Occupational therapists who are not involved in the primary care of neuromusculoskeletal disorders of the upper extremity will be categorically credentialed. When occupational therapists are working in subspecialty areas where additional skills are required, other clinical privileges will be granted. Examples of subspecialty areas are neurodevelopmental, intervention with children, and community mental health activities.

    Chapter 4, Paragraph 4-1 delineates similar expanded roles for Army physical therapists. Additional Army physical therapist subspecialty practice areas include inhibitive casting, early intervention with high-risk infants, stress testing, and percent body fat measurement. Both professions are privileged, under their "expanded roles," to write medication prescriptions from a limited formulary, order rest from and limitations on work, order diagnostic radiographic studies, and refer patients to other specialty clinics (including to physician-specialists). *AR*, Paragraphs 4-2, 5-2.

38. Hayward, R.S., Wilson, M.C., Tunis, S.R., et. al. "How to Use Clinical Practice Guidelines: Are the Recommendations Valid?" *Journal of the American Medical Association*, 1995; 274:570–574.

39. Garnick, D.W., Hendricks, A.M., Brennan, T.A. "Can Practice Guidelines Reduce the Number and Costs of Malpractice Claims?" *Journal of the American Medical Association*, 1991; 266:2856–2891.

40. *Greening by Greening* v. *School District of Millard*, 393 N.W. 2d 51 (Neb. 1986).

41. *Piccarillo*, note 18.

42. Prosser, W.L. *Handbook of the Law of Torts*, 4th ed. St. Paul, MN: West Publishing Company, 1971, pp. 888–897.

43. Restatement (Second) of Torts, Section 520.

44. *Karibjanian* v. *Thomas Jefferson University Hospital*, 717 F. Supp. 1081 (E.D. Pa. 1989).

45. *Escola* v. *Coca-Cola Bottling Company*, 150 P. 2d 436 (Ca. 1944).

46. Under the 1976 Medical Device Amendments to the Food, Drug and Cosmetic Act (21 United States Code Section 360(c)(a)(1)), medical devices are classified as either Class I (normally safe without ongoing quality controls, e.g., non-motorized wheelchairs), Class II (safe with ongoing quality controls, e.g., surgical staples), or Class III (devices unavoidably unsafe, yet necessary to sustain life or limit dysfunction, e.g., contact lenses). The administrative Code of Federal Regulations (21 C.F.R. Ch. 1, Section 801.109) requires that all prescription medical devices have the statement: "Federal law restricts this device to sale by or on the order of a physician, dentist, veterinarian, or other appropriate health care professional." For more information on specific legal cases involving Class III medical devices, see Wilson, R.M. "Products Liability: Medical Device Manufacturers May Avoid a Potential Torrent of Litigation as Some Courts Exempt Certain Devices from Strict Liability for Design Defect." *National Law Journal*, October 17, 1994, pp. B6–7, 11–12.

47. Gerlin, A. "Surgeons Feel Trapped by Implant Suits." *Wall Street Journal*, March 30, 1995, p. B8.

48. Scott, R.W. "Overview of Legal and Ethical Issues Related to Health-Care Malpractice for Prosthetists and Orthotists." *Journal of Prosthetics and Orthotics*, 1995; 8(1):17–20.

49. *Winona Memorial Foundation* v. *Lomax*, 465 N.E. 2d 731 (Ind. App. 1984).

50. *St. Paul Fire and Marine Insurance Company* v. *Prothro*, 590 S.W. 2d 35 (Ark. App. 1979).

51. *Emig*, note 32.

52. Robitzek, W.D. "Is There a Potential Lawsuit Brewing in Your Office?" *Physician's Management*, April 1992, pp. 131–138.

53. *Winona*, note 49, at 734, footnote 4.

54. Keeton, W.P. *Prosser and Keeton on Torts*, 5th ed. St. Paul, MN: West Publishing Company, 1984, pp. 386–434.

55. Kearney, K.A., McCord, E.L. "Hospital Management Faces New Liabilities." *Health Lawyer*, 1992; 6(3):1,3–5.

56. Winslow, R. "Hospitals' Weak Systems Hurt Patients, Study Says." *Wall Street Journal,* July 5, 1995, pp. B1,6.

57. Johnson, G. "Statute of Limitations." *United States Department of Justice 1989 Federal Tort Claims Act Litigation Seminar Handbook*, p. N3.

58. *O'Neal* v. *Throop and Rehab Works*, 596 N.E. 2d 984 (Ind. App. 1992).

59. *Myers* v. *Woodall*, 592 P. 2d 1343 (Colo. Ct. App. 1979).

60. Under the Restatement (Second) of Torts, Section 524, contributory negligence is a viable defense in a strict liability case when a plaintiff knowingly and unreasonably subjects him- or herself to risk of harm. Similarly, intentional, unreasonable misuse of a product by a plaintiff may create a valid defense to a strict product liability legal action. *Daly* v. *General Motors Corp.*, 20 Cal. 3d 725 (1978).

61. *Davis* v. *Sykes*, 121 S.E. 2d 513 (Va. 1961).

62. *Schneider* v. *Revici*, 817 F. 2d 987 (2d Cir. 1987).

63. Federal Tort Claims Act, 28 United States Code Sections 1346(b) and 2671–2680.

64. Federal Employees Liability Reform and Tort Compensation Act, 28 United States Code Section 2679, reads in pertinent part:

    (b)(1) The remedy against the United States provided by Sections 1346(b) and 2672 of this title for injury or loss of property, or personal injury or death arising or resulting from the negligent or wrongful act or omission of any federal employee of the Government while acting within the scope of his office or employment is *exclusive* [emphasis added] of any other civil action or proceeding for monetary damages by reason of the same subject matter against the employee whose act or omission gave rise to the claim or against the estate of such employee. Any other civil action or proceeding for monetary damages arising out of or relating to the same subject matter against the employee or the employee's estate is precluded without regard to when the act or omission occurred.

65. Furrow, B.R., Johnson, S.H., Jost, T.S., Schwartz, R.L. *Health Law: Cases, Materials and Problems*, 2nd ed. St. Paul, MN: West Publishing Company, 1991, p. 294 (Arizona, Florida, Georgia, Illinois, Maine, South Carolina, and Virginia).

66. *Guide for Professional Conduct*, Section 8.1 (Pro Bono Service) reads:

    Physical therapists should render pro bono publico (reduced or no fee) services to patients lacking the ability to pay for services, as each physical therapist's practice permits.

67. *Occupational Therapy Code of Ethics*, Principle 1.D reads:

    Occupational therapy personnel shall strive to ensure that fees are fair, reasonable, and commensurate with the service performed and are set *with due regard for the service recipient's ability to pay* [emphasis added].

68. *Tunkl* v. *Regents of the University of California*, 383 P. 2d 441 (Ca. 1963).

69. California Civil Code Section 1668.

70. *Leidy* v. *Deseret Enterprises*, 381 A. 2d 164 (Pa. Super. Ct. 1977).

71. *Meiman* v. *Rehabilitation Center, Inc.*, 444 S.W. 2d 78 (Ky. 1969).

72. Health Care Quality Improvement Act of 1986, 42 United States Code Sections 11101 to 11152.

73. Section 11111(a) reads in pertinent part:

    SUBCHAPTER 1—PROMOTION OF PROFESSIONAL REVIEW ACTIVITIES

    (1) Limitation on damages for professional review actions

If a professional review action . . . of a professional review body meets all the standards specified . . .

(A) the professional review body,

(B) any person acting as a member or staff to the body, and

(C) any person who participates with or assists the body with respect to the action, shall not be liable in damages under any law of the United States (or political subdivision thereof) with respect to the action. . . .

(2) Protection for those providing information to professional review bodies

Notwithstanding any other provision of law, no person (whether as a witness or otherwise) providing information to a professional review body regarding the competency or professional conduct of a physician shall be held, by reason of having provided such information, to be liable in damages under any law of the United States or of any State (or political subdivision) unless such information is false and the person providing it knew that such information was false.

74. SUBCHAPTER II—REPORTING OF INFORMATION reads in pertinent part:

Section 11131. Requiring reports on medical malpractice payments

(a) In general

Each entity (including an insurance company) which makes payments under a policy of insurance, self-insurance, or otherwise in settlement (or partial settlement) of, or in satisfaction of a judgment in, a medical malpractice action or claim shall report . . . information respecting the payment and circumstances thereof.

(b) Information to be reported

The information to be reported under subsection (a) of this section includes—

(1) the name of any physician or licensed health care practitioner for whose benefit the payment is made,

(2) the amount of the payment,

(3) the name (if known) of any hospital with which the physician or practitioner is affiliated or associated,

(4) a description of the acts or omissions and injuries or illnesses upon which the action or claim was based. . . .

75. Mullan, F., Politzer, R.M., Lewis, C.T., et. al. "The National Practitioner Data Bank: Report From the First Year." *Journal of the American Medical Association*, 1992; 268:73–79.

76. Reports to National Practitioner Data Bank, Department of Health and Human Services, September 1, 1990–August 31, 1991.

77. "Using the National Practitioner Data Bank." *Medical Staff Briefing*, December 1991, pp. 9–10.

78. 42 United States Code Section 11135(a)(2).

79. Felsenthal, E. "Doctors Oppose Publicizing Legal Claims." *Wall Street Journal*, May 18, 1993, p. B8.

80. "Group Lists 'Questionable Doctors,' Seeks Action on 80,000 Annual Deaths." *PT Bulletin*, 1995; 9(25):1.

81. "Guidelines for Occupational Therapy Documentation." *American Journal of Occupational Therapy*, 1986; 40:830–832.

82. "Application of Uniform Terminology to Practice." *Uniform Terminology for Occupational Therapy*. Bethesda, MD: American Occupational Therapy Association, 1989.

83. "Guidelines for Physical Therapy Documentation." *Journal of the American Physical Therapy Association*, 1995; 75:762–764.

84. *Hearsay* evidence includes out-of-court statements offered as evidence in legal proceedings for the truth of the matter asserted in them (*Black's Law Dictionary*, 5th ed. St. Paul, MN: West Publishing Company, 1979, p. 649.) The hearsay rule, in effect in every state, and in the federal legal system, prevents hearsay evidence from being admitted in legal proceedings, absent a recognized exception, such as a confession (in a criminal case) or admission (in a civil case), or a dying declaration (statement made by someone near to the time of death).

85. Clifton, D.W. "'Tolerated Treatment Well' May No Longer Be Tolerated." *PT: Magazine of Physical Therapy*, 1995; 3(10)24–27.

86. Guarino, K.S. "Developing a Comprehensive Records Management Plan." *Health Lawyer*, 1994; 7(3):15–16, at 16.

87. *Community Hospitals of Indianapolis v. Medtronic, Inc, Neuro Div.*, 594 N.E. 2d 448 (Ind. App. 1992).

88. *Gonzales v. Fairfax Hospital*, 389 S.E. 2d 458 (Va. 1990).

89 *Hodo v. Basa*, 449 S.E. 2d 523 (Ga. App. 1994).

90. *Augustine v. Frame*, 425 S.E. 2d 296 (Ga. App. 1992).

91. *Flores v. Center for Spinal Evaluation*, 865 S.W. 2d 261 (Tex. App. 1993).

92. Winslow, R. "Sometimes, Talk Is the Best Medicine." *Wall Street Journal*, October 5, 1989, p. B1. ("Many medical [and other health professions?] schools pay only lip service to the subject.")

93. "Poor Communication Often a Prelude to Litigation." *Hospital Risk Management*, September 1992, pp. 117–120.

94. "Remind Physicians of the '12 R's' of Malpractice Prevention." *Hospital Risk Management*, March 1991, pp. 34–35.

95. Scott, R.W. *Legal Aspects of Documenting Patient Care*. Gaithersburg, MD: Aspen Publishers, Inc., 1994, pp. 153–155.

96. Brennan, T.A., Hebert, L.E., Laird, N.M., et. al. "Hospital Characteristics Associated With Adverse Events and Substandard Care." *Journal of the American Medical Association*, 1991; 265:3265–3269.

97. *Garnick*, note 39.

Suggested Readings

1. "A Guide for Physical Therapist Practice, Volume I: A Description of Patient Management." *Journal of the American Physical Therapy Association*, 1995; 75:707–764.

2. *Army Regulation 40-48: Non-Physician Health Care Providers*. Washington, DC: Department of the Army, 1986.

3. Bashi, H.L., Domholdt, E. "Use of Support Personnel for Physical Therapy Treatment." *Journal of the American Physical Therapy Association*, 1993; 73:421–436.

4. Beauchamp, T.L., Childress, J.F. *Principles of Biomedical Ethics*, 4th ed. New York: Oxford University Press, 1994.

5. Brushwood, D.B. "Hospital Pharmacist's Duty to Question Clear Errors in Prescriptions." *American Journal of Hospital Pharmacy*, 1994; 51:2031–2033.

6. Clifton, D.W. "'Tolerated Treatment Well' May No Longer Be Tolerated." *PT: Magazine of Physical Therapy*, 1995; 3(10)24–27.

7. Coile, R. *The New Governance: Strategies for an Era of Health Care Reform*. Ann Arbor, MI: Health Administration Press, 1994.

8. *Commonalities and Differences Between the Professions of Physical Therapy and Occupational Therapy*. Alexandria, VA: American Physical Therapy Association, 1994.

9. Furrow, B.R., Johnson, S.H., Jost, T.S., Schwartz, R.L. *Health Law: Cases, Materials and Problems*, 2nd ed. St. Paul, MN: West Publishing Company, 1991.

10. Guarino, K.S. "Developing a Comprehensive Records Management Plan." *Health Lawyer*, 1994; 7(3):15–16.

11. *Guide for Professional Conduct*. Alexandria, VA: American Physical Therapy Association, Judicial Committee, 1995.

12. "Guidelines for Occupational Therapy Documentation." *American Journal of Occupational Therapy*, 1986; 40:830–832.

13. "Guidelines for Physical Therapy Documentation." *Journal of the American Physical Therapy Association*, 1995; 75:762–764.

14. Hayward, R.S., Wilson, M.C., Tunis, S.R., et. al. "How to Use Clinical Practice Guidelines: Are the Recommendations Valid?" *Journal of the American Medical Association*, 1995; 274:570–574.

15. Jacobson, P.D. "Medical Malpractice and the Tort System." *Journal of the American Medical Association*, 1989; 262:3320–3327.

16. Kearney, K.A., McCord, E.L. "Hospital Management Faces New Liabilities." *Health Lawyer*, 1992; 6(3):1,3–5.

17. Keeton, W.P. *Prosser and Keeton on Torts*, 5th ed. St. Paul, MN: West Publishing Company, 1984.

18. *Occupational Therapy Code of Ethics*. Bethesda, MD: American Occupational Therapy Association, Commission on Standard and Ethics, 1994.

19. "Poor Communication Often a Prelude to Litigation." *Hospital Risk Management*, September 1992, pp. 117–120.

20. Prosser, W.L. *Handbook of the Law of Torts*, 4th ed. St. Paul, MN: West Publishing Company, 1971.

21. Robitzek, W.D. "Is There a Potential Lawsuit Brewing in Your Office?" *Physician's Management*, April 1992, pp. 131–138.

22. Scott, R.W. "For the Public Good." *PT: Magazine of Physical Therapy*, 1993; 1(1):82–85.

23. Scott, R.W. *Health Care Malpractice: A Primer on Legal Issues for Professionals*. Thorofare, NJ: Slack, Inc., 1990.

24. Scott, R.W. *Legal Aspects of Documenting Patient Care*. Gaithersburg, MD: Aspen Publishers, Inc., 1994.

25. Scott, R.W. "Lessons From Court." *Aon Direct Group Risk Advisor*, 1995; 1(1):5.

26. Scott, R,W. "Malpractice Update." *PT: Magazine of Physical Therapy*, 1993; 1(12):62–64.

27. "Standards of Practice for Occupational Therapy." *American Journal of Occupational Therapy*, 1994; 48:1039–1043.

28. Standards of Practice for Physical Therapists. HOD 06-91-25, 1991.

29. *1993 APTA State Licensure Reference Guide*. Alexandria, VA: American Physical Therapy Association, 1993.

Chapter 3

Liability for Intentional Conduct

This chapter introduces the concept of civil liability for intentional conduct. Legally actionable intentional conduct can consist of either affirmative actions, or omissions when one has the duty to act. The range of conduct that can give rise to intentional tort liability in health care settings includes assault and battery (including sexual assault and battery, a growing concern in the health professions), defamation of character, false imprisonment, fraud, and invasion of privacy, among other conduct.

There are recognized defenses to intentional tort legal actions, including, with defamation, reporting suspected child, spousal, or elder abuse. Clinicians, managers, and administrators must take responsibility for preventing the occurrence of intentional misconduct in health care delivery environments.

Introduction

Intentional wrongs committed against individuals or property are referred to as *intentional torts*. As the phrase implies, legally actionable intentional conduct requires some kind of injury to a person or to a person's property. The "injury" can be something seemingly as innocuous as interfering with a person's right to exclusive use of his or her tangible property or touching someone in such a way that may reasonably be construed as offensive.

The word "wrong" associated with "intentional wrong" may be a bit misleading as used here, in that the person committing an intentional tort need not have any specific intent to injure a victim (or the victim's property). The tortfeasor merely has to act with intent, or volition,

> **Intentional tort:** conduct in which a person intends that the resulting consequences of the act or omission occur, or where the person engaging in the conduct knows with substantial certainty that the occurrence of certain results are probable, with resultant injury to a person or to a person's property.

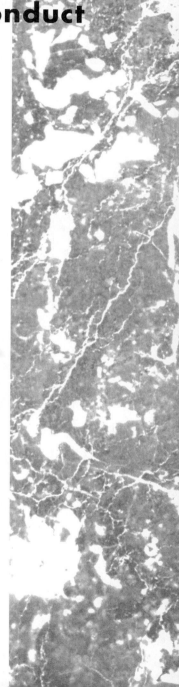

to effect a desired or probable result through his or her conduct. When that conduct results in injury to a person or to a person's property, an intentional tort action may arise.

A legally actionable intentional tort may exist even where the party whose conduct is in question did not intend to do an act that results in personal injury. It is often sufficient that the person intentionally engaging in some type of conduct knew that the conduct was substantially certain to cause a legally actionable result.

There is normally no intentional tort where a person engaging in conduct is either unconscious or acts reflexively. For example, consider the following hypothetical case examples.

1. A physical therapist assistant, acting under proper supervision of a licensed physical therapist and in compliance with the applicable state practice act, applies electrode pads from a neuromuscular stimulation device to a patient's lateral forearm musculature to effect extensor muscle re-education. As the assistant activates the device, it malfunctions, sending a surge of electrical current into the control box of the device. In a purely reflexive act, the assistant flails her arm into the air. Her moving arm strikes the patient in the left side of the face, resulting in a deep scratch to the patient's cheek, and a corneal abrasion to the patient's left eye. Does the physical therapist assistant's "harmful and offensive" touching of the patient constitute the intentional tort of battery?

   Answer: Probably not. Although the physical therapist assistant would be legally responsible for unintended patient injury if she had been flailing her arms in response to being told about a pay raise, for example, here, her conduct was unintentional. It also cannot be said that she knew with substantial certainty that, by turning on the neuromuscular stimulator device, it would surge and her arm would flail into the air, striking and injuring the patient. It would be a different case if the stimulator device had failed in a similar manner in the recent past, and physical therapist assistant was using it anyway—knowing with substantial certainty that a surge of electricity would probably cause her to flinch reflexively. The law will not impose intentional tort liability for a non-volitional act, unless it was reasonable to assume that the non-volitional act would take place.

2. X, an occupational therapist employed by ABC Community Hospital enters the break room and observes Y, an aide, sleeping in a chair. X applies a hand to Y's shoulder, gently shaking Y awake. Startled by being awakened suddenly, Y lashes out a fist, striking X in the face, knocking off X's glasses. Has either X or Y committed an intentional tort, i.e., battery? (Battery, as discussed later in this chapter, involves the intentional harmful, offensive, or otherwise impermissible touching of another person.)

> Answer: Probably neither *X* nor *Y* committed the tort of battery upon one another. *X* presumably acted reasonably as a representative of management in awakening *Y* during working hours. A certain amount of physical contact between people—even in the "intimate zone"[1] of contact—is a reasonable consequence of normal social relations. A different conclusion would result if *X*'s touching of *Y* was unreasonable—either by applying excessive force to *Y*'s shoulder, or by touching *Y* in a private zone of contact. *Y*'s act of striking *X* is considered legally to be an unconscious act, for which *Y* normally is not legally responsible.

In a legally actionable intentional tort action, then, there is no requirement for the injured party-plaintiff to prove *malicious* intent. That is, there is no requirement that a defendant's intention was to commit wrongdoing. It is sufficient that the defendant's conduct was volitional and intended (or substantially certain) to cause some even innocent result that causes injury to another person. If a defendant is proven to have had malicious intent incident to an intentional tort, then a court is more likely to permit the award of punitive damages against the wrongdoer.

One legal concept related to intent is the transferred intent doctrine. Under *transferred intent*, a defendant intends to direct conduct toward one person, but unintentionally affects another person. For example, consider the following hypothetical scenario.

> During a staff Christmas party in the cafeteria at Anywhere Medical Center, a food fight spontaneously erupts, involving several employees. Within seconds, it escalates to the point where one of the participants reaches into a punch bowl and retrieves a small piece of ice. The employee, *C*, throws the ice cube at *D*, who is engaged in the fray. *D* ducks, and the ice cube strikes *E*, another employee who is just entering the cafeteria to attend the party, in the right eye. Even though *C* had no intent to strike *E*, *C* is liable under the concept of transferred intent for injuries sustained by *E*, because *C* acted with intent toward *D*.

Why would a patient allegedly injured by a physical or occupational therapist in the course of a professional-patient relationship bring a civil legal action for an intentional tort vs. ordinary or professional negligence? There are several advantages to the patient in labeling a malpractice case as an intentional wrong case instead of as a negligence case. In proving an intentional wrong case (as with an ordinary negligence case), the patient normally does not have to introduce (expensive) expert testimony about the professional standard of care, since a lay jury or a judge normally can discern the nature and consequences of intentional conduct without the need for expert witness assistance. Also, if the court finds the defendant's conduct to have been egregious, it may allow for the award of punitive (or punishment) damages in the case. Punitive damages are over and above the normal compensatory monetary damages designed to make a tort plaintiff "whole."

The main disadvantage to a plaintiff in bringing a health care malpractice lawsuit as an intentional tort case is that a defendant-health care professional's liability insurer may not be legally obligated to indemnify the insured for liability for malicious intentional torts or for punitive damages, necessitating *execution of the judgment* (collection of monetary damages) from the defendant personally, a prospect that is less certain than collecting the award from the defendant's professional liability insurer.

Acts vs. Omissions

The kinds of conduct that can give rise to intentional tort liability—in the health care delivery setting (or any other setting)—are affirmative *acts*, and legally actionable *omissions*. Acts involve affirmative, volitional, intended conduct in furtherance of a specific result. For example, the application of non-therapeutic touch during a massage is an example of an affirmative act giving rise to potential intentional tort liability. So is striking a person without legal justification or excuse (i.e., committing battery). By definition, affirmative acts of battery designed to arouse or gratify the sexual desires of the aggressor or of the victim constitute sexual battery. Sexual battery, a subset of the tort of battery, will be discussed later in this chapter.

Legally actionable omissions involve the intentional and wrongful failure to act when one has the legal duty to act. As was discussed in Chapter 2, once a health care professional has assumed a legal duty of care for a patient, the provider is obligated by law to act reasonably toward the patient until the professional-patient relationship is properly terminated. When a provider leaves a patient under care without supervision, or improperly refuses to treat a patient, the *intentional* tort of patient *abandonment* becomes an issue. Similarly, where a health care professional intentionally fails to communicate critical patient information to others having an official need to know, an intentional tort issue arises. Consider the following hypothetical example.

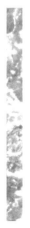

A surgical nurse is assisting an operating room technician in setting up a surgical suite for an orthopedic case. In the course of depositing sterile instruments onto the sterile back table, the nurse, in haste, knowingly drops an unsterile electrocautery cable onto the field, contaminating the sterile field and the "scrub" technician, who begins to touch instruments on the field. The orthopedic surgeon and the anesthesiologist are already visibly furious about routine delays in starting the case and would be incensed if the nurse revealed that the sterile field was contaminated. The field would have to be broken down to start over again. The nurse elects not to admit that the cable that was placed on the table was unsterile. If the surgical patient becomes infected as a result of the nurse's intentional (mis)conduct, then the patient will have an actionable claim for battery. (In this case, the harmful touching would be indirect, involving the unsterile electrocautery device that infects the patient.)

Assault and Battery

Assault and battery are terms that, although used interchangeably by lay people, really define two separate torts. The torts of assault and battery often go hand-in-hand in a real-life case; however, it is possible to have one tort occur without its complimentary intentional wrong. They will be discussed separately below.

Assault

Assault involves a situation where a victim reasonably anticipates, or has apprehension or fear about, an impending battery. Although both apprehension and fear are possible elements of the tort of assault, they are really two different concepts. A victim can apprehend (or sense) that harmful, offensive, or otherwise impermissible physical contact (i.e., battery) is imminent, yet not be in fear of it. Such might be the case when a patient knows that a health care provider is about to kiss the patient without permission. But, assault may also involve a fear of a touch, such as when a person flinches or winces in anticipation of an impending blow by another. In either case, the victim is displaying a normal reaction to an unwanted wrongful touch.

Another excellent example of assault is represented by a scene in the feature film, *The Hand That Rocks the Cradle*,[2] in which the female protagonist finds herself at the beginning of the film in her gynecologist's examining room with her legs placed in stirrups. Sensing that the gynecologist's imminent touch is improper, the protagonist flinches in disgust. This conduct alone on the part of the gynecologist gives rise to a legally actionable assault. The patient would have a cause of action, or case, even if the gynecologist had noticed that the patient was aware of his malicious intent and arrested his movement toward her without ever touching the patient.

In making the tort of assault legally actionable, the legal system serves to protect a person's privacy right to carry out activities of daily living free of the fear or anticipation of a battery at the hands of another. Considering the large number of reported assault and battery cases in society,[3] one may wonder how effective the legal system really is in protecting the rights of citizens to be free from the threat of violence. Because of the availability and threat of legal redress, every act of assault and battery carries with it a potentially high cost in terms of civil and criminal liability and adverse administrative consequences for the offender.

> **Assault:** reasonable anticipation or fear by a person of an impending battery.

Battery

Battery involves unjustified and unexcused harmful, offensive, or otherwise impermissible intentional contact by a tortfeasor with another person. Harmful contact includes volitional actions by the offender that cause pain, impairment, or disfigurement of a victim. Offensive contact includes direct and indirect acts of touching that offend a person's sense of dignity, such as when a health care profession inappropriately touches a patient's breasts or genitals.

A victim may be the subject of a battery without experiencing a prior assault. In the hypothetical example involving the nurse who contaminated a sterile surgical field, the patient, who was the victim of a battery, could not have apprehended the harmful touch (by the unsterile instruments), because the patient was sedated, and the patient's view obscured by a drape sheet. Similarly, when a patient is asleep, the patient cannot sense an impending battery (e.g., from a kiss or from touching of a sexual nature), so the patient becomes the victim of a battery without an assault.

There are several recognized *complete defenses* to the torts of assault and battery. The first recognized defense is consent. If a person who otherwise would be a victim of assault and/or battery knowingly and voluntarily consents to harmful or offensive contact, then there is no legally actionable assault or battery. For example, a customer of a prostitute solicits sadomasochistic sex with the prostitute, and the prostitute complies, tying and beating the customer. Even if the customer is injured, there may be no actionable assault or battery claim against the prostitute or the prostitute's employer if the customer consented to the beating.

In health care delivery, public policy considerations normally preclude consent by a patient or client to an assault or battery. So, even if a patient nominally consents to some socially impermissible contact such as sexual relations with the patient's health care provider, an action for assault and battery may be viable, on the grounds that the patient's "consent" is invalid as a matter of law. A patient cannot consent to sexual contact incident to routine health care delivery (with limited exceptions for situations such as legitimate sexual therapy), because the patient's consent would violate public policy.

Battery: unjustified and unexcused harmful, offensive, or otherwise impermissible intentional contact by a tortfeasor with another person.

Another legitimate defense to assault and battery is self-defense. Even in the health care treatment setting, a provider has the legal right to defend him- or herself from harmful or offensive contact by another person, including a patient. A health care provider may be privileged to use whatever physical force (or threat of force) is necessary to repel an attack, even to the point of meeting deadly force with deadly force.

The same legal rules apply for legitimate defense of others. Consider the following hypothetical example (based on a real case).

 A patient with a diagnosis of bipolar manic-depressive psychosis suddenly attacks a neurosurgical resident who is examining the patient at bedside. The patient begins to choke the resident, and the resident cries for help. Two licensed practical nurses and one patient come to the resident's aid and attempt in vain to pry the psychotic patient's fingers from the resident's neck. As the resident begins to lose consciousness, one of the nurses and the good Samaritan patient begin to strike the aggressor hard in the face. The other nurse draws and administers an ampule of Thorazine

intramuscularly into the aggressor's arm. After a few seconds, the psychotic patient releases his grip on the resident's neck and falls to the ground, unconscious. Did the nurse and patient who struck the aggressive patient commit battery?

Answer: No. The nurse and patient had the legal right to use reasonable force to protect the neurosurgical resident, who was in real danger of losing his life.

Defamation

Definition

Defamation includes legally actionable untrue communication(s) of purported fact about a person that harm the victim's positive personal reputation in the eyes of a significant number of other people in the victim's community. Defamatory communications cause other people to hold the target of the defamation up to ridicule, disgust, or scorn. *Business disparagement* [also called *trade libel*] involves verbal or other communications that harm a target person's business, rather than exclusively personal, reputation in the relevant community. Business disparagement will be discussed in greater detail in Chapter 10.

There are two primary classifications of defamation: slander and libel. *Slander* is a defamatory communication that is transmitted orally or through signing. *Libel* includes defamatory communications transmitted by all other means including writings, film, video and audiotape, and computer transmissions. Slanderous communications are transitory in nature, while libelous communications are considered to be of a more permanent nature.

A special category of defamation is *defamation per quod*. Under this concept, a communication made to others is not, on its face, defamatory. In fact, the communication may even appear to be complimentary of the target person. However, a defamation results once the negative implication of the primary communication (called the *innuendo*) is realized, after the communication is coupled with extrinsic facts (called the *inducement*) that make the communication defamatory. Consider the following hypothetical example:

> **Defamation:** false communication(s) of purported fact about a person that harm the victim's positive personal reputation in the eyes of a significant number of other people in the victim's community.
>
> **Slander:** a defamatory communication transmitted orally or through signing.
>
> **Libel:** a defamatory communication transmitted by all other means including writings, film, video and audiotape, and computer transmissions.
>
> **Business disparagement:** [also called **trade libel**] verbal or other communications that harm a target person's business reputation in the community.

A, a physical therapist working in a comprehensive outpatient rehabilitation facility, announces to the assembled rehabilitation team at a weekly meeting that *B*, an occupational therapist (who is not present at the meeting), became "certified" today in psychiatric therapy. Later that day, it is discovered that *B* was hospitalized for a nervous breakdown. Everyone then realizes that *A* meant to ridicule *B* by inferring that *B*'s certification was as a psychiatric patient. The original statement—seemingly innocent—then becomes a legally actionable defamation under defamation per quod.

To win a defamation lawsuit, a target person of a defamatory communication must normally prove special damages specific to the victim, not just generalized pain and suffering damages. One exception involves communications that constitute *defamation per se*. Under defamation per se, certain comments about people are actionable without proof of any damages, such as statements ascribing a loathsome, communicable disease—such as venereal disease—falsely to another person.

There are several complete defenses to a legal action for defamation. The first is the defense of truth, i.e., that what was said or otherwise communicated about a defamation plaintiff was, in fact, true. Although proof of the truth of a purportedly defamatory communication brings an end to a defamation legal action, it may give rise to another intentional tort action for wrongful *invasion of privacy*. (Invasion of privacy is discussed below.)

Another defense to defamation is *privilege*. Certain members of society—rightfully or not—are afforded by law an absolute (or complete) privilege to make defamatory statements about others. These include sitting judges in legal proceedings from the bench, congresspersons, and high-level executive officials acting in their official capacities.

Health care professionals, like prosecutors and defense attorneys in legal proceedings, have, under certain circumstances, a qualified privilege to make statements believed in good faith to be true about others, but that in fact are false and therefore defamatory. For health care professionals, for example, there is a qualified privilege under federal statute to give good-faith testimony in credentialing administrative actions about the competency of a physician under inquiry, without fear of defamation liability.[4] Health care professionals also are normally immune from defamation liability incident to good-faith official reporting of suspected child, spousal, or elder abuse (discussed below).

Constitutionally Protected Speech

One other defense to defamation related to privilege involves communications that are protected from suppression under the federal Constitution. Since the landmark U.S. Supreme Court decision in *New York Times* v. *Sullivan*[5] in 1964, it may be permissible for one person (particularly if that person is from the media) to "publish" (i.e., communicate to others) defamatory information about a target person who is either a public official or a public figure. In order to enjoy constitutional immunity from defamation liability, the person making a false statement about a public official or public figure must prove that he or she acted without actual knowledge of the falsity of the statement and did not communicate the defamatory information in reckless disregard of the truth.

Public officials, while not encompassing all public employees, includes policy-making governmental officials at all levels—federal, state, and local, and from all three branches—executive, legislative, and judicial. Examples of public officials also include, among others, persons who are political appointees to policy-making positions, such as heads of governmental task forces. As has become evident in recent political campaigns and appointment hearings, seemingly every aspect of these public officials' public and private lives is open to investigation and dissemination.

Public figures are not subject to the same degree of permissible scrutiny under law as public officials. Public figures are those persons who have achieved some degree of public fame or recognition incident to some pursuit, or who have voluntarily injected themselves into the public eye regarding some subject of public interest. Only areas related to their fame or reputation are permissible areas of scrutiny, not their entire lives or life histories. Examples of public figures include, among others, the leaders of major health professional associations.

Why should the legal system shield from defamation liability false communications made about public officials or public figures? The stated rationale for this constitutional privilege to defame is that the press's and public's right to know important information about public officials and public figures outweighs the privacy rights of those who have voluntarily placed themselves in the public eye.

Reporting Statutes and Requirements

Health care professionals in most or all states are required by statute to report certain findings incident to patient care activities. Included among these reportable findings is objective, credible evidence of possible child, spousal, and elder abuse.

Child Abuse

A recent Rand Corporation survey revealed that as many as 40 percent of health care professionals and educational professionals admit to not reporting suspected child abuse.[6] The primary stated rationale given for failing to report child abuse as required by law was that professionals were disillusioned with what they perceived as overtaxed and understaffed child protection service agencies. Another rationale for not reporting was that professionals stated that they were uncertain about the nature of their legal duty to report suspected child abuse.

Perhaps an unstated reason for failing to report suspected child abuse is the fear of liability exposure. Health care and other professionals have been subjected to liability exposure both for reporting and failing to report suspected child abuse.[7,8] Even when a health care or other professional is vindicated in a defamation lawsuit involving a report of suspected child abuse, the cost in terms of stress, injury to personal and professional reputation, and monetary outlays may be very high.

Domestic (Spousal) Abuse

Each year, as many as four million women (accounting for 90 to 95 percent of total domestic abuse cases) may be victims of domestic violence at the hands of their partners.[9] The continuum of types of spousal abuse range from battering with or without weaponry to sexual assault and battery to prolonged torture and murder. Health care professionals in all but five states are required by law to report suspected acts of spousal abuse to law enforcement authorities.[10]

The duty incumbent on health care professional clinicians is formidable. Providers are expected to be able to identify indices of possible abuse. Providers also routinely and expressly make inquiries of patients about possible domestic abuse, make reports when indicated, to appropriate agencies, and provide professional support and empathy. Imparting information about options to affected patients, addressing immediate safety concerns of patients and their children, properly documenting suspected abuse, and making appropriate client referrals to support agencies and other providers, is part of the duty indicated.[11]

The reporting spousal or other abuse in the face of client resistance to reporting creates an ethical dilemma, with the ethical principles of confidentiality and compliance with legal mandates in opposition. The reluctance to report is even stronger when the provider knows or reasonably believes that law enforcement or social service agencies will not protect the patient, exposing him or her to further violence.

Sexual assaults and batteries of female victims are estimated to number more than 700,000 per year.[12] Health care providers must be cognizant of overt and even subtle signs of sexual abuse in patients, including among other considerations, reticence, lack of eye contact, reluctance to shake hands or allow other physical contact, inappropriate dress, unexplained injuries, panic attacks during examination or conversation, and crying.

Elder Abuse

The phenomenon of elder abuse is less well recognized than child abuse or spousal domestic violence. Yet, elder abuse is a growing problem in the United States, Great Britain, and other countries, and is a problem that health care clinicians may fail to recognize and address.[13]

Health care providers should screen for elder abuse, just as they should for child or spousal abuse. There are noted physical findings and behavioral characteristics of elder abuse that are identifiable in the client and the elder's caregiver that should be watched for.

Physical warning signs of possible abuse in the elder abuse or neglect victim may include:

- untreated injury
- unexplained injury
- pain or withdrawal from touch
- seemingly minor skin bruising, lacerations, and/or burns

- malnutrition and/or dehydration
- unexplained weight loss
- pallor, sunken eyes and/or cheeks
- poor personal hygiene
- soiled clothing; clothing inappropriate for the season

The following, among others, are commonly noted behavioral characteristics of patients who are victims of elder abuse or neglect:

- anxiety, nervousness, apparent fear
- reticence, failure to make eye contact, withdrawal
- allowing a caregiver to answer when questioned about health-related complaints
- refusal of treatment intervention
- depression
- anger, hostility, belligerence
- inappropriate apparent euphoria
- lethargy

The abused elder patient's caregiver may display the following behavioral characteristics:

- intoxication, drug use
- aggression and/or history of violence
- indifference to caregiver education efforts
- verbal abuse of the patient
- answering questions for the elderly patient
- verbal and physical cues of a sexual nature that may indicate sexual abuse of the elderly patient, such as inappropriate touching of the patient and inappropriate patient dress for the clinical environment

Health professionals are urged to educate themselves about both the common and subtle indices of possible elder abuse, and to take appropriate action to prevent further abuse, including client and family/significant other education and reporting suspected abuse to social service entities or law enforcement authorities, as required by law. Failure to recognize and act on obvious signs of likely abuse, on the part of health care providers, constitutes professional negligence, for which liability may attach.

Other Reporting Requirements

Other forms of mandatory reporting requirements include the reporting to appropriate state health agencies of suspected or known infectious diseases[14] and enumerated occupational diseases[15] under state statutes. Non-physician health care professionals who evaluate and treat patients without physician referral have the same duty to recognize and report disease, injury, and abuse as physicians have.

False Imprisonment

False imprisonment, as it applies in the health care delivery environment, involves an allegation that a health care professional or someone employed by the provider acted intentionally to unlawfully restrict a patient's movement. False imprisonment allegations can arise from such actions as the involuntary commitment to hospitals of a patient with a psychiatric diagnosis and the unjustified physical restraint of a patient.

Another basis for false imprisonment liability exposure involves a situation in which a health care professional is alleged to have compelled a patient to remain in a specific location to undergo treatment, against the patient's will. There have also been cases in the reported legal literature involving allegations of false imprisonment involving health care professionals either attempting to stop, or actually prohibiting, patients from leaving the clinic area pending resolution of outstanding billing charges.

> *False imprisonment:* an intentional act to unlawfully restrict a patient's movement.

There are certain nuances and qualifiers to false imprisonment liability that warrant elaboration. False imprisonment is an intentional tort, therefore, any allegedly wrongful act on the part of a defendant-health care provider would have to have been done with the specific intent to confine a plaintiff-patient's free movement. Negligent, or careless, action that results in the confinement of a patient would not normally be sufficient to give rise to false imprisonment liability. Consider the following hypothetical scenario.

A certified occupational therapy assistant is treating a hospital patient in the patient's room on a ward. The patient requires a chair or her walker at one side of her bed, in order to rise and ambulate to the bathroom. The patient's chair and walker are moved away from bedside during the ADL treatment session. Despite the patient having told the occupational therapy assistant of this fact, and the assistant promising to reposition the chair and walker after treatment, the assistant forgets to do so and leaves the room. Because of this oversight, the patient cannot get up to use the toilet. The patient calls in vain for nursing assistance to help her get up, and finally urinates in bed, soiling her clothing and the bed linen. Is the certified occupational therapy assistant liable for false imprisonment? No. Although the intentional actions of the certified occupational therapy assistant resulted in the confinement of the patient to a limited area, i.e., the patient's bed, the certified occupational therapy assistant did not act with the specific intent to confine the patient. The assistant's actions constituted negligence, at worst.

Another nuance to false imprisonment liability is that verbal threats of physical force directed at a patient or threats of harm to a patient's property, resulting in a patient electing to limit volitional movement, may also constitute wrongful false imprisonment. False imprisonment liability, unlike most other torts, normally does not require proof of special damages, such as incurring additional medical expenses or resultant lost wages, in order for a plaintiff-patient to prevail.

One qualifier to false imprisonment liability is that a victim must be conscious of the fact that he or she is being confined or threatened with force if he or she moves. Therefore, legally, comatose, or perhaps even disoriented patients, cannot be "falsely imprisoned" by restraint, threats, or involuntary hospitalization.

Often, an act that constitutes false imprisonment (or assault or battery) also gives rise to another tort action—*intentional infliction of emotional distress*. Intentional infliction of emotional distress occurs when a defendant intentionally engages in extreme, outrageous conduct (such as unlawful false imprisonment of a patient) that results in severe emotional distress to a plaintiff.

Fraud

Black's Law Dictionary defines fraud, in part, as "an intentional perversion of the truth."[16] The intentional tort of *fraud* may be defined as the intentional false representation (or concealment) of a material fact designed to deceive another person, which causes that person to act (or not act) in some manner to the victim's legal detriment. Fraud is often thought of as being synonymous with "misrepresentation"; however, the latter term is used to describe fraudulent conduct that involves affirmative action by a wrongdoer.

> **Fraud:** the intentional false representation (or concealment) of a material fact designed to deceive another person, which causes that person to act (or not act) in some manner to the victim's legal detriment.

The subject of health care fraud has been widely reported in the recent professional literature.[17–34] Defraudation by health care providers of federal programs, such as Medicare and Medicaid, and of private insurers, account for at least ten percent of all health care expenditures.[35] Defraudation primarily takes place as a result of fraudulent billing for services, the receipt of bribes and kickbacks for patient referrals, and self-referral. Self-referral has decreased dramatically as a result of enactment and implementation by Congress of *Stark I and II*,[36] which prohibit physician self-referral of Medicare and Medicaid patients for the following types of services, among others, in which the physician has a financial interest:

- clinical laboratory services
- physical therapy
- occupational therapy
- durable medical equipment suppliers
- prosthetics
- orthotics

In addition to the *Stark* laws, another federal statute, the Fraud and Abuse Act,[37] enacted in 1972, prohibits the offer or receipt of payment of bribes, kickbacks, and rebates in exchange for Medicare or Medicaid patient referrals. By federal regulation, there are a limited number of "safe harbors"[38] under which providers may be immune from prosecution or civil liability for health care fraud, based on their good faith attempts to comply with the law. The existence of safe harbors from prosecution and liability are particularly important to providers in managed care environments, who must have a certain degree of practice flexibility.

Civil legal action against health care professionals for defraudation of federal health care programs can take place under a federal statute entitled the False Claims Act.[39] Under that statute, the intentional submission of a false claim to the federal government, which results in reimbursement by the federal government, may subject an offender to mandatory civil penalties of between $5,000 and $10,000 for every false claim submitted, plus *treble* (triple) damages. Either the federal government or a private citizen (under the *qui tam* [Latin for "who as well"] provisions of the statute) may initiate civil legal action against an alleged offender. If a private citizen initiates a qui tam action for fraud against an offender and the action is successful, the private citizen receives between ten and thirty percent of the government's recovery, plus the award of reasonable legal expenses.[40]

The federal government is making significant headway in battling health care fraud. In 1994 alone, the Department of Justice recovered some $587 million in judgments and penalties against providers and others in health care fraud legal actions.[41] Senator Cohen (R-Maine) introduced Senate Bill 245, the Health Care Fraud Prevention Act of 1995, which would greatly expand federal jurisdiction over health care fraud and abuse, to encompass all health care providers and all health care services—governmental and private. The proposed law would create a new federal criminal offense—health care fraud, boost civil monetary penalties against offenders, and result in program exclusion at both federal and state levels.[42]

Invasion of Privacy

There is perhaps no environment (except the military service) in which individual privacy is sacrificed to so great a degree as in health care delivery settings. In fact, one recent article in the medical professional literature, referring to the growing state of government encroachment on the privacy of the provider-patient relationship, was titled "How the Doctor Got Gagged: The Disintegrating Right of Privacy in the Physician-Patient Relationship."[43]

As part of their fiduciary duty owed to patients under their care, health care professionals are obligated by law and ethics to jealously safeguard patient confidences, except where they are required by law to disclose them, or where disclosure is made to other health care professionals having a need to know the information disclosed. Occasionally, health care providers, administrators, and support personnel unlawfully fail to respect patient privacy, resulting in the intentional tort of *invasion of privacy*.

As in defamation cases, invasion of privacy legal actions are premised on an allegation of wrongful disclosure of information to third parties. There are four principal forms of legally actionable invasion of privacy in the health care delivery environment. They are:

- intrusion upon a patient's seclusion or solitude
- "false light" publicity about a patient
- misappropriation of a patient's name or likeness
- public disclosure of private facts about a patient

Unreasonable Intrusion Upon Patient Solitude

To be liable for invasion of privacy under the *unreasonable intrusion* prong of this tort, a defendant must (1) intentionally intrude, physically or otherwise, upon the seclusion or solitude of another person, (2) in such a way that is deemed highly offensive to an ordinary, reasonable person (i.e., the fact-finder in litigation). Everyone—even patients—have the right to reasonable privacy or seclusion. Of course, for patients—especially inpatients—there are few areas where seclusion can be experienced.

There are many scenarios involving intrusion on a patient's solitude that take place in the health care setting. One involves the opening of a patient's mail or a private drawer of a nightstand, in order to peruse a patient's private property. Another is the unauthorized photographing of a sleeping or comatose patient—even if the photo is never shown to anyone. Consider another hypothetical example:

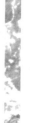

X is a male physical therapy aide, employed at HMO Health Care Center. *Y* is a female outpatient under care in the physical therapy clinic. During one treatment session, *X* suddenly opens the curtain to *Y*'s cubicle while *Y* is undressing, in order to see her in a state of partial undress. Does *X*'s act constitute a tort? Yes. *X* is liable for invasion of *Y*'s privacy, by intruding on her reasonable seclusion. (Note that *X* might also be liable for other torts, such as intentional infliction of emotional distress and sexual harassment. There would probably be no liability if exigent, or emergency, circumstances (such as a fire in the clinic) existed that required *X* to enter the cubicle where *Y* was undressing.

False-Light Publicity

False-light invasion of privacy, like the remaining two prongs of the intentional tort of invasion of privacy, involve situations where a defendant violates a plaintiff's privacy rights in some way and disseminates private information about the plaintiff to third parties who do not have a right to know, or legitimate need for, the information. There are three classic elements to actionable false-light invasion of privacy:

- The defendant disseminates private information to others about a plaintiff and somehow casts the information conveyed in such a way as to place the plaintiff in a false public light.
- The defendant's actions are objectively unreasonable and highly offensive.
- The information disclosure is done with *malice* (knowledge of the fact that the disclosure would place the plaintiff in a false public light or reckless disregard for the consequences of the act).

Consider the following hypothetical example:

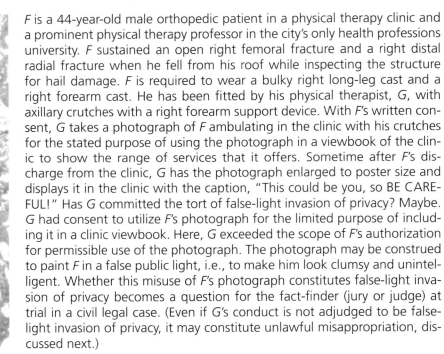

F is a 44-year-old male orthopedic patient in a physical therapy clinic and a prominent physical therapy professor in the city's only health professions university. *F* sustained an open right femoral fracture and a right distal radial fracture when he fell from his roof while inspecting the structure for hail damage. *F* is required to wear a bulky right long-leg cast and a right forearm cast. He has been fitted by his physical therapist, *G*, with axillary crutches with a right forearm support device. With *F*'s written consent, *G* takes a photograph of *F* ambulating in the clinic with his crutches for the stated purpose of using the photograph in a viewbook of the clinic to show the range of services that it offers. Sometime after *F*'s discharge from the clinic, *G* has the photograph enlarged to poster size and displays it in the clinic with the caption, "This could be you, so BE CAREFUL!" Has *G* committed the tort of false-light invasion of privacy? Maybe. *G* had consent to utilize *F*'s photograph for the limited purpose of including it in a clinic viewbook. Here, *G* exceeded the scope of *F*'s authorization for permissible use of the photograph. The photograph may be construed to paint *F* in a false public light, i.e., to make him look clumsy and unintelligent. Whether this misuse of *F*'s photograph constitutes false-light invasion of privacy becomes a question for the fact-finder (jury or judge) at trial in a civil legal case. (Even if *G*'s conduct is not adjudged to be false-light invasion of privacy, it may constitute unlawful misappropriation, discussed next.)

Misappropriation

Misappropriation invasion of privacy involves the unauthorized use of a plaintiff's name and/or likeness, usually, but not always, for a defendant's commercial gain. Misuse of a plaintiff's name or likeness for non-commercial purposes is also legally actionable as misappropriation.

This branch of invasion of privacy is particularly applicable to health care delivery, since health care professionals are frequently asked by commercial product manufacturers and others to involve patients in research studies. In addition to the ethical considerations surrounding the use of patients in clinical research, clinicians are urged to remember that misuse, or "overuse" of patient information may give rise to misappropriation liability.

Public Disclosure of Private Patient Facts

There are three elements to the tort of *public disclosure of private facts* invasion of privacy. They are:

- The defendant publicizes information about a person that is of a personal nature.
- The disclosure is highly offensive from the viewpoint of an ordinary, reasonable person.
- The subject matter of the disclosure is not legitimately in the public interest.

Every person has constitutional (federal and state), statutory, and common law rights to legitimate privacy and intimacy. These rights are perhaps the most fundamental in American society, a nation which prides itself on respect for individual rights and freedom. The constitutional right of privacy is the only judicially-recognized personal freedom that is not enumerated in the Constitution. This implied right was added to those enumerated in the Constitution by the U.S. Supreme Court in 1965[44] and was based on language from multiple enumerated rights in the Bill of Rights.

Examples of actionable public disclosure-invasion of privacy abound in the health care setting. It is frequently said by health care attorneys at continuing education courses that any lawyer could discover almost any private fact about a patient just by walking through the corridors of a hospital and listening to what others say. Hopefully, this assertion is not factual. However, actions such as the release of patient information from medical records without patient authorization,[45] revelation of a patient's HIV status or sexual preferences, and disclosure of other private facts about a patient, among other actions, may give rise to public disclosure invasion of privacy litigation. Consider the following hypothetical example.

> *B* is a 32-year-old female patient with a diagnosis of a right quadratus lumborum muscle strain. *B* is being evaluated for treatment by *C*, a physical therapist. During the course of evaluation, *C* notices that *B* has significant prominent stretch marks on her abdomen from her two previous pregnancies, a fact that *B* struggles to keep private. After *B*'s initial treatment session, she leaves the hospital and is scheduled to return the next day for follow-up. While in the cafeteria with fellow staff professionals later that day, *C* reveals, in the course of a conversation about pregnancy, that *B* has prominent stretch marks on her abdomen. This revelation— even though factual and even if considered trivial by those who hear it— constitutes actionable public disclosure invasion of privacy.

Sexual Misconduct

The incidence of allegations of sexual misconduct involving professionals is disproportionately high in the health care environment. The fact that sexual misconduct involving health care professionals and patients occurs at alarmingly high rates tarnishes the reputation of all health care disciplines. This section describes sexual misconduct that constitutes sexual assault and battery and other impermissible forms of sexual contact, such as meretricious consensual sexual relations between providers and patients. The discussion in this section does not extensively address the topic of sexual harassment. Sexual harassment is discussed in greater detail in Chapter 8.

Rehabilitation professions, including physical and occupational therapy, prosthetics, and orthotics, are frequently referred to as "hands-on" professions. In fact, in physical therapy, one popular slogan is, "If it's physical, it's therapy." Physical and occupational therapists experience some of the most intense professional relationships with their patients—largely because of the length of time spent in close physical contact with patients during their rehabilitation.

Health care professionals, especially in the rehabilitation setting, elicit and assess a great deal of personal information about patients during the course of patient evaluation and assimilate this information into care plans. In the ensuing professional relationships, rehabilitation health care professionals become privy to many intimate details about patients' private lives. And—just as in psychotherapy, law, and religion—patients who share their intimate thoughts may experience *transference* with their health care providers, within the therapeutic relationships.

A patient may be vulnerable to abuse because of the trust that the patient places in his or her health care professional. The patient may develop intense affection for his or her treating clinician and may sense an urgent need for approval, creating a kind of parent-child relationship. Romantic feelings may develop as well. These transference emotions are normal phenomenon in a patient and must not be exploited by health professionals responsible for the patient's care.

A physical or occupational therapist is a fiduciary to his or her patient, meaning that the therapist has both a legal and ethical duty to act principally in the patient's best interests. It is therefore one of the highest duties incumbent upon a physical or occupational therapist to ensure that the professional-patient relationship does not turn into an intimate, personal, or sexual relationship. Any reciprocal counter-transference feelings that arise in the clinician must be sublimated in order to prevent the sexual abuse of the patient. Even when not prohibited by law, sexual relations with patients during the pendency of the therapist-patient professional relationship are always wrong.

From a legal perspective, there are two possible classifications of sexual abuse involving health care professionals and patients. The first type of health-care-related sexual abuse is *sexual assault* or *battery*, which can be defined as:

> any nonconsensual touching of a patient's or health care provider's sexual or other body parts (or clothing) by the other party, for the purpose of arousing or gratifying the sexual desires of either party to the relationship, or for the purpose of sexually abusing a patient.[46]

Commission, by a health care professional, of sexual assault or battery upon a patient can give rise to civil liability, not only for the tort of malicious intentional sexual assault or battery, but also for intentional infliction of emotional distress and professional negligence. Concomitant legal and adverse administrative actions may also ensue in criminal court, before state licensure entities, before judicial committees of professional associations of which the offender is a member, and before credentials committees at institutions where the offender holds clinical privileges.

A finding of civil liability against a health care professional for sexual assault or battery may result in a civil court award of punitive (punishment) damages against the wrongdoer and in favor of the patient-victim in addition to the normal compensatory damages for lost wages, medical expenses, and pain and suffering incurred by the victim. A finding of liability for a malicious intentional tort and the award of punitive damages may mean that the defendant-provider's professional liability insurer is relieved of the legal responsibility for indemnifying the provider for the judgment, making the provider personally liable for the monetary judgment rendered against him or her.

The second type of health-care-related sexual abuse involves meretricious and specious provider-patient intimate relationships labeled *consensual*. In such relationships, a patient falls in love with his or her health care provider, and the provider reciprocates. Because of transference emotions, the inherent vulnerability of patients dependent upon their providers for care and support, and providers' fiduciary duty of good faith and trust toward their patients, the concept of "consent" on the part of patients to sexually intimate meretricious relationships with health care professionals responsible for their care has no real meaning. It is the health care professional who is always singularly responsible for the creation of such a relationship. Patients, on the other hand, are not bound by professional ethical or legal standards for their behavior in provider-patient intimate relationships.

> **Hint** *The concept of "consent" on the part of patients to sexually intimate meretricious relationships with health care professionals responsible for their care has no real meaning.*

In 1991, the State Bar of California attempted to fashion a regulation that expressly sanctions sexual relations between California-licensed attorneys and their clients, so long as the attorney does not "employ coercion, intimidation, or undue influence in entering into sexual relations with a client."[47] From the viewpoint of many legal commentators, this official position by the California bar failed to recognize the fact that any sexual relationship between a professional and client is inherently potentially exploitative, and therefore to be avoided at all costs.

A more reasoned approach to both nonconsensual and putative "consensual" sexual relationships between professionals and their clients or patients is one that, considering the fragile psychological and emotional status of patients (and legal and other clients) and the actual impropriety or appearance of impropriety of such relationships, prohibits them altogether. The American Physical Therapy Association's *Guide for Professional Conduct*, Section 1.3, governing the conduct of member-physical therapists, states that:

> Physical therapists shall not engage in any sexual relationship or activity, whether consensual or nonconsensual, with any patient while a physical therapist/patient relationship exists.[48]

The American Physical Therapy Association's *Guide for the Conduct of the Affiliate Member*, Standard 2.4, governing the conduct of member-physical therapist assistants, similarly requires that:

> Physical therapist assistants shall not engage in any sexual relationship or activity, whether consensual or nonconsensual, with any patient while a physical therapist assistant/patient relationship exists.[49]

The American Occupational Therapy Association's *Occupational Therapy Code of Ethics*, Principle 1B, governing the conduct of all occupational therapy professionals and support personnel, states that:

> Occupational therapy personnel shall maintain relationships that do not exploit the recipient of services *sexually* [emphasis added], physically, emotionally, financially, socially, or in any other manner. Occupational therapy personnel shall avoid those relationships or activities that interfere with professional judgment and objectivity.[50]

What should a health care professional do when an intimate relationship with a patient cannot be avoided? Because most health professional ethics codes prohibit an intimate relationship simultaneously with a professional-patient relationship, a provider who is about to enter into an intimate relationship with a patient, despite this prohibition, must expeditiously disengage from further care of the patient and take appropriate steps to transfer the patient, with appropriate coordination, to another competent health care professional. The American Physical Therapy Association's *Guide for Professional Conduct*, Principle 3.3D states that:

> In the event of elective termination of a physical therapist/patient relationship by the physical therapist, the therapist should take steps to transfer the care of the patient, as appropriate, to another provider.[51]

Not addressed in the above professional ethics standards is any guidance about recommended or mandatory waiting periods after severance of provider-patient professional relationships, before commencing intimate relationships. Some authorities suggest a minimum six-month waiting period.[52]

Health care clinical professionals and managers and administrators have the legal and ethical duty to take all appropriate measures to both prevent allegations of, and actual sexual abuse of, patients in the health care delivery environment. Simple risk-management measures that can be implemented include the following:

- Provide a same-sex chaperone for observation of patient evaluation and treatment, available either upon patient request or when a health care provider believes that the chaperone's presence is required.

- Implement a "knock-and-enter" clinic policy, under which any staff member having a need to open a closed door to a room in which a patient and provider are located may do so after giving due warning by knocking.

- Establish an informed consent policy that ensures that patients understand the nature of all therapeutic procedures—especially those which are intensively "hands-on"—and always give informed consent to treatment.

- Provide ongoing continuing education to professional and support staff on how to prevent sexual abuse and harassment (see Box 3-1).

3-1 Sexual Abuse

The incidence of sexual abuse of patients is well-documented and publicized in the professional and popular literature. Sexual abuse is estimated to occur in seven to eleven percent of encounters between patients and psychotherapists, family practice physicians, gynecologists, internists, and surgeons. A similar prevalence is estimated for attorneys, clergy, educators, and social workers. Sexual abuse of these patients ranges from verbal abuse to sexual intimacies (including kissing and fondling) to sexual intercourse. Of the total number of reported cases of sexual abuse involving psychiatrists and patients, 80 percent are estimated to involve male therapists and female patients; 13 percent, female therapists and female patients; five percent, male therapists and male patients; and two percent, female therapists and male patients.

Although studies have not been conducted to provide detailed statistics on sexual relationships between physical or occupational therapists and patients, the number of reported incidents of sexual abuse in these fields is clearly on the rise, as evidenced by cases brought before the courts,[53] state licensure boards,[54] and the Judicial Committee (APTA), and Standards and Ethics Commission (AOTA), for adjudication. In physical therapy, many allegations of sexual abuse arise from intensively hands-on evaluative and treatment techniques, where misunderstandings are more likely to occur, such as myofascial release and strain-counterstrain and where physical therapists' hands may come into close proximity to patients' breasts, buttocks, and genitals.

Chapter Summary

Liability for intentional conduct may have more serious adverse consequences for health care professionals than does liability for professional or ordinary negligence. For intentional acts that are found to be malicious, such as sexual battery, health care professionals may face loss of licensure and professional association membership, as well as personal monetary liability for an adverse judgment, since insurers are generally not legally obligated to indemnify their insured against such losses.

The types of tortious conduct that can give rise to intentional tort liability range from assault and battery to defamation of character to fraud, among other volitional conduct. Allegations and the commission of sexual assault and battery by health care providers against patients pose a serious threat to the professional reputations of all "hands-on" health care disciplines. Clinicians, managers, and administrators must work together, proactively and aggressively, to prevent such allegations from arising in all health care practice settings.

Regarding defamation of character, one important exception to intentional tort liability involves compliance with statutory reporting requirements, under which health care professionals are obligated to report to authorities suspected child, domestic (spousal), and elder abuse. A good faith report by a health professional, grounded in reasonable suspicion, will not result in defamation liability, even if the report is unsubstantiated by authorities.

Because one must act consciously and deliberately in order to be held liable for intentional conduct, careful thought before taking any official action incident to patient care delivery is perhaps the best, as well as the simplest, risk management measure that health care professionals can undertake to dampen intentional tort liability.

Cases and Questions

1. A physical therapist attending a risk management seminar inquires about risk management measures that should be taken to prevent misunderstandings about the nature of therapeutic touch in an intensively hands-on orthopedic physical therapy practice. What would you advise the audience to do?

2. You are an occupational therapist in a multi-specialty outpatient rehabilitation clinic. The clinic's manager and co-owner of the private group practice directs you to bill Medicare for patient no-shows, at one-half the billing rate of normal clinic visits. Can you legally and ethically comply with the manager's order?

Suggested Answers to Cases and Questions

1. In all settings, patients should clearly understand the nature of therapeutic touch. Thorough education about procedures to be used and relevant anatomical structures, including the use of anatomical models, should help patients understand recommended treatments, such as orthopedic mobilization and myofascial release. Patients must be given legally sufficient disclosure information about recommended treatments so that they can make valid, voluntary, and intelligent elections of treatment. Considerations of modesty, privacy, and common sense require that therapists, assistants, and aides adequately drape patients undergoing evaluation and treatment. Patients have the absolute right to request and have present a same-gender chaperone during evaluation and treatment. Clinics that cannot comply with this requirements must take immediate steps to rectify their noncompliant practice.

1. No. Billing for care that is not delivered under false pretenses constitutes actionable intentional fraud. A finding of defraudment against Medicare or Medicaid, known as "program-related misconduct," results in automatic exclusion from participation in these programs for five years. See footnote 18. Additional adverse action in federal (criminal) court and before licensure boards and professional associations may also result. Commission of an illegal and unethical act is not legally justified because a superior orders an employee to carry it out.

References

1. There are four potential physical areas of social interaction between people. The public zone includes distances where physical contact is unlikely, such as in a concert hall or across a public street. The social zone includes distances of between about four and twelve feet, and encompasses normal business relations between colleagues in an office or university environment. The personal zone involves arms-length business transactions between two or more people and includes encounters such as an interview between a health care clinic's receptionist or provider and a patient. The intimate zone involves hands-on or skin-to-skin contact between people. Certain health care professionals, including physical and occupational therapists, are privileged as part of their professional licensure to enter patients' intimate zones for legitimate professional purposes. For more on social distances, see Purtilo, R. *Health Professional and Patient Interaction*, 4th ed. Philadelphia, PA: W.B. Saunders Company, 1990, p. 149.

2. *The Hand That Rocks the Cradle.* Hollywood Pictures, November, 1992.

3. In 1992, there were 742,130 arrests nationwide for violent crimes. Of that total number, 507,210 arrests were made for aggravated assault and battery, and 39,100 arrests were made for forcible rape. *Information Please Almanac.* Boston, MA: Houghton Mifflin Company, 1995, p. 853.

4. 42 United States Code Section 11111(a)(2).

5. *New York Times* v. *Sullivan*, 376 U.S. 254 (1964).

6. "40% of Health Professionals Admit Not Reporting Abuse." *PT Bulletin*, February 21, 1990, pp. 6, 40.

7. *Landeros* v. *Flood*, 551 P.2d 389 (Cal. 1976) (addressing potential physician liability for failure to diagnose and report battered child syndrome).

8. *Kempster* v. *Child Protective Services*, 515 N.Y.S. 2d 807 (App. Div. 1987) (addressing potential liability on the part of health care professionals for making reports of suspected child abuse).

9. Sassetti, M.R. "Domestic Violence." *Primary Care*, 1993; 20:289–305.

10. Hyman, A., Schillinger, D., Lo, B. "Laws Mandating Reporting of Domestic Violence." *Journal of the American Medical Association*, 1995; 273:1781–1787. (Especially noteworthy is the table listing all state reporting statutes on page 1782.)

11. *Ibid.* at 1781.

12. Saltus, R. "Doctors Urged to Learn Signs of Sexual Abuse." *Houston Chronicle*, November 7, 1995, p. 5A.

13. Kingston, P., Penhale, B. "Elder Abuse and Neglect: Issues in the Accident and Emergency Department." *Accident and Emergency Nursing*, 1995; 3:122–128.

14. Chorba, T.L., Berkelman, R.L., Safford, S.K., et al. "Mandatory Reporting of Infectious Diseases by Clinicians." *Journal of the American Medical Association*, 1989; 262:3018–3026.

15. Freund, E., Seligman, P.J., Chorba, T.L., et al. "Mandatory Reporting of Occupational Diseases by Clinicians." *Journal of the American Medical Association*, 1989; 262:3041–3044.

16. *Black's Law Dictionary*, 5th ed. St. Paul, MN: West Publishing Company, 1979, p. 594.

17. "Accuracy of Therapists' Documentation Questioned at Two Florida Nursing Homes." *PT Bulletin*, August 18, 1995, p. 15.

18. "ALJ Holds Physical Therapist Responsible for Billing for 'No Show' Patients." *Civil Money Penalties Reporter: Medicare/Medicaid Fraud & Abuse*, January 1993, p. 5. (In this adverse administrative federal action before an administrative law judge, a physical therapist, who previously had pleaded guilty in a state criminal trial to knowingly filing false Medicaid claims for "no show" patients, was excluded from participation in Medicare and Medicaid programs [officially referred to as "program exclusion"] for five years.)

19. Crane, T.S., "The Problem of Physician Self-Referral Under the Medicare and Medicaid Antikickback Statute." *Journal of the American Medical Association*, 1992; 268:85–91.

20. "Fraud Among Health Care Providers Costs $44 Billion Annually." *PT Bulletin*, April 7, 1995, pp. 1, 6.

21. "Fraud Crackdown in Health Care." *Advance for Physical Therapists*, July 17, 1995, pp. 4, 17.

22. "Federal Grand Jury Returns Indictment Against Physical Therapist." *PT Bulletin*, April 27, 1994, p. 2.

23. Harlan, C. "He Apparently Succeeded Better Than Most of Us at Avoiding Work." *Wall Street Journal*, March 14, 1991, p. B1.

24. "Health Care Fraud Convictions Up 73 Percent." *Advance for Physical Therapists*, March 27, 1995, p. 20.

25. Jesilow, P., Geis, G., Pontell, H. "Fraud by Physicians Against Medicaid." *Journal of the American Medical Association*, 1991; 266:3318–3322.

26. Kusserow, R. "Health Care Fraud Prevention Act of 1995." *Biomechanics*, April 1995, p. 96.

27. MacKelvie, C., McGuire, M.L. "Fraud, Abuse and Inurement: The Growing Impact on Provider-Physician Relations." *Journal of Health and Hospital Law*, 1990; 23(1):1–9.

28. Olsen, G.G. "Fraud and Abuse in Health Care." *Rehab Management*, August/September 1994, pp. 111–113.

29. Peregrine, M.W., Nodzenski, T.J. "Expanded Enforcement of the Fraud and Abuse Laws." *Journal of Health and Hospital Law*, 1990; 23(1):10–14.

30. Salcido, R. "HHS' Voluntary Disclosure Program: How to Obtain Benefits Under the Program While Minimizing Risk." *The Health Lawyer*, 1995; 10(4):1, 3–8.

31. Stevens, C. "Curbing Insurance Fraud and Abuse." *Rehab Management*, December 1995/January 1996, pp. 62–63, 116.

32. "The Justice Department Plans to Step Up Enforcement Action to Decrease Fraud, Abuse." *PT Bulletin*, September 8, 1995, p. 12.

33. Wakeman, N., "Georgia, P.T. Arrested on Fraud Charges." *PT Bulletin*, March 30, 1994, pp. 3, 40.

34. "$90 Billion Lost to Fraud, Health-Care Experts Say." *PT Bulletin*, March 23, 1993, p. 6.

35. See 62 *Fed. Const. Rep.* 373-274. BNA, October 17, 1994.

36. 42 United States Code Section 1395nn.

37. Section 1128B(b) of the Social Security Act, 42 United States Code Section 1320a-7(b) (7).

38. 42 Code of Federal Regulations Section 1001.952, 56 *Federal Register* 35952-87. See also Scott, R.W. *Legal Aspects of Documenting Patient Care*. Gaithersburg, MD: Aspen Publishers, Inc., 1994, p. 200, note 30.

39. 31 United States Code Section 3729 *et seq.*

40. *Ibid.* at Section 3730(d).

41. See 62 *Fed. Const. Rep.* 373-274. BNA, October 17, 1994.

42. Kusserow, note 26, at 96.

43. Sugarman, J., Powers, M. "How the Doctor Got Gagged: The Disintegrating Right of Privacy in the Physician-Patient Relationship." *Journal of the American Medical Association*, 1991; 266:3323–3327.

44. *Griswold* v. *Connecticut*, 381 U.S. 479 (1965).

45. See *Industrial Foundation of the South* v. *Texas Industrial Accident Board*, 540 S.W. 2d 668 (Texas 1976), *cert. denied*, 430 U.S. 931 (U.S. Supreme Court 1977).

46. Adapted as a composite definition of sexual assault and battery from the following criminal law codes: The Model Penal Code, Section 213.4, American Law Institute, Proposed Official Draft, 1962, and Colorado Revised Statutes, Section 18-3-401(4).

47. "Defined, Barred: Sex with Clients." Rule 3-120, State Bar of California. *National Law Journal*, May 6, 1991, p. 6.

48. *Guide for Professional Conduct*, Section 1.3 (Patient Relations). Alexandria, VA: American Physical Therapy Association, January 1996.

49. *Guide for Conduct of the Affiliate Member*, Standard 2.4 (Patient Relations). Alexandria, VA: American Physical Therapy Association, January 1996.

50. *Occupational Therapy Code of Ethics*, Principle 1.A (Occupational therapy personnel demonstrate a concern for the well-being of the recipients of their services [beneficence]). Bethesda, MD: American Occupational Therapy Association, July 1994.

51. *Guide for Professional Conduct*, Section 3.3D (Provision of Services). Alexandria, VA: American Physical Therapy Association, January 1996.

52. Stromber, C.D., Haggarty, D.J., Leibenluft, R.F., et al. "Physical Contact and Sexual Relations with Patients." *The Psychologist's Legal Handbook*. Washington, DC: The Council for the National Register of Health Service Providers in Psychology, 1988, p. 463.

53. The case of *Oslund* v. *United States*, Civ. No. 4-88-323, (U.S. Dist. Court, District of Minnesota, Oct. 23, 1989), involved a Federal Tort Claims Act lawsuit initiated by an occupational therapy patient at a Veterans Administration Hospital, who allegedly was simultaneously involved in a professional and a meretricious sexual relationship with an occupational therapy intern. Allegedly, herpes was transmitted between the alleged paramours during the intimate relationship. The patient sued the United States (since the occupational therapy intern possessed personal immunity from suit under federal law) for battery and intentional infliction of emotional distress. The district court ruled, in part, that the occupational therapy intern's medical records were subject to release to establish when she developed and received medical treatment for herpes.

54. Licensure boards and professional associations legally may take adverse action against respondent-health professionals for consensual sexual relationships with active patients. See "Physician May Be Disciplined for Consensual Sexual Relationship with Patient." *Journal of Health and Hospital Law*, 1993; 26(3):86.

Suggested Readings

1. Campbell, M.L. "The Oath: An Investigation on the Injunction Prohibiting Physician-Patient Sexual Relations." *Perspectives on Biological Medicine*, 1989; 32(2):300–308.

2. Council on Ethical and Judicial Affairs, American Medical Association. "Sexual Misconduct in the Practice of Medicine." *Journal of the American Medical Association*, 1991; 266:2741–2745.

3. Gabbard, G.O. *Sexual Exploitation in Professional Relationships*. Washington, DC: American Psychiatric Press, Inc., 1989.

4. *Guide for Professional Conduct*. Alexandria, VA: American Physical Therapy Association, January 1996.

5. *Guide for Conduct of the Affiliate Member*. Alexandria, VA: American Physical Therapy Association, January 1996.

6. Hyman, A., Schillinger, D., Lo, B. "Laws Mandating Reporting of Domestic Violence." *Journal of the American Medical Association*, 1995; 273:1781–1787.

7. Kingston, P., Penhale, B. "Elder Abuse and Neglect: Issues in the Accident and Emergency Department." *Accident and Emergency Nursing*, 1995; 3:122–128.

8. *Occupational Therapy Code of Ethics*. Bethesda, MD: American Occupational Therapy Association, July 1994.

9. Pitulla, J. "Unfair Advantage." *Journal of the American Bar Association*, November 1992, pp. 78–80.

10. Purtilo, R. *Health Professional and Patient Interaction*, 4th ed. Philadelphia, PA: W.B. Saunders Company, 1990.

11. Samuelson, R.J. "Sex and Psychotherapy." *Newsweek*, April 13, 1992, pp. 52–57.

12. Sherman, C. "Behind Closed Doors: Therapist-Client Sex." *Psychology Today*, 1993; 26(3):67.

13. Schunk, C., Parver, C.P. "Avoiding Allegations of Sexual Misconduct." *Clinical Management*, 1989; 9(5):22.

14. Scott, R.W. *Health Care Malpractice: A Primer on Legal Issues for Professionals.* Thorofare, NJ: Slack, Inc., 1990; Ch. 4.

15. Scott, R.W. *Legal Aspects of Documenting Patient Care.* Gaithersburg, MD: Aspen Publishers, Inc., 1994.

16. Scott, R.W. "Sexual Misconduct." *PT Magazine*, 1993: 1(10):78–79.

17. Sugarman, J., Powers, M. "How the Doctor Got Gagged: The Disintegrating Right of Privacy in the Physician-Patient Relationship." *Journal of the American Medical Association*, 1991; 266:3323–3327.

Chapter 4

Informed Consent

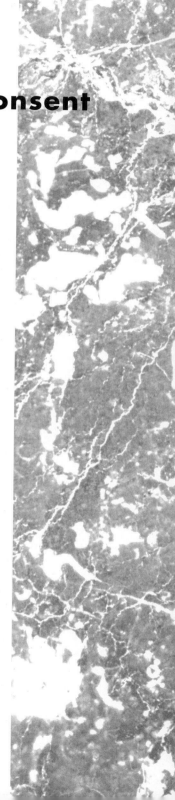

*T*his chapter outlines the requirements of the legal and ethical duty to obtain patient and human subject research informed consent. The right of patients and research subjects to receive sufficient disclosure information to enable them to make knowing, intelligent, voluntary, and unequivocal decisions about whether to accept or reject care or inclusion in studies is based on respect for patient or subject autonomy.

There are two principal exceptions to the requirement to obtain patient informed consent to treatment: the emergency treatment doctrine and therapeutic privilege (authority to withhold diagnostic or prognostic information that patients cannot psychologically handle). Surrogate decision makers receive disclosure information, and give informed consent, on behalf of minors and legally-adjudicated incompetent adult patients and subjects, in accordance with legal precedent. Documentation requirements for informed consent vary according to setting, law, custom, and purpose of the intervention.

Introduction

Informed consent to treatment is probably the most important mixed legal-ethical clinical issue impacting on a health care providers' practice. Every health care clinician has the ethical duty, and in most cases, the legal duty, to obtain patient (or *surrogate*) informed consent for health care interventions. This obligation is incumbent not only on physicians and surgeons, but also on all other licensed health care professionals, especially including physical and occupational therapists. The obligation to obtain patient informed consent applies irrespective of whether a nonphysician health care professional evaluates and treats a patient with, or without, physician referral.

> **Hint** *Every licensed health care professional has an ethical and legal duty to obtain patient informed consent to evaluation and treatment intervention.*

Ethical Duty to Obtain Patient Informed Consent

The ethical obligation to universally obtain patient or surrogate informed consent to health care evaluation and treatment is based on the foundational ethical principle of *autonomy.*[1] Making relevant disclosure of information about evaluation and treatment and involving the patient in health care decision making evidences respect for patient self-determination. All competent adult patients have the right to control the health care treatment decision making process under the foundational ethical principle of autonomy.[2] Those patients not considered legally competent to make such decisions—those patients who are legally adjudicated as incompetent, and minors, in some cases—have the right to have a surrogate decision maker or other legal representative receive the same disclosure information that would be imparted to a competent patient, and make decisions for them.

For many centuries, the foundational ethical principle of respect for patient autonomy was not the preeminent guiding ethical principle governing health care delivery. Rather, physicians and other primary health care professionals conformed their conduct to another foundational ethical principle, *beneficience*, under which health care professionals formulated and executed professional judgments that they believed to be in patients' best interests, but did not involve patients in decision making regarding interventions.[3]

The history of the development of the law and ethics of patient informed consent reveals that, until very recent times, health care professionals practiced their professions largely without involving their patients in treatment-related decision making. Many explanations—some seemingly reasonable—were proffered by medicine and other health professions to justify unilateral decision making regarding health care interventions. The ancient Greeks believed that to involve patients in medical decision making would impair patients' confidence in the ability of their health care providers to make professional judgments. By the Middle Ages, it was widely believed that the use of deception was necessary to ensure patient compliance with prescribed medical treatment that was deemed to be in patients' best interests.[4] Now, there is legitimate concern among health care professionals that patients will not understand, and will be confused by, the myriad of complex bits of information that must be imparted as part of informed consent disclosure. Finally, with streamlined managed heath care delivery, there is even a sense among some health care providers that routinely obtaining patient consent to treatment is just too time-consuming.

The customary professional health care practice of not including patients as partners in health care decision making began to change in the early to mid-1900s. Several phenomena accelerated the rise in importance of respect for patient autonomy in health care decision making. First, courts began to mandate that health care professionals respect patient autonomy and impart "legally sufficient" disclosure to permit patients to make knowing, intelligent, voluntary, and unequivocal elections of recommended treatment. The advent of this trend in judicial activism is exemplified by the 1914 New York case, *Schloendorf* v. *Society of New York Hospital,*[5] which expanded intentional tort liability in battery of health care providers who failed to respect the right of patients to knowingly consent to treatment. In 1965 in *Natanson v. Kline*,[6] the Kansas Supreme Court held:

> *The courts frequently state that the relationship between the physician and his patient is a fiduciary one, and therefore the physician has the obligation to make a full and frank disclosure to the patient of all pertinent facts related to his illness. We are here concerned with a case where the physician is charged with treating the patient without consent on the ground that the patient was not fully informed of the nature of the treatment or its consequences, and therefore, and "consent" obtained was ineffective. . . .*

In another leading informed consent case in 1972, *Canterbury v. Spence*,[7] Judge Spotswood Robinson III of the U.S. Court of Appeals for the District of Columbia further refined the nature of the ethical duty owed by health care professionals toward their patients. He stated:

> *The patient's reliance upon the physician is a trust of the kind which traditionally has exacted obligations beyond those associated with arms length transactions. [The patient's] dependence upon the physician for information affecting his well-being, in terms of contemplated treatment, is well-nigh abject. . . .*

Other twentieth-century developments that furthered the recognition of patient autonomy over decision making and the need for patient informed consent in health care service delivery include: the growth in post-secondary education after World War II and the concomitant rise of the consumerism movement in the United States, Canada, and later in Western Europe. As consumers became more aware of their power over merchants in the retail industry, the age-old adage, *caveat emptor* (Latin for "let the buyer beware") became whittled away as the public lobbied federal and state legislators forcefully for the enactment of consumer protection laws. As a result of consumer protection legislation, the doctrine of *caveat emptor* largely came to have little meaning in retail consumer business transactions. About the same time, it was realized that this doctrine was even less appropriately applied in the delivery of health services to patients.

Many health professional association codes of ethics expressly recognize an ethical duty on the part of professional members to make sufficient disclosure of pertinent information to patients under their care to permit patients to make informed elections about treatment. For example, the *Guide for Professional Conduct*, governing ethical behavior for physical therapist-members of the American Physical Therapy Association, states in pertinent part: "Physical therapists shall obtain patient informed consent before treatment."[8] Similarly, the *Occupational Therapy Code of Ethics*, governing the ethical conduct of occupational therapist-members of the American Occupational Therapy Association, states in pertinent parts: "Occupational therapy personnel shall fully inform [patients] of the nature, risks, and potential outcomes of any intervention;"[9] "Occupational therapy personnel shall respect the individual's right to refuse professional services or involvement in research or educational activities."[10]

Legal Aspects of Patient Informed Consent to Treatment

Failure to Obtain Patient Informed Consent Constitutes Health Care Malpractice

Failure on the part of health care professionals to make necessary disclosure of evaluative and treatment-related information, so as to enable patients to make informed decisions about treatment options, constitutes professional negligence. Until very recently, lack of informed consent tort cases in the health care setting were treated as intentional tort actions and processed as battery cases.[11] The rationale for labeling lack of informed consent health care malpractice cases as battery cases was that physicians and other health care professionals charged with such malpractice actions were considered by law to have had physical contact with their patients without any consent. By 1965, when the *Natanson* v. *Kline*[12] decision was announced, courts began to realize that there was a fundamental distinction between consent-related cases that involved intentional wrongs (lack of authorization) and those that involved unintentional wrongs (lack of understanding). The courts and began to correctly classify lack of informed consent health care malpractice cases as professional negligence actions, since patients treated without informed consent probably had at least have given nominal (albeit uninformed) consent to the treatment that led to injury.

Certain consent-related actions still are properly brought as intentional battery cases. For example, when a surgeon operates on a patient and amputates the wrong limb, or excises the wrong breast during a mastectomy, or when a nurse administers the wrong medication to a patient and causes patient injury, the proper designation for the ensuing legal actions is "battery." This is so because the defendant-health care professionals involved had absolutely no authorization from such patients to carry out incorrect harmful treatment.

The professional negligence designation for lack of informed consent health care malpractice cases takes into account the fact that patients injured in such cases probably gave nominal consent to treatment, but their health care providers failed to conform with acceptable practice standards by neglecting to respect patient autonomy by involving the patients in treatment-related decision making. Therefore, failure to obtain patient informed consent to treatment equates to substandard care.

Only one state's legal system, Pennsylvania, still considers lack of informed consent to be a battery.[13] As will be illustrated in the next section, Pennsylvania also apparently is the only state whose courts have ruled that health care providers in nonsurgical settings have no legal obligation under state law to even obtain patient informed consent for health care interventions.

Hint *Failure to obtain patient informed consent to treatment equates to substandard care.*

116

Legal Recognition of the Obligation to Obtain Patient Informed Consent

Except perhaps under Pennsylvania law, the right of patients to give informed consent to health care interventions is recognized as a fundamental legal right, by statute, by case law, and/or by customary professional health care practice, in every jurisdiction in the United States. This legal obligation is reflected in health professional written practice standards, such as those of the American Physical Therapy Association.[14]

The Pennsylvania courts have repeatedly held that informed consent in the health care setting is a concept reserved exclusively for surgical and operative procedures—not for routine health care delivery.[15,16] In *Spence* v. *Todaro*, the Federal District Court for the Eastern District of Pennsylvania, interpreting Pennsylvania state law, specifically held that the doctrine of informed consent to treatment does not apply to post-operative physical therapy care. This case concerned a post-operative orthopedic patient who was referred to physical therapy for rotator cuff rehabilitation. The patient claimed injury incident to physical therapy and sued his physical therapist for malpractice, citing a lack of informed consent as the basis for his lawsuit. The federal court held that, under Pennsylvania statutory law, the doctrine of patient informed consent to treatment applies only to surgical interventions—not to routine (nonsurgical) health care delivery. The court went on to reject the plaintiff-patient's contention that, because his physical therapy followed directly from his rotator cuff repair, it was legally part of the surgery, thereby making his lack of informed consent issue a valid one for judicial review.

In all other health care legal cases, however, the doctrine of patient informed consent to treatment has been found applicable, either expressly or by implication, to nonsurgical cases and to non-physician primary health care providers. Consider, for example, *Flores* v. *Center for Spinal Evaluation*,[17] a physical and occupational therapy malpractice case involving an allegation of professional negligence incident to post-injury rehabilitation. The court held in dismissing the case that, despite a "paucity" of law on physical and occupational therapy malpractice, these health care professionals should be treated exactly like their physician colleagues as malpractice defendants.

Recent U.S. Supreme Court case decisions interpreting the Constitution have reflected the Court's deference to and respect for patient self-determination regarding important health care decision making. For example, U.S. Supreme Court case decisions (and those of state supreme and appellate courts) based on the fundamental right of privacy have favored patients in their decisions to compel removal of life support apparatus and even the withdrawal of nutrition and hydration.[18,19,20]

In many states (including Florida, Georgia, Idaho, Iowa, Louisiana, Maine, Nevada, North Carolina, Ohio, Texas, Utah, and West Virginia), state legislatures have enacted statutes that mandate for surgical procedures and anesthesia administration the exact elements of informed consent disclosure required as a matter of law. In these states, compliance with the statutory disclosure mandates, coupled with the signature of a patient on a statutory form, creates a rebuttable presumption that the patient gave informed consent to care. The burden of persuasion to dispute or rebut that presumption in litigation then shifts to the patient.

Another (federal) statute, the Patient Self-Determination Act[21] (discussed in greater detail in Chapter 10) codifies the rights of hospitalized inpatients and nursing home residents to participate in treatment decision making and to control the use of extraordinary treatment measures, such as artificial life support. The Patient Self-Determination Act, although not creating any new substantive legal requirements, binds all health care facilities that receive Medicare or Medicaid funding to inform patients about their substantive rights under state law regarding treatment decision making, and respect patients' advance directives concerning treatment. Regarding informed consent, the law provides in pertinent part[22] that:

[A] provider [must] maintain written policies and procedures with respect to all adult individuals receiving medical care. . .to provide written information to each such individual concerning an individual's rights under state law (whether statutory or as recognized by the courts of the state) to make decisions concerning. . .medical care, including the right to accept or refuse medical or surgical treatment.

Another source of legal obligation to obtain patient informed consent is the American Hospital Association's Patient Bill of Rights,[23] a document customarily posted in reception areas in all health care clinics across the United States. The Patient Bill of Rights states:

We consider you a partner in your hospital care. When you are well-informed, participate in treatment decisions, and communicate openly with your doctor and other health professionals, you help make your care as effective as possible. This hospital encourages respect for the personal preferences and values of each individual.

While you are a patient in the hospital, your rights include the following:

- You have the right to considerate and respectful care.
- You have the right to be well-informed about your illness, possible treatments, and likely outcome and to discuss this information with your doctor. You have the right to know the names and roles of people treating you.
- You have the right to consent to or refuse a treatment, as permitted by law, throughout your hospital stay. If you refuse a recommended treatment you will receive other needed and available care.
- You have the right to have an advance directive, such as a living will or health care proxy. These documents express your choices about your future care or name someone to decide if you cannot speak for yourself. If you have a written advance directive, you should provide a copy to the hospital, your family, and your doctor.
- You have the right to privacy. The hospital, your doctor, and others caring for you will protect your privacy as much as possible.
- You have the right to expect that treatment records are confidential unless you have given permission to release information or reporting is required or permitted

by law. When the hospital releases records to others, such as insurers, it emphasizes that the records are confidential.

- You have the right to review your medical records and to have the information explained, except when restricted by law.

- You have the right to expect that the hospital will give you necessary health services to the best of its ability. Treatment, referral, or transfer may be recommended. If transfer is recommended or requested, you will be informed of risks, benefits, and alternatives. You will not be transferred until the other institution agrees to accept you.

- You have the right to know if this hospital has relationships with outside parties that may influence your treatment and care. These relationships may be with educational institutions, other health care providers, or insurers.

- You have the right to consent or decline to take part in research affecting your care. If you choose not to take part, you will receive the most effective care the hospital otherwise provides.

- You have the right to be told of realistic care alternatives when hospital care is no longer appropriate.

- You have the right to know about hospital rules that affect you and your treatment and about charges and payment methods. You have the right to know about hospital resources, such as patient representatives or ethics committees, that can help you resolve problems and questions about your hospital stay and care.

You have responsibilities as a patient. You are responsible for providing information about your health, including past illnesses, hospital stays, and use of medicine. You are responsible for asking questions when you do not understand information or instructions. If you believe you can't follow through with your treatment, you are responsible for telling your doctor.

This hospital works to provide care efficiently and fairly to all patients and the community. You and your visitors are responsible for being considerate of the needs of other patients, staff, and the hospital. You are responsible for providing information for insurance and for working with the hospital to arrange payment, when needed.

Your health depends not just on your hospital care but, in the long term, on the decisions you make in your daily life. You are responsible for recognizing the effect of life-style on your personal health.

A hospital serves many purposes. Hospitals work to improve people's health; treat people with injury and disease; educate doctors, health professionals, patients, and community members; and improve understanding of health and disease. In carrying out these activities, this institution works to respect your values and dignity.

The Joint Commission on the Accreditation of Healthcare Organizations (JCAHO), like other similar private accreditation entities, imposes similar requirements on its member health care organizations. Specifically, JCAHO standards require appropriate evidence in patient health records of informed consent to treatment, as well as institutional policy statements on patient informed consent.[24]

Finally, health care organizations and networks can create legally binding standards regarding patient informed consent in their organizational procedures manuals, protocols, and clinical practice guidelines, over and above those otherwise required by law. Administrators and clinical managers are urged to review these types of documents to ensure that what is written therein reflects what is the desired practice standard for the organization.

When Is Lack of Patient Informed Consent Legally Actionable?

Even though every single unexcused and unjustified omission of patient informed consent is an example of professional negligence, only a limited number of instances practically are legally actionable. Professional negligence malpractice litigation premised on a lack of informed consent is legally actionable only when:

- an undisclosed risk materializes, resulting in patient injury, and

- the plaintiff-patient can establish (i.e., prove) that he or she would not have consented to the treatment intervention in issue had full disclosure been made.

The court in *Canterbury*[25] clearly spelled out the requirement for a causal connection between the negligent omission on the part of a health care clinician to make legally sufficient disclosure to a patient and resultant patient injury:

No more than breach of any other legal duty does nonfulfillment of the physician's obligation to disclose alone establish liability to the patient. An unrevealed risk that should have been made known must materialize, for otherwise the omission, however unpardonable, is legally without consequence. Occurrence of the risk must be harmful to the patient, for unrelated to injury is nonactionable. *And, as in malpractice actions generally, there must be a causal relationship between the physician's failure to adequately divulge (information) and damage to the patient [emphasis added].*

A causal connection exists when, but only when, disclosure of significant risks incidental to treatment would have resulted in a decision against it . *The patient obviously has no complaint if he would have submitted to the therapy notwithstanding awareness that the risk was one of its perils. On the other hand, the very purpose of the disclosure rule is to protect the patient against the consequences which, if known, he would have avoided by foregoing the treatment [emphasis added].*

Litigation over informed consent to treatment should never occur, if health care professionals remember that disclosure of treatment-related information is a requisite part of the provider-patient communication process. The disclosure elements (discussed below) are relatively straightforward, and the process, if made a routine part of provider-patient communications, is neither unduly burdensome nor time-consuming. Health care professionals are strongly advised to universally make the informed disclosure process an integral part of their patient evaluation processes.

Obviously, open and thorough communication between health care providers and patients is key to minimizing health care malpractice liability exposure. The word *consent* itself literally means that the provider and patient jointly should agree on a recommended treatment intervention before it is implemented.[26] Decades of medical research have shown that patients achieve optimal treatment outcomes when they are informed partners in their own care.[27]

One confounding factor to the health care provider-patient communication process is the fact that some patients, especially elderly patients, may wish not to participate in the treatment decision making process with their providers. Rather, some patients—even though they are fully competent to do so—prefer to leave treatment decision making to family members or trusted others. Regarding revelation of terminal illnesses, this impediment to provider-patient communications may be race- or ethnicity-related. One study revealed that while African-Americans and white elderly Americans generally believe that it is appropriate for providers to discuss terminal illnesses with their patients, Korean-Americans and Mexican-Americans more often do not.[28] In complicated fact scenarios like those presented in this study, providers are strongly encouraged to consult with facility and/or personal legal advisors for advice on how to proceed and to document their actions.

Disclosure Elements for Legally Sufficient Disclosure of Information to Patients

Although legal requirements differ from state to state for what constitutes legally sufficient information disclosure in the provider-patient informed consent communication process, the following elements are commonly included in most or all states. For specific advice on what must information must be imparted to patients under a specific state's laws, consult with legal counsel.

For patient consent to treatment to be legally "informed," the following items of disclosure information should be addressed:

Diagnosis and pertinent evaluative findings. A health care clinician should always discuss with a patient the patient's diagnosis and pertinent evaluative findings (unless the patient effectively waives disclosure or another exception applies). Although it may be particularly difficult for a health care professional to avoid the use of health professional jargon in communications because of his or her training and continuing education, the professional must remember to speak to a patient in lay person's language, at the level of understanding appropriate for each patient.

Nature of the treatment intervention recommended. After patient evaluation is completed, and a diagnosis is made, a clinician formulates a proposed treatment plan designed to optimize function or achieve some other therapeutic result. That recommended treatment intervention must be disclosed to the patient before its implementation, and the patient must agree to treatment. If specific treatment has been prescribed by a physician or other provider privileged to legally make referrals, then the prescribed treatment must likewise be described to the patient. In either case, the patient must consent to treatment.

Material (decisional) risks of serious harm or complications. Any credible risk of possible serious harm or complication associated with a proposed treatment intervention must be disclosed to a patient before treatment commences. The term *material* refers to a risk of harm that would cause an ordinary reasonable patient to think seriously about whether he or she will accept or reject the proposed treatment intervention. (In some cases, the term *material* has been construed by courts to mean the risk of harm that a particular patient would *subjectively* consider to be serious, even if that particular patient was not an "ordinary reasonable person.")

It is often said that there are few material risks of serious harm or complication associated with physical and occupational therapy treatment interventions. This is probably true, however, there are some material risks associated with physical and occupational therapy treatment that should be disclosed to patients. One non-obvious material risk associated with physical therapy involves axillary crutch gait instruction. Unless a physical therapist warns a patient about the material risk of possible axillary nerve and vessel injury associated with leaning on the soft axillary pads on the top portions of the crutches, a patient might reasonably believe that the soft pads are designed to be leaned upon. By disclosing this potential risk, a physical therapist may prevent patient injury and malpractice litigation. The law generally recognizes that the only material risks that need to be disclosed to patients are those that are non-obvious to ordinary reasonable people. Obvious risks, such as the risk of being cut by a sharp needle or of being burned by an extremely hot thermal treatment modality, generally are commonly understood by adult lay patients and are not required to be discussed. However, patients may not fully comprehend the gravity of the risk of harm associated with seemingly obvious risk scenarios. Consider the following hypothetical example:

A 68-year-old male patient, with a medical diagnosis of diabetes mellitus and a left lateral malleolar diabetic ulcer on his ankle, is referred to physical therapy for "evaluation and hydrotherapy, as appropriate." After evaluation and initial treatment, the physical therapist advises the patient to soak his left

foot in very warm water at home for 20 minutes, b.i.d. The patient asks, "How warm should the water be?" to which the therapist replies, "As warm as you can tolerate the temperature on the unaffected part of your left foot." Unfortunately, the physical therapist had neglected to evaluate the patient's whole foot, which was severely desensitized as a result of peripheral neuropathy. The next day, the patient returns to the clinic with third-degree thermal burns to his left foot. The patient had boiled water, poured it into a basin, and placed his left foot into the scalding water, resulting in serious injury. The patient's left foot was amputated several weeks later.

Out of concern for patient welfare and as a matter of prudent risk management, always discuss even seemingly obvious risks of serious harm or complications of treatment with patients to prevent needless patient injury and liability exposure.

Expected benefits of treatment. It is incumbent upon health care clinicians to establish functionally-relevant, objectively measurable short- and long-term treatment goals for patients under their care. As an integral part of the informed consent process, health care clinicians must also reveal and discuss the goals established for patients with them. If patients understand the treatment goals made on their behalf and take an "ownership" interest in the treatment goals, then they will be more motivated to achieve better functional outcomes.

Reasonable alternatives to the proposed treatment. If there are any reasonable alternatives to a proposed treatment intervention, then these must be disclosed to and discussed with the patient. In addition to describing reasonable alternatives to proposed treatments, clinicians must also discuss their attendant material risks (if any) and expected benefits. This disclosure element may pose a problem under a managed care model of health care, in that alternative treatments or interventions, even if more efficacious than the proposed treatment, may not be available under the patient's managed care plan. This fact does not, however, obviate the need for discussion of alternative treatments or interventions.

After disclosing all of the above informed consent parameters to a patient: diagnosis/evaluative findings, nature of recommended treatment, material risks, expected benefits, and reasonable alternatives, a health care clinician is obliged to take one further step. The provider must ensure that the patient understands all of the information conveyed, by asking for and satisfactorily answering patient questions related to treatment. If the patient's primary language is one other than English, then the provider must provide for translation, as needed, and ensure that all information conveyed was understood by the patient (see Box 4-1).

4-1 Informed Consent to Treatment: Disclosure of Relevant Treatment-Related Information

- patient diagnosis, or evaluative findings
- nature of the treatment or intervention recommended or ordered
- material (decisional) risks of serious harm or complication associated with the proposed treatment
- expected benefits, or goals, of treatment
- reasonable alternatives, if any, to the proposed treatment

Occasionally, a patient will refuse recommended or ordered treatment, even after informed disclosure has been made. Certain additional steps must be taken by a health care provider when a patient refuses care. The clinician must first ensure that the patient understands the disclosure information conveyed and solicit any further questions or comments about the proposed treatment that the patient may have to offer. If this reiteration and summarization of the informed consent process does not resolve the problem, then the clinician should explain, in a caring and objective manner, the expected consequences to the patient's health status of refusal of treatment. Discussion with the patient should be interactive and participative, rather than directive, and the clinician should display both sincere empathy for the patient and respect for patient autonomy over decision making.

If the patient persists in his or her refusal to allow recommended treatment, then this fact and a summarization of the "informed refusal" processes employed on the patient's behalf should be well-documented in the patient's health record. In addition, the clinician is legally responsible to coordinate expeditiously with any referring entity and other key health care professionals having a need to know of the patient's refusal of care.

Legal Standards for Adequacy of Informed Consent

There are two possible legal standards used to determine whether a health care professional made sufficient disclosure of treatment-related information in order to permit a patient to make an informed decision about care. The states are nearly equally divided in their use of each available standard, however, a slight majority of jurisdictions use a *professional standard* for disclosure.[29] In states employing this standard, a health care professional is required to disclose to a patient that information that another professional from the same discipline, who is acting under the same or similar circumstances, would disclose. Health care malpractice litigation involving informed consent issues in states using the professional standard requires the introduction of expert testimony concerning: (1) the propriety of information actually disclosed by a defendant-provider, and (2) what information would be appropriate for disclosure generally.

A slight minority of states employ a *lay person's standard* for disclosure. In these jurisdictions, a health care professional is required to disclose all relevant information that an ordinary, reasonable patient, under the same or similar circumstances as the patient in issue, would consider material to make an informed decision about treatment. Obviously, the lay standard imposes greater responsibility on health care providers, who must carefully contemplate what information an ordinary, reasonable lay patient would deem to be "material" for each and every possible treatment or intervention.

The court in *Canterbury* enunciated, in a very reasoned manner, the rationale for and the parameters of the (ordinary reasonable) *lay person's standard* for the first time, as follows:

> *We do not agree that the patient's cause of action is dependent upon the existence and nonperformance of a relevant professional tradition. There are, in our view, formidable obstacles to acceptance of the notion that [a health care professional's] obligation to disclose is either germinated or limited by medical practice. To begin with, the reality of any discernible custom reflecting a professional consensus on communication of option and risk information to patients is open to serious doubt. We sense the danger that what in fact is no custom at all may be taken as an affirmative custom to maintain silence, and that [health professional-witnesses] to the so-called custom may state merely their personal opinions as to what they or others would do under given conditions.*
>
> . . .
>
> *The decision to unveil the patient's condition and the chances for as to remediation. . . .is ofttimes a non-medical judgment and, if so, is a decision outside the ambit of the special standard. . . . Prevailing medical practice. . . does not. . . define the standard.*
>
> . . .
>
> *In our view, the patient's right of self-decision shapes the boundaries of the duty to reveal. That right can be effectively exercised only if the patient possesses enough information to enable an intelligent choice. The scope of the [provider's] communication to the patient, then, must be measured by the patient's need, and that need is the information material to the decision. Thus the test for determining whether a particular peril must be divulged is its materiality to the [ordinary reasonable] patient decision: all risks potentially affecting the decision must be unmasked.*

One advantage of the lay person standard for assessing disclosure to parties to an informed consent lawsuit is that normally, expert testimony on health professional discipline-specific disclosure standards is unnecessary, since it will be the responsibility of lay jurors to decide what an ordinary reasonable patient would need to know in order to make an informed decision about treatment. This fact results in a monetary savings at trial, which inures to the benefit of both parties to the lawsuit. Additionally, when expert witnesses are not utilized in a case, substantial time is usually also saved in litigating the material issues in the case.

Exceptions to the Requirement to Obtain Patient Informed Consent

There are several well-established exceptions to the requirement to otherwise universally obtain patient informed consent before carrying out health care treatment interventions. The two most important ones are: the *emergency doctrine* and *therapeutic privilege*.[30]

Under the emergency doctrine, whenever a patient presents for evaluation and treatment in a life-threatening emergency situation and is unable to communicate his or her wishes regarding treatment (such as when the patient is unconscious), it is generally presumed that the patient would consent to reasonable, life-saving medical intervention. Consider the following hypothetical case scenario.

A senior physical therapist student on a clinical affiliation is treating a 65-year-old male rehabilitation patient, who is status-post left CVA, with proprioceptive neuromuscular facilitation exercises on a mat in the physical therapy clinic. Suddenly, the patient suffers a myocardial infarction and grasps his chest. The patient is initially unable to speak because of pain and shortness of breath and then becomes unconscious. What action should the student therapist take? (At the time of the incident, there is no one else—including the supervisory clinical instructor—in the clinic area.)

Answer: This scenario presents an example of a situation in which the emergency doctrine exception to the law of patient informed consent is applicable. In such a situation, it is generally presumed, as a matter of law, that an ordinary reasonable person would wish to avail him- or herself of life-saving treatment intervention. Absent clear evidence of contrary patient desires, the student should immediately call for help and commence cardiopulmonary resuscitation.

There are, of course, exceptions to the exception of a presumption favoring rendition of care in life-threatening emergencies. For example, if a patient's desire not to receive life-saving care in the event of an emergency have been memorialized in a valid patient advance directive (discussed in detail in Chapter 10), then health care professionals and supportive personnel are obligated to respect the patient's autonomy and not initiate life-saving treatment. A similar exception applies when a valid "do not resuscitate" order appears in a patient's medical record.

"Do not resuscitate" (DNR) orders preclude the otherwise automatic initiation of cardiopulmonary resuscitation efforts for a patient in cardiorespiratory arrest. A DNR order does not affect the provision of any other substantive care, such as life support, nutrition, and hydration. A DNR order may be appropriate either to respect the prior choice of a patient regarding treatment, or when, in the professional judgment of a patient's attending physician (normally with the concurrence of at least one other physician), resuscitative efforts for a patient would be medically futile. DNR orders are written for patients who are terminally ill or living in a persistent vegetative state.[31] Because of complex legal and ethical issues surrounding DNR orders and other decisions involving life support, nutrition, and hydration of patients, health care professionals confronting these situations are urged to expeditiously consult with facility legal counsel and institutional ethics committees for advice.

Therapeutic privilege is the other major exception to informed consent law.[32] Under therapeutic privilege, a physician may be justified in withholding from a patient information about the patient's diagnosis or prognosis when, in the physician's professional judgment, the patient cannot deal psychologically with the information. The exercise of a therapeutic privilege by a physician to withhold information from a patient does not excuse the physician (or other health care professionals treating the patient) from disclosing all other required information to the patient.

Therapeutic privilege is relatively rarely invoked, and even less often, accepted by the courts as legitimate. This is so because the exercise of the privilege derogates from the foundational ethical principle of respect for patient autonomy and self-governance.

What course of action can a health care professional treating a patient take when he or she disagrees with a physician's invocation of therapeutic privilege? Consider the following hypothetical case example.

An occupational therapist treating a 32-year-old female patient diagnosed with terminal, end-stage metastatic breast cancer, meets with the other rehabilitation team members for a weekly team conference. At the meeting, the patient's attending physician advises the team members that he is discharging the patient to home in order to allow her to die in peace with her family. The attending physician tells the team treating the patient that he is invoking therapeutic privilege concerning the patient's prognosis. (The patient already knows her diagnosis.) The occupational therapist knows, from her recent conversations with the patient, that the patient wishes to know about her prognosis and apprises the rest of the team of this fact. The physician becomes angry and states that *he* is the patient's physician and the leader of the rehabilitation team. The physician ends the discussion by imposing a "gag order" on the entire treatment team, ordering all to remain silent if asked by the patient about her prognosis.

Is this the end of the matter? No. In this case, the occupational therapist is unable to abide by the physician's decision as a matter of principle. What can she do? There are several acceptable options open to the occupational therapist. First, the occupational therapist should consider requesting a private meeting with the physician in order to express her concerns about the gag order. Assume that she does this and poignantly states her position. Assume further that her resistance to his edict enrages the physician, who summarily ejects the occupational therapist from his office, stating, "Just do what I ordered!"

At this point, there are three options open to the occupational therapist. She may resign herself to acceptance of the physician's order. However, in this case, the patient, who has become accustomed to confiding in the occupational therapist, might pressure her for information about her prognosis.

The occupational therapist's second option is to excuse herself from the patient's treatment team if she cannot abide by the physician's order, and allow another occupational therapist, who can accept the gag order, to continue to care for the patient. However, in this case, the occupational therapist believes that this option is an unacceptable "cop-out."

The last option available to the occupational therapist is perhaps the best one. After exercising all reasonable efforts to discuss the situation civilly with the physician, she may formally request an ethics consultation from the *institutional ethics committee* in the facility. The institutional ethics committee is a multidisciplinary committee of health care and other professionals that offers consultative services and convenes to hear and make recommendations about cases involving ethical dilemmas (among other roles—see Chapter 11). There should always be a mechanism for licensed and certified health care professionals and others to avail themselves of the advice and intervention of the institutional ethics committee. There should never be any stigma associated with requesting consultation from the institutional ethics committee. Similarly, the fact that the occupational therapist acted reasonably in requesting an ethics consultation should not cause her to suffer retribution from the physician whose judgment is challenged. It may be necessary for facility administrators to educate physicians and other health professionals about the role(s) of the institutional ethics committee on a regular basis, so that misunderstandings and anger over its intervention do not occur.

Two other scenarios—involving the treatment of incompetent and minor patients—may seem to present as possible exceptions to the requirement to obtain patient informed consent to treatment, however, such is not the case. When a patient is legally incompetent to consent to treatment—either because the patient cannot understand information conveyed and is a legally adjudicated incompetent, or because the patient is a minor and cannot consent as a matter of law—a health care professional must obtain informed consent from a *surrogate* (or substitute) *decision maker*.

The disclosure of information made to a surrogate decision maker is exactly the same as would be made to a competent patient. The surrogate decision maker, appointed either by the patient or by law, acts on the patient's behalf and has the same right to have questions answered to the surrogate's satisfaction before treatment commences.

One exception to the general rule that parents or guardians normally consent on behalf of their minor children is that minors—especially when they are nearing the age of majority (age 18)—may have the right under applicable state law to exercise autonomy to personally consent (usually without revelation to their parents) to treatment in cases involving elective abortion, treatment of drug (including alcohol) abuse, and the treatment of sexually-transmitted diseases. These exceptions to the general rule of substituted consent for minors vary from state to state, and providers must consult proactively with legal counsel to remain current on the state of the law, so as to protect the rights of all parties.

Another difficult dilemma involving incompetent patients centers around informed consent involving patients who, practically, but not legally, are incompetent to make knowing, intelligent, voluntary, and unequivocal decisions about treatment. While the determination of patient competence to make decisions about health care interventions is a question for physicians and jurists, other health care professionals involved in the care of particular patients can offer important input into competency decisions based on their observations and interactions with patients.

There is relatively little guidance in the literature for physicians and other health care professionals on mental competence assessment,[33] however, an excellent article on the topic that presents a framework for patient treatment decision making competency assessment (including dimensions of competence and a series of questions to assess competence), is Searight, H.R. "Assessing Patient Competence for Medical Decision Making." *American Family Physician*. 1992; 45:751–759. In cases of questionable patient competence to make treatment-related decisions, health care professionals are urged to raise the issue expeditiously with physicians, facility administrators, and legal counsel, so that a competency determination can be undertaken, if appropriate. Where a question about patient competence exists, a competency assessment is required in order to comply with legal requirements concerning consent to care and to meet foundational ethical standards, including respect for patient autonomy and dignity, beneficence, and nonmaleficence.

Documentation of Patient Informed Consent

Like all other issues in the law concerning patient informed consent, the legally correct form for documenting a patient's informed consent to treatment varies from state to state. Some jurisdictions have specific statutory disclosure requirements that must be followed for specific interventions (normally only for surgical procedures). In these states, the required use of statutory "consent forms" may give rise to presumptive, or even conclusive, evidence of patient informed consent for the named procedures. Most states permit the use of a wide range of variegated methods for documenting patient informed consent—especially for nonsurgical, routine health care interventions, including occupational and physical therapy. (The specific disclosure, informed consent, and documentation requirements for your practice can and should be evaluated for legal sufficiency by your institutional and/or personal legal advisor.)

In general, there are at least four acceptable ways to document patient informed consent to routine health care interventions. These include the use of (1) direct documentation in the form of consent forms, both short and long versions, (2) direct documentation in patient health records, (3) indirect documentation in memoranda for record that are maintained in office files, like other ordinary business records, and (4) indirect documentation in clinic procedures manuals and/or in quality improvement manuals, with or without brief documentation in individual patient treatment records. Each method is discussed below. (For more detailed information on documentation formats, including examples of the various formats, see Scott, R.W. *Legal Aspects of Documenting Patient Care.* Gaithersburg, MD: Aspen Publishers, Inc., 1994, Chapter 4.)

The Use of "Boilerplate" Informed Consent Forms

There are two general types of "boilerplate," or standardized, consent forms: a short version and a long version. The formats differ only in the amount of detail regarding disclosure information that they contain. Both formats include patient signatures. An example of a short version informed consent form is shown in Figure 4-1.

A long version consent form may either be a generic, boilerplate form (as most surgical consent forms are) or may be customized to include specific information about individual patients and/or more detailed information about each required disclosure element.

There are several potential problems associated with the use of customized long version consent forms. There is an inference, or even a presumption, in law that what appears on such a form represents exactly the specific information that was conveyed by a health care professional to a patient. If an element of disclosure was in fact related to a patient during the informed consent process, but inadvertently omitted from the form, it would be very difficult to prove that the contested disclosure item was in fact conveyed to the patient. In fact, it would probably be more difficult to try to convince a judge or jury that an omitted disclosure item from a long consent form was conveyed to a patient than it would be to convince the fact-finder that an item was disclosed if there were no documentation of informed consent at all. Another consideration weighing against using a customized long version consent form is the fact that it is relatively time-consuming to generate.

Documentation of Informed Consent in Patient Treatment Records

Documentation of informed consent in a patient's treatment record may also appear in short and long versions. The key distinction between treatment record informed consent documentation and the use of consent forms is that the patient's signature typically does not appear in the treatment record entries.

Figure 4.1

My diagnosis (or evaluative findings), the therapist's recommendations regarding treatment, the expected benefits or goals of treatment, and reasonable alternatives to recommended treatments, have all been explained to me and my questions about care answered to my satisfaction. I consent to the recommended course of treatment.

_____

Patient signature

_____

Therapist signature

_____

Witness signature

_____

Date

Documentation of Patient Informed Consent in Office Memoranda

Documentation of patient informed consent in an office memorandum normally occurs as an exception to policy, rather than as a matter of routine practice. The generation of an office memo is time-consuming, and its storage as a business document is cumbersome. However, in cases where clinicians do not routinely otherwise document patient informed consent for each and every patient, clinicians may want to selectively memorialize the exact disclosure and informed consent processes for selected patients, such as litigation or potential litigation patients. The consent memo may contain little or much detail, and is commonly signed by the health care provider (and perhaps a witness), but not by the patient. Such a memo is principally a self-protective risk management document.

Documentation of Patient Informed Consent in Policies Manuals

Perhaps the simplest and most convenient way to document a health care clinic's policies and procedures regarding patient informed consent to treatment is to spell out in detail the requirements of health care clinicians in policy or quality management manuals. These requirements, then, are conveyed to new clinicians upon employment, and it is made known to them then (and at subsequent clinical continuing education experiences) that they are required to follow these policies as a matter of routine practice.

There is nothing that normally precludes a health care professional from testifying in a legal proceeding about the professional's (or clinic's or institution's) customary practice regarding the processes involved in obtaining patient informed consent, even when there is no evidence of individualized documentation of patient informed consent in patient treatment records. It is probably sound documentation risk management to retain copies of outdated clinical procedures manuals and other important policy manuals indefinitely to use as evidence of the existence of some policy on issues such as documentation of patient informed consent.

The Air Force uses a system of documentation of patient informed consent to routine health care interventions that does not require individualized patient treatment record documentation. This system is described as follows:

> **Routine Informed Consent Briefings.** Once the appropriate scope and form of informed consent has been established, practitioners should develop a consistent patient disclosure and discussion for the treatment concerned. This is a professionally appropriate [method] to ensure adequate patient understanding of the treatment. In addition, litigation experience reflects that customary disclosure plus a handwritten note (even though general in nature) by the practitioner in the patient's health record are the most important evidence in the defense of an informed consent case. This is primarily because the handwritten note is credible evidence (more so than a printed form) that the communication occurred, and because the Federal Rules of Evidence allow the practitioner to testify to what he or she *customarily* discloses to

patients for a given procedure. That is, the practitioner need not have recall of the specific conversation if the [provider] makes consistent customary disclosures to patients concerning that procedure.[34]

Professional Association Informed Consent Documentation Standards

The American Physical Therapy Association promulgated (based largely on input from this author) informed consent documentation standards for member-physical therapists in 1993 (revised in 1995). The standards areas are as follows:

Guidelines for Physical Therapy Documentation

I. General Guidelines

    A. All documentation must comply with the applicable jurisdictional/regulatory requirements.

        1. All handwritten entries should be made in ink.

        2. Informed consent shall be obtained as required by the APTA Standards of Practice.

            2.1. The Physical therapist has the sole responsibility for providing information to the patient and for obtaining the patient's informed consent in accordance with jurisdictional law before initiating physical therapy.

            2.2. Those [patients] deemed competent to give [informed] consent are competent adults. When the adult is not competent, and in the case of minors, a parent or legal guardian consents as the surrogate decision maker.

            2.3. The information provided to the patient should include the following: (a) a clear description of the treatment ordered or recommended, (b) material (decisional) risks associated with the proposed treatment, (c) expected benefits of treatment, (d) comparison of the benefits possible with and without treatment, and (e) reasonable alternatives to the recommended treatment. The physical therapist should solicit questions from the patient and provide answers. The patient should be asked to acknowledge understanding and consent before treatment proceeds.

      Examples of ways in which to accomplish this documentation:

            2.3.1. Signature of patient/guardian on long or short consent form.

            2.3.2. Notation/entry of what was explained by the physical therapist or the physical therapist assistant[35] in the official record, and

            2.3.3. Filing of a completed consent checklist signed by the patient.[36]

133

Informed Consent Issues in Research Settings

The informed consent of human research subjects is a fundamental requirement of, and prerequisite to, carrying out clinical research involving people. The process of obtaining research subject informed consent is more complex than for obtaining patient informed consent to routine health care interventions. Research-related consent is subject to greater institutional, administrative, and legal oversight than treatment-related informed consent, because research-related subject consent normally must be documented in long form, according to strict, rather than flexible, standards.

The intense regulation of human subject research resulted in large part from testimony from the Nuremburg trials that followed World War II. In those trials, approximately 20 prominent German physicians were tried for human rights violations involving cruel and inhumane medical experimentation on prisoners of war. Most were convicted, and several were hanged.

Subsequent to the Nuremberg trials, the Nuremberg Code of 1947 was drafted and adopted. This code, in part, established as codified international law that, "the voluntary consent of the human subject is absolutely essential" [to legally and ethically permissible medical research].[37] The Nuremberg Code was augmented in 1975 by the Helsinki Declarations of 1964 (I) and 1975 (II), which established the international law requirement of independent review of research proposals involving human subjects, as follows: "The design and performance of each experimental procedure involving human subjects should be clearly formulated in an experimental protocol which should be transmitted to a specially appointed independent committee for consideration, comment, and guidance."[38]

Based in large part of these international treaties and on human rights abuses in the American Tuskegee Syphilis Study, the Department of Health and Human Services (then the Department of Health, Education and Welfare) adopted human subject research guidelines in 1975 that delineated the permissible scope of, and procedures for, human subject research activities that use federal funding. These guidelines also established the requirement for independent review of human subject research protocols by institutional review boards (IRBs). The federal guidelines were amended in 1981 to delete the requirement for IRB approval of a limited class of very-low-risk human subject research protocols.[39]

There are special federal guidelines regarding required elements that must be included in human subject research informed consent forms. These guidelines include the following parameters:

- The consent form must impart sufficient information about a proposed study, its procedures, expected benefits, material risks, and reasonable alternatives to enable a potential subject to make a knowing, intelligent, and voluntary decision about whether or not to agree to participate.

- The investigator (or approved designee) must personally explain the parameters stated above to the potential subject.

- The consent form must be written in the first person and must be in lay-person's language, without significant technical medical "jargon." If the potential subject's language of comprehension is other than English, a translation of the consent form is required.

- In general, consent forms from other institutions may not be used to obtain human subject research consent.

- The consequences of subject injury must be clearly spelled out, including therapeutic measures to be taken in the event of subject injury, and who bears the cost of such care.

- Any compensation or benefit that the subject will received for participation in a research study must be clearly stated in the informed consent form.

- A copy of the signed form must be given to the subject. If the subject is also a patient, then a copy of the research consent form must be filed in the patient's medical treatment record. The original copy of the consent form must be retained for at least five years after completion of the study.

- The consent form must be witnessed. The witness or witnesses attest only to a subject's signature, not to the subject's comprehension of disclosure elements or comprehension of them.

- The informed consent form must state contact phone numbers for the principal investigator, where the subject can personally reach the investigator 24 hours a day.

Additional safeguards for research subject protection include:

- No person may be excluded from consideration as a research subject because of race, ethnicity, or language. The equitable inclusion of women and minorities in research is strongly encouraged.

- The subject's confidentiality and autonomy enjoy absolute respect and protection. The subject has the right to review all data collected from and about him or her and to withhold permission for their use by the researcher.

- The subject may withdraw consent at any time, without prejudice.

- The subject may not be prejudiced in receiving necessary and equitable care based on a decision not to participate in a research study.

Chapter Summary

Informed patient consent to health care evaluation and treatment intervention is a legal and ethical prerequisite to care. Health care clinicians responsible for patient evaluation and treatment—including physical and occupational therapists—bear primary responsibility for obtaining patient informed consent. Informed consent to physical or occupational therapy intervention is not the responsibility of referring physicians at one end of the continuum, nor of assistants carrying out therapists' directives at the other end of the continuum.

While the elements of legally sufficient patient informed consent vary from state to state (according to state or federal law, as applicable), the following disclosure elements must normally be imparted to patients (or their surrogate decision makers) before health care commences:

- diagnosis and pertinent evaluative findings

- nature of the intervention(s) recommended or ordered

- risk of potential harm or complications material to the patient's decision whether to accept or reject treatment

- expected benefits (i.e., goals) of treatment

- reasonable alternatives to the proposed treatment or intervention

In addition to the above disclosure elements, a health care professional must also solicit and satisfactorily answer any patient questions before the informed consent process is consummated. There are a variety of legally acceptable ways to document patient informed consent to treatment.

There are two principal exceptions to the requirement to obtain patient informed consent: the emergency doctrine and therapeutic privilege. In life-threatening emergency situations, it is generally presumed that patients grant implied consent to medical interventions designed to save their lives. (There may be exceptions to the exception, such as where a specific patient's prior contrary wishes are known.) Therapeutic privilege allows a physician to withhold diagnostic and/or prognostic information from a patient who is deemed to be psychologically incapable of dealing with the information. It is rarely allowed, because the exception derogates from respect for patient autonomy and control over treatment-related decision making.

Human subject research informed consent is normally more formal and complex than patient informed consent, in part because of the substantial federal, state, and institutional oversight over human subject research activities, and in part because of the (very recent) history of horrific abuse of human subjects in medical research. The details of the processes of human research subject informed consent are governed at the operative level by independent institutional review boards (IRBs).

Cases and Questions

1. You are an occupational therapist who has been assigned to evaluate and care for a 14-year-old male patient with a diagnosis of Dupuytren's contracture of the right hand. The patient is accompanied to the evaluation by his parents. The patient and his parents consent to evaluation. At the end of the evaluation, you design a plan of care, based on your evaluative findings, that includes stretching techniques and appropriate exercises. At this point, the patient—who also has psychological problems, but is mentally alert—states that he does not consent to treatment. The parents, however, are insistent that the proposed treatment plan proceed. How do you resolve this dilemma?

2. You are a staff physical therapist at ABC Community Hospital. Your clinic manager has asked you to develop a clinical indicator of quality measurement that will assess whether patients seen in the clinic for evaluation and treatment truly give informed consent to the care that they receive. A protocol already exists (and is universally complied with) that spells out in detail the disclosure elements of informed consent by staff physical therapists. What measures might you employ to adjudge whether patient informed consent is valid?

Suggested Answers to Cases and Questions

1. While normally, the parents or legal guardians of a minor patient consent to treatment involving routine care for their children, there may be a legal and ethical problem with carrying out the treatment on an adolescent patient who objects to care. The objection to proceeding without the concurrence of the older minor patient is based on respect for the minor's fledgling autonomy. The occupational therapist facing this dilemma may wish to review anew the informed consent disclosure elements with the patient and his parents to ensure that the patient understands them. The therapist might also ask permission to discuss with the patient his reluctance to accept care, outside of the presence of the parents. The therapist might wish to involve a supervisor or another professional colleague in the process, and should consult with the facility's legal counsel for advise before proceeding with care delivery.

2. There are many ways to test patient's knowledge of the disclosure information imparted by health care clinical professionals as part of the informed consent process. Some of these methods have been reported recently in the professional literature. Perhaps the most important point to remember from the outset is that patient informed consent is an active, participative process, not the mechanical completion of a paper form.[40] Methods to evaluate whether patients truly understand what is imparted during informed consent briefings by their providers include: (1) short, simple-question, multiple-choice tests on facts that patients should reasonably be expected to know by the end of an informed consent briefing session,[41,42] (2) patient interviews by professionals acting as monitors

after disclosure and informed consent briefing processes are completed, and (3) retrospective records reviews of disclosure and informed consent content in cases where detailed documentation of informed consent processes is customarily done.

References

1. Beauchamp, T.L., Childress, J.F. *Principles of Biomedical Ethics*. 4th ed. New York: Oxford Press, 1994, p. 120.

2. In an early leading case on informed consent, *Schloendorf* v. *Society of New York Hospital*, 105 N.E. 2d 92 (N.Y. 1914), Justice Benjamin Cardozo wrote, "Every human being of adult years and sound mind has a right to determine what shall be done with his [or her] own body, and a surgeon who performs an operation without [a] patient's consent commits an assault for which he [or she] is liable in money damages."

3. According to Jay Katz, author of *The Silent World of Doctor and Patient* (New York: Free Press, 1984), "disclosure and consent, except in the most rudimentary fashion, are obligations alien to medical thinking and practice."

4. Furrow, B.R., Johnson, S.H., Jost, T.S., Schwartz, R.L. *Health Law: Cases, Materials and Problems*, 2nd ed. St. Paul, MN: West Publishing Company, 1991, p. 322.

5. See note 2, above.

6. *Natanson* v. *Kline*, 350 P.2d 1093 (Kansas 1960).

7. *Canterbury* v. *Spence*, 464 F.2d 772 (D.C. Cir. 1972), *cert.* [U.S. Supreme Court appeal] *denied*, 409 U.S. 1064 (1974).

8. *Guide for Professional Conduct*, Section 1.4 (Informed Consent). Alexandria, VA: American Physical Therapy Association, 1996.

9. *Occupational Therapy Code of Ethics*, Principle 2B. Bethesda, MD: American Occupational Therapy Association, 1994.

10. *Occupational Therapy Code of Ethics*, Principle 2D. Bethesda, MD: American Occupational Therapy Association, 1994.

11. See *Schloendorf* v. *Society of New York Hospital*, note 2.

12. "The fundamental distinction between assault and battery on one hand, and [professional] negligence such as would constitute malpractice, on the other, is that the former is intentional and the latter unintentional. . . ." *Natanson* v. *Kline*, note 2.

13. Furrow, B.R., Johnson, S.H., Jost, T.S., Schwartz, R.L. *Health Law: Cases, Materials and Problems*, 2nd ed. St. Paul, MN: West Publishing Company, 1991, p. 327, note 7; *Foflygen* v. *Zemel*, 615 A.2d 1345 (Pa. 1992).

14. Standards of Practice for Physical Therapy, Provision of Care, X, *Informed Consent*, reads: "The physical therapist obtains the patient's informed consent in accordance with jurisdictional law before initiating physical therapy." HOD Policy 06-91-21-25. Alexandria, VA: American Physical Therapy Association, 1991.

15. *Spence* v. *Todaro*, No. 94-3757 (E.D. Pa. October 14, 1994).

16. *Friter and Friter* v. *Iolab Corp.*, 607 A.2d 1111 (Pa. Sup. Ct. 1992).

17. *Flores* v. *Center for Spinal Evaluation and Rehabilitation*, 865 S.W. 2d 261 (Texas App. 1993).

18. In re *Quinlan,* 355 A.2d 647 (N.J. 1976).

19. *Bouvia* v. *Superior Court*, 179 Cal. App. 3d 1127, 225 Cal. Rptr. 297 (Cal. App. 1986).

20. *Cruzan v. Director, Department of Health*, 497 U.S. 261 (1990).
21. Patient Self-Determination Act, 42 United States Code Sections 1395, 1396.
22. 42 United States Code Section 1395cc(f)(1)(A)(i).
23. *Patient Bill of Rights and Responsibilities*. Chicago, IL: American Hospital Association, 1992.
24. *Accreditation Manual for Hospitals*. Chicago, IL: Joint Commission on the Accreditation of Healthcare Organizations, current edition.
25. *Canterbury v. Spence*, note 7.
26. Curtin, L.L. "Ethics in Management: Informed Consent: Cautious, Calculated Candor." *Nursing Management*, 1995; 24(4):18–20.
27. "How Is Your Doctor Treating You?" *Consumer Reports*, February 1995, pp. 81–88.
28. Tanner, L. "Study Asks How Much Patients Want to Know." *Senior News*, October 1995, p. 15.
29. Furrow, B.R., Johnson, S.H., Jost, T.S., Schwartz, R.L. *Health Law: Cases, Materials and Problems*, 2nd ed. St. Paul, MN: West Publishing Company, 1991, p. 336.
30. *Canterbury v. Spence*, note 7.
31. "Council on Ethical and Judicial Affairs, American Medical Association, Guidelines for the Appropriate Use of Do-Not-Resuscitate Orders." *Journal of the American Medical Association*, 1991; 265:1868–1871.
32. Somerville, M.A. "Therapeutic Privilege: Variation on the Theme of Informed Consent." *Law, Medicine & Health Care*, 1984; 12(1):4–12.
33. Searight, H.R. "Assessing Patient Competence for Medical Decision Making." *American Family Physician*. 1992; 45:751–759.
34. Air Force Regulation 160-12, *Medical Service: Professional Policies and Procedures*, paragraph 55c, Routine Informed Consent Briefings, May 6, 1988, p. 38.
35. Remember that the legal responsibility to obtain patient informed consent to physical therapy rests with the patient's physical therapist.
36. "Guidelines for Physical Therapy Documentation, I.A.2." *Journal of the American Physical Therapy Association*, 1995; 75:762.
37. "Principle 1, Nuremberg Code of 1947." *Trials of War Criminals Before the Nuremberg Military Tribunals under Control Council Law No. 10*, Vol. 2. Washington, DC: U.S. Government Printing Office, 1949, pp. 181–182.
38. "Principle 2, World Medical Association Declaration of Helsinki." Adopted by the 18th World Medical Assembly, Helsinki, Finland, June 1964; and amended by the 29th World Medical Assembly, Tokyo, Japan, October 1975; 35th World Medical Assembly, Venice, Italy, October 1983; and the 41st World Medical Assembly, Hong Kong, September 1989.
39. "Protection of Human Subjects." *Title 45, Code of Federal Regulations, Part 46*. Washington, DC: U.S. Government Printing Office, 1983.
40. Hudson, T., *citing* Rozovsky, F.A. "Informed Consent Problems Become More Complicated." *Hospitals*, March 20, 1991, p. 38.
41. Hutson, M.M., Blaha, J.D. "Patients' Recall of Preoperative Instruction for Informed Consent for an Operation." *Journal of Bone and Joint Surgery*, 1991: 73A:160–162.
42. Winslow, R. "Videos, Questionnaires Aim to Expand Role of Patients in Treatment Decisions." *Wall Street Journal*, February 25, 1992, p. B1.

Suggested Readings

1. *Accreditation Manual for Hospitals*. Chicago, IL: Joint Commission on the Accreditation of Healthcare Organizations, current edition.

2. Beauchamp, T.L., Childress, J.F. *Principles of Biomedical Ethics*, 4th ed. New York: Oxford Press, 1994.

3. *Canterbury* v. *Spence*, 464 F.2d 772 (D.C. Cir. 1972), *cert.* [U.S. Supreme Court appeal] *denied*, 409 U.S. 1064 (1974).

4. Curtin, L.L. "Ethics in Management: Informed Consent: Cautious, Calculated Candor." *Nursing Management*, 1995; 24(4):18–20.

5. Furrow, B.R., Johnson, S.H., Jost, T.S., Schwartz, R.L. *Health Law: Cases, Materials and Problems*, 2nd ed. St. Paul, MN: West Publishing Company, 1991.

6. *Guide for Professional Conduct*. Alexandria, VA: American Physical Therapy Association, 1996.

7. "Guidelines for Physical Therapy Documentation, I.A.2," *Journal of the American Physical Therapy Association*, 1995; 75:762.

8. "How Is Your Doctor Treating You?" *Consumer Reports*, February 1995, p. 81–88.

9. Hudson, T. "Informed Consent Problems Become More Complicated." *Hospitals*, March 20, 1991, pp. 38–40.

10. Hutson, M.M., Blaha, J.D. "Patients' Recall of Preoperative Instruction for Informed Consent for an Operation." *Journal of Bone and Joint Surgery*, 1991: 73A:160–162.

11. Katz, J. *The Silent World of Doctor and Patient*. New York: Free Press, 1984.

12. *Occupational Therapy Code of Ethics*. Bethesda, MD: American Occupational Therapy Association, 1994.

13. *Patient Bill of Rights and Responsibilities*. Chicago, IL: American Hospital Association, 1992.

14. Patient Self-Determination Act, 42 United States Code Sections 1395, 1396.

15. Portney, L.G., Watkins, M.P. *Foundations of Clinical Research: Applications to Practice*. Norwalk, CT: Appleton & Lange, Publishing, 1993, pp. 27–37.

16. "Protection of Human Subjects." *Title 45, Code of Federal Regulations, Part 46*. Washington, DC: U.S. Government Printing Office, 1983.

17. Rozovsky, F.A. *Consent to Treatment*, 2nd ed. Boston, MA: Little, Brown & Company, 1990.

18. Searight, H.R. "Assessing Patient Competence for Medical Decision Making." *American Family Physician*, 1992; 45:751–759.

19. Scott, R.W. *Legal Aspects of Documenting Patient Care*. Gaithersburg, MD: Aspen Publishers, Inc., 1994.

20. Somerville, M.A. "Therapeutic Privilege: Variation on the Theme of Informed Consent." *Law, Medicine & Health Care*, 1984; 12(1):4–12.

21. Tanner, L. "Study Asks How Much Patients Want to Know." *Senior News*, October 1995, p. 15.

22. Timm, K. "Informed Consent in Clinical Research." *Orthopaedic Practice*, 1995; 7(3):14–15.

23. Winslow, R. "Videos, Questionnaires Aim to Expand Role of Patients in Treatment Decisions." *Wall Street Journal*, February 25, 1992, p. B1.

Chapter 5

Contract Law

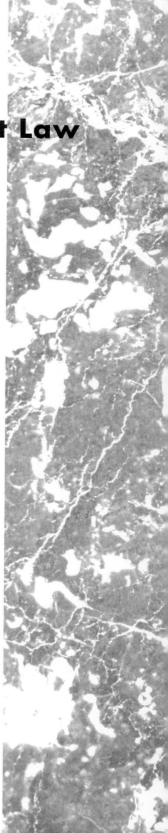

A contractual promise is one that the legal system will enforce. Every day, tens of millions of business contracts are consummated, most of which are not reduced to writing. Health care professional-patient interactions involve at least implied contracts, under which the provider promises to utilize his or her best clinical judgment to effect an optimal therapeutic result, and under which the patient promises to cooperate with the treatment and to pay for services. This chapter explores many (but certainly not all) of the terms, issues, and nuances associated with health care contracts.

Introduction

The study of contract law, and particularly, familiarization with basic contract law terms and concepts, is critically important for health care professionals—whether they are employed by an entity or self-employed. This is especially true in the current managed care environment, under which health care delivery is becoming ever more businesslike.

Contract law forms the foundation for all commercial transactions, including purchases of goods and services (including patient care services) and employment relationships. A majority of civil legal cases involve, not health care malpractice, but commercial, contractual disputes. An important introductory point that may not be obvious now, but will become so in this chapter, is that **a binding contract does not necessarily have to be in writing in order to be enforceable**.

As much as with any area of law, issues involving commercial contracts have business, legal, and ethical considerations. For example, beyond the legalities of, say, a student physical therapist accepting multiple interview opportunities in exotic locations (even though the student has already accepted a position locally and has no intention of accepting one of those positions), there are also ethical concerns to address. Is this sort of practice right or fair, and does it reflect favorably or disfavorably on the profession? In addition, a business consideration associated with the practice of accepting multiple job interviews for positions that a candidate has no intention of pursuing is that this practice may have adverse employment consequences, in that the candidate's professional reputation may be tarnished by the practice. Also, the sojourner may find him- or herself without important future networking opportunities with professional colleagues.

This chapter begins with an introduction to the nature of contractual obligations between people or business entities and then moves into an analysis of the differences between oral and written contractual agreements. A discussion of clinical affiliation agreements follows. The chapter ends with a discussion of contracts involving continuing educational experiences and the special considerations for presenters, sponsors, and participants associated with them.

The Nature of Contracts and Contractual Obligations

The right of individuals and corporations (also legally considered to be "persons") to contract is fundamental in American law. In fact, this right is one of only a few private rights that are enumerated in the body of the U.S. Constitution. Article I, Section 10 of the Constitution states:

> No state shall . . . pass any . . . Law impairing the Obligation of Contracts. . . .[1]

The freedom of individuals to create contracts gives private citizens and corporations immense power over private business affairs. In essence, parties to business contracts are virtually free to create their own "private law," which the civil courts will enforce with few exceptions. Those exceptions to enforcement of private, contractual law generally involve agreements that either involve illegal subject matter or contain provisions that violate public policy considerations.

As has been stated throughout this book, every professional interaction between a health care professional and a patient involves at least an *implied contract*. Even when there are no written or otherwise formally stated contractual terms to the patient care agreement, i.e., an *express contract*, the law imposes certain obligations upon both the health care provider and the patient.

When does a health care provider begin to owe a duty of special care to a patient? The special, implied contractual duty of special care arises when the health care provider agrees to accept the patient for evaluation and possible treatment. In simplified contractual terms, the patient presents him- or herself for care and makes an *offer* to become a patient. The health care professional, then, is normally free to accept or reject the patient's offer. *Acceptance* of the patient by the health care provider for care completes the *bilateral contract*, in which both parties incur legally enforceable obligations.

The health care professional has (at least) the following contractual obligations: to exercise sound professional judgment in order to reach a correct diagnosis and effect an optimal therapeutic result for the patient; to maintain a professional demeanor throughout the relationship; to refer the patient to other health care (or other) professionals, when warranted; and to safeguard confidential patient information, unless required by law to breach patient confidentiality.

The patient, too, has legally binding contractual obligations associated with the health care professional-patient relationship. These normally include the obligation to pay for services rendered (either personally or through a third-party intermediary) and to cooperate with the health care professional in charge of the patient's care, as well as the support staff carrying out the clinician's directives.

The Definition of a "Contract"

A contractual promise, in its simplest terms, is one that a person (or corporation) makes that is legally enforceable. The American Law Institute formally defines a contract as "a promise or set of promises for the breach of which the law gives a remedy, [and] the performance of which the law in some way recognizes as a duty."[2] By a "promise," the legal system defines a contractual obligation as one that binds a party to a contract to perform some action, or refrain from action, presently or at some future time.

> **Contract:** a promise enforceable as a legally-binding obligation.

Bilateral vs. Unilateral Contracts

Most business contracts are *bilateral contracts*, meaning that there are two or more parties to an agreement who are legally bound to perform (or refrain from acting) in some way. In a bilateral contract, both parties exchange mutual contractual promises, which, by virtue of *consideration* (discussed below), create legally binding obligations upon the parties. Contracts between health care professionals and patients for health care service delivery are examples of bilateral contracts.

A *unilateral contract* (relatively uncommon in business settings) is one in which one party can consummate a binding contract only by completing some action (or omission) requested by another party. In a unilateral contract, then, there is no formal exchange of contractual promises, only a contractual offer made by one person to another, that demands specific action on the part of the latter party. Consider the following hypothetical situation.

It is a Wednesday. *A*, a contract physical therapist working in a home-health setting, is obligated to come to the home of *B*, a bedridden patient, for a treatment session on Saturday. *A*, however, is suddenly called away for an emergency out-of-town professional association meeting and knows that she cannot return by Saturday. *A* wants to ensure that she provides physical therapy coverage for her home patients, including *B*. *A* telephones *C*, a competent, licensed physical therapist colleague, to whom she has made frequent referrals in the recent past. When *A* calls *C* at *C*'s office, *A* is already at the airport, ready to board a flight for her meeting. *C* is not in, so *A* leaves the following message on *C*'s answering machine: "If you make the home visit to *B* for me on Saturday for treatment, I will pay you $50.00." *C* returns to her office at the end of the day and hears the message. Once *C* completes performance of the patient visit to *B*, the unilateral contract is consummated, and *A* becomes legally bound to fulfill her promise to pay *C* for *C*'s services.

Under a unilateral contract, then, only the party making a contractual promise (*A*, in the hypothetical example above) is contractually bound to act in a certain way (in this case, to pay money to *C* for *C*'s services). The person to whom the offer and promise to perform are made (*C*) has no legal obligation to do anything. Only if the party to whom the offer and promise are made completes the requested performance does a contract exist. At that point, the promisor's duty is to perform as promised (e.g., by paying for what was requested or by performing a service in return).

The Basic Elements of a Binding Contract

There are four basic required elements that are common to all contracts. They are: (1) contractual agreement between or among the parties, (2) mutual consideration in support of parties' contractual promises, (3) recognized legal capacity on the part of the parties to enter into a binding contract, and (4) legality of the subject matter of the agreement.[3]

Parties to a Contract

There are several legal terms commonly used to describe the parties to a contract. These terms initially may appear somewhat confusing, but, once learned, aid in simplifying the discussion of contract issues with readers' business advisors and legal counsel. In either a bilateral or unilateral contract, the party making an offer to be contractually bound to some performance is called the *offeror*, or *promisor*. The party to whom an offer is directed is called the *offeree*, or *promisee*.

Agreement

Agreement of the parties in a bilateral contract to be legally bound to perform their mutual promises is a fundamental element in the contractual process. The mutual agreement of parties to a bilateral contract to be bound to performance is often referred to as *mutuality of assent*.[4]

An offeror virtually controls the scope of duty that he or she incurs to an offeree by the way in which the offeror phrases the contractual offer. An offeror can restrict acceptance of the offer to specifically named persons. Restrictions can also be placed on acceptable timeframes for accepting a contractual offer. Restrictions can even be placed on the permissible modes and forms of acceptance of an offer.

Special conditions can be attached to an offer as the offeror sees fit (within the bounds of law and public policy), and the occurrence (or nonoccurrence) of such conditions may discharge one or both parties' duty to perform under the contract. For example, an offeror can expressly condition his or her performance under a contract to the happening of some precondition, such as receipt of favorable financing for a business loan. Such a condition is called a *condition precedent*.

In the health care setting, it is generally illegal to condition patient care on the patient's signing of a waiver or limitation of liability. These *exculpatory releases* are generally unenforceable as conditions precedent, because they violate public policy.[5] Bargained-for agreements that require providers and patients to resolve grievances through arbitration, rather than through litigation, however, are generally valid and enforceable.

Parties to a bilateral contract may also require simultaneous performance of their contractual obligations, such as might be the case in a contract between a health care continuing education course sponsor and presenter. Simultaneous performance conditions are called *conditions concurrent*.

Finally, the parties may condition their continuing performance under a contract to some future event, such as is exemplified by a "military relocation" discontinuance clause in a military health care provider's off-duty employment contract with a civilian health care agency. Such conditions are referred to as *conditions subsequent*.

Once an offer, whose terms are reasonably certain, is properly accepted by an offeree, there is *mutuality of assent*, and a binding contract is formed. Remember that the making of a *counteroffer* by an offeree to an offer is normally considered as a *rejection* of the initial offer, not a conditional acceptance. The counteroffer then becomes a new offer, which the original offeror may be able to accept and thus form a bilateral contract.

Generally, certain basic elements must be present in every oral and written business contract. These are:

- identification of the parties to the contract
- identification of the subject matter of the contract
- the consideration, or value, given by each party to the other
- timeframes for performance of the parties and payment, when indicated

Consideration

Consideration can be thought of as the inducement that causes a party to a contract to allow him- or herself to become legally bound to perform under the agreement. Consideration does not always equate to money. Many health care and other business contracts (especially under the so-called barter system) call for mutual performance of professional services, rather than the payment of any money.

Another common explanation for consideration in support of a party's contractual promise is that it can be construed as some *legal detriment* to the promisee or some *legal benefit* to the promisor.[6] That is, the party promising performance must be legally benefited in some way by the other party for having made a contractual promise, or the party to whom performance is promised must incur some legal detriment (such as foregoing another business opportunity).

> **Consideration:** value given in exchange for another person's contractual promise.

In short, consideration is value given in exchange for another person's contractual promise. Courts will not normally critique whether what is exchanged is equivalent, but rather will normally leave contractual parties free to bargain as they see fit.

Capacity

Contractual *capacity* refers to the legal ability of prospective parties to enter into contracts that are enforceable. Most prospective parties to business contracts display obvious capacity to contract. Those who do not include minors, persons incapacitated by alcohol or psychotropic drugs, and persons who have been legally adjudicated as incompetent. The consequences of contracting with a person with no legal capacity, or with limited capacity, to contract include (1) the purported contract may be null and *void*, (2) the contract may be unilaterally *voidable* at the option of the party lacking capacity, or (3) the contract may be valid, if an exception to lack of contractual capacity applies.

As a general rule, minors in most states have the limited legal capacity to contract for any goods or services that adults may contract for. However, also in most cases, minors are permitted by law to *disaffirm*, or disavow, their contractual obligations any time before they reach the legal age of majority (18–21) and even for a limited time thereafter. To validate a contract made by a minor, the minor normally must continue to perform under a contract after the minor achieves the age of majority. This is called contract *ratification*.

When a minor properly disaffirms a contract, the minor normally only has to give back to the other party to the contract that property (including money) that the minor presently has in his or her possession. A minor may even disaffirm most contracts when the minor has misrepresented his or her age.

A minor, however, may be obligated by law to repay the reasonable value of necessary goods and services received under contract. Necessities, which require repayment for value, include food, health care services, and shelter.

Intoxicated or otherwise impaired persons have limited protection under law from contractual obligations, similar to those granted to minors. In most cases, an impaired person may elect to void a contract made while impaired, however, unlike minors, the impaired person must repay, in *restitution*, the reasonable value of any goods or services received.

Only those persons who are legally adjudicated as incompetent fully lack capacity to contract. For such persons, such as institutionalized patients with mental illnesses, contracts must be entered into with the incompetent persons' surrogate decision makers, i.e., court-appointed conservators or guardians. A purported contract with a legally adjudicated incompetent person is *void*, i.e., no contract exists.

Legality

In addition to all of the other requirements of a valid, enforceable contract discussed above, the subject mater of a contract must be legal and must not violate public policy. For example, a written contract among several health care professionals to provide health care services to patients that includes an unwritten understanding that the parties will defraud the Medicare and Medicaid programs is illegal and therefore, null and void.

The law will not countenance an illegal contractual agreement. This is so because, under its equity, or fairness powers, a court will only come to the aid of a contractual party who comes to court "with clean hands." This concept is known as the equitable *clean hands doctrine*.

> **Hint** *The law will not countenance an illegal contractual agreement nor one that violates public policy.*

Examples of contracts that are void because they violate public policy considerations include agreements grounded in immoral (but legal) or unconscionable behavior, or unprofessional conduct. For example, a managed care contract that requires of participating health care providers that all outpatient physical and occupational therapy care be limited to a maximum of four visits, irrespective of patient diagnosis, might very well be declared unconscionable by a court and thereby void as violative of public policy (see Box 5-1).

Quasi-Contract

It was previously stated in the chapter that every health care professional-patient interaction involves at least an implied contract for service delivery. Such an implied contract is referred to in law as an *implied-in-fact* contract. The contract and its terms are implied from the conduct of the health care professional and of the patient. Certain other types of interaction are referred to legally as contracts *implied-in-law*. In such an arrangement, one party believes—reasonably or otherwise—that a contract exists with another party. However, there is no agreement or assent to be bound by the other party. Such a scenario is also called *quasi-contract* (Latin for "analogous to a contract").

Because there is no assent to be contractually bound by one side in a quasi-contractual situation, a court cannot award contractual damages for non-performance by a party. However, using its equitable powers, a court can prevent unjust enrichment on the part of a party by compelling the party who receives goods or services from another to pay the fair value of the goods or services. Consider the following hypothetical example.

5-1 The Four Basic Elements of a Binding (Bilateral) Contract

- *agreement* of the parties (mutuality of assent)
- *consideration* (mutuality of obligation)
- *capacity* (recognized legal status to contract)
- *legality* of subject matter

A, a trauma surgeon, is driving along a country road when she comes upon a one-automobile crash victim, *B*, on the side of the road. *A* renders emergency medical treatment to *B*, who is unconscious. Under quasi-contract principles, *A* is entitled to recover the reasonable value of her medical services to *B*.

Oral and Written Agreements

Only specific types of contracts must be in writing in order to be legally enforceable. State laws requiring that certain contracts be in writing to be enforceable are called *statutes of frauds*. In this case, the word "fraud" does not refer to deceptive misrepresentation.

Although statutes of frauds differ from jurisdiction to jurisdiction, there are common types of contracts that usually require a writing. These include:

- a contractual promise to serve as a surety (or *guarantor*) for another person's debts, i.e., a cosigner
- contracts for the transfer of long-term interests in real property
- promises in consideration of marriage, i.e., prenuptial agreements
- contracts for the sale of goods (under the Uniform Commercial Code) for purchases over $500[7]
- contracts that cannot be performed (*executed*) within one year from the making of the agreement

The provision requiring contracts that cannot objectively be performed within one year to be in writing is called the *one-year rule*. Consider the following hypothetical examples.

1. It is June 1st. *Q*, a student physical therapist who will graduate on June 15, receives an offer of employment from *R*, a human resources manager at XYZ Hospital, for a period of one year commencing on June 16. *Q* accepts the offer without condition.

2. It is June 1st. *O*, an occupational therapist, receives an employment offer from *R* for a period of one year commencing immediately. *O* accepts the offer without condition.

    In which example, if either, is the statute of frauds applicable?

    The statute of frauds's one-year rule requires that the employment offer in example 1 be in writing in order to be enforceable. In example 2, no writing is required to enforce the agreement, because the one-year period does not begin to run until the next calendar day (June 2), and the employment contract in this example will be fully executed within one year.

Interpretation of Contracts

While contracts that are not required to be in writing by the statute of frauds or other laws may be either written or oral, the existence and interpretation of an agreement is certainly easier to ascertain and make if the contract is in writing. One admonition that readers should take from this chapter is that **all business agreements should be reduced to writing.**

As a general rule, courts asked to interpret written contracts will only interpret the understandings memorialized by the parties to the agreement in writing. This is often referred to as the *four-corners doctrine*. Like the adage concerning patient care documentation that "if it isn't written, it wasn't done," with contracts one can say, "if it isn't written, it wasn't part of the agreement," with limited exceptions.

A corollary rule to the four-corners rule is the *parol* ("spoken") *evidence rule*. Under this rule of interpretation of a written contract, a court will not normally permit the introduction into evidence of any purported prior or contemporaneous "understandings" by the contractual parties that were not incorporated into the written agreement. The parol evidence rule exists, in part, to protect the integrity of written contractual agreements, and, in part, to give legal effect to the clear meaning of the parties as stated in their written agreement.

Many written agreements contain (usually at the end of the contract) an *integration clause*, which restates that there are no contractual understandings or obligations that are not included in the written agreement. Check out the bill of sale for your next new car for an excellent example of an integration clause.

Defenses to Performance of Contractual Obligations

Contracts may be *executed*, or fully performed, in one of several ways. Most often, parties to contracts complete their contractual obligations by legal *performance*. For example, a physical therapist contracts with a home health agency to render home physical therapy services to specified patients for a three-month period. The contractual duties of the parties are fully discharged when (1) the physical therapist performs the duties under the contract for three months, and (2) the agency pays for professional services rendered by the physical therapist.

Occasionally, full or even substantial performance of contractual obligations by parties is made impossible by circumstances such as the death or bankruptcy of one of the parties, or unforeseeable destruction of equipment necessary to complete the contract. Such circumstances are referred to as *impossibility of performance*, and discharge contractual obligations *by operation of law*.

Finally, a contract may be terminated by agreement (Get it in writing!) of the parties, or by the *material breach*, or failure of even substantial performance, of one of the contractual parties. A material breach of contract equates to a lack of legal consideration and normally excuses the non-breaching party from further performance under the contract.

Breach of Contract and Contractual Remedies

In addition to a material breach of contract, a contractual party may commit a minor breach of contract. In the case of a minor breach of contract, the party in compliance may often have the right to suspend his or her continued performance until the minor breach has been corrected. Consider the following hypothetical example.

D, an occupational therapist and bioethicist, lectures extensively on biomedical ethics to occupational therapy professional students across the country. As part of one contract to lecture, *D* agrees with *E*, the full-time instructor in a management course in an occupational therapy program, to lecture to *E*'s students for a four-hour period. *D* finishes with the lecture after two hours and releases the students on a break. Is *D*'s breach of contract a minor or a material breach? The answer probably depends on whether *D* can cure the breach by calling the students together and substantially completing the four-hour period of instruction.

Remedies for Breach of Contract

In addition to suspending performance under an existing contract, an aggrieved party in a breach of contract situation can sue for monetary damages, as well as other legal and equitable remedies. Consider the case of *Sullivan* v. *O'Connor*,[8] a medical malpractice contract-based lawsuit concerning a surgeon's alleged breach of promise to improve the plaintiff-patient's facial appearance with a rhinoplasty. The court in this case distinguished three possible ways to calculate monetary damages in contractual lawsuits. These three types of contract damages are *restitution* damages, *reliance* damages, and *expectancy* damages.

An award of restitution damages provides sufficient monetary recovery only to restore the aggrieved party to the *status quo ante*, or the position he or she occupied before beginning performance under the contract. Restitution damages, then, compensate a plaintiff only for labor and materials expended in support of the plaintiff's performance under the contract.

Reliance damages operate, not only to restore a contract plaintiff to the status quo ante, but also give the aggrieved party reasonable monetary damages to compensate for the breach. The court in *Sullivan* endorsed reliance damages as the most appropriate measure of contractual monetary damages in health care cases.

Expectancy (or compensatory) damages give a contract plaintiff the full "benefit of the contractual bargain," as contemplated by the parties when they formed the contract. That is, expectancy damages serve to place the plaintiff in exactly the same position that he or she would have been in had the defendant not breached the contract. Elements of damages included in expectancy recoveries include (1) *incidental* (direct) *damages* and (2) *consequential* (indirect) *damages*. Incidental damages include such things as travel and other out-of-pocket expenses. Consequential damages include lost profits (provable to a reasonable certainty) and pain and suffering. Subtracted from an expectancy award is the sum that the plaintiff saved by not having to perform further under the contract after the defendant's breach of contract.

In addition to monetary damages, or *damages at law*, contract plaintiffs may seek *equitable remedies* in litigation. The most common types of equitable contract remedies are (1) injunctions and (2) orders for specific performance of contractual obligations.

An injunction is an order issued by a court to a defendant to cease some offensive activity. By way of example, a health care professional-presenter of continuing education courses, who is under an exclusive contract with an educational group to make presentations, may be *enjoined* by a court from comparing his independent, but competitive courses, to those sponsored by the plaintiff.

Specific performance involves an equitable order by a court directed to a party, ordering that party to perform as required under a contract. Courts will not order specific performance of personal services contracts (including health care services delivery contracts), on the ground that such an order violates the Thirteenth Amendment to the Constitution, which reads:

Section 1. Neither slavery nor *involuntary servitude* [emphasis added], except as a punishment for crime whereof the party shall have been duly convicted, shall exist within the United States, or any place subject to their jurisdiction.
Section 2. Congress shall have the power to enforce this article by appropriate legislation.[9]

Two final points about contractual damages warrant mention. First, punitive (or punishment) damages, are seldom, if ever, awarded or appropriate in contract litigation cases. The concept of punitive damages is a tort concept, reflecting public policy considerations other than respect for the lawful private law made by parties to contracts. In contract litigation, punitive damages are normally only awarded when there is egregious misconduct by a defendant that constitutes a mixed tort-contract action. Second, *liquidated damages*, pre-agreed default damages specified in a contract, may be enforced by a court, provided that they are adjudged as reasonable and bargained for.

Breach of Warranty

Breach of warranty involves contractual liability for the failure of a product to meet reasonable or expressly agreed performance standards. In most states, an injured party has the right to sue any distributor (including health care professionals) along the chain of commercial distribution. Courts disfavor imposing breach of warranty liability on health care professionals, because courts view health care principally as a professional service. Normally only when health care professionals regularly market products in clinical practice, such as orthotists and prosthetists (and others who sell equipment in their clinical practices), will courts allow breach of warranty cases to proceed.

Types of warranties include express and implied warranties. Express warranties involve statements of purported fact about a product's performance or potential, which become part of the consideration, or benefit of the bargain. There is no legal requirement that express warranties be made, and they may be expressly disclaimed in contracts.

Implied warranties are of two types: implied warranties of merchantability and implied warranties of fitness for particular purposes. Merchantability means that products are generally suitable for expected uses. Fitness for particular purposes implies that products are especially appropriate for buyers' stated needs. The laws of many states prohibit the disclaimer of implied warranties of merchantability.

Clinical Affiliation Agreements

Relevant clinical experiences are integral component parts of professional health care education programs. Contracts between academic institutions and clinical sites for student placement are known as *clinical affiliation agreements*. Such agreements normally spell out in varying detail the major rights and responsibilities of the respective parties. One principal duty incumbent upon academic institutions is to certify that professional students participating in clinical experiences have had appropriate academic preparation for their particular assignments prior to arriving at clinical sites. A principal duty of clinical sites is to provide relevant learning experiences for affiliates, under appropriate guidance and supervision, consistent with individual student competency and agreed learning objectives.

Clinical affiliation agreements may or may not delineate who bears vicarious legal responsibility for student malpractice or ordinary negligence over and above that covered by student liability insurance. For many reasons, clinical sites may refuse to accept financial responsibility for professional student affiliates. Similarly, many public academic institutions are immune from liability under state sovereign immunity. It is incumbent upon all parties to clinical affiliation contracts to have them thoroughly reviewed before signing them.

In the absence of express provisions fixing financial responsibility for student conduct in clinical affiliation agreements, courts may utilize a legal concept called the *borrowed servant rule* to affix vicarious liability for student conduct. Under this ancient rule of law, liability attaches to the party whose interests are most being served by the student at the time of legally actionable conduct. For health care professional students, vicarious liability under the borrowed servant rule might logically attach to the academic institution early in a student's education (when the student is primarily serving the academic institution's objectives) and to the clinical site late in a student's education (when the student is primarily serving the clinic's needs).

Continuing Education Courses: A Special Case of Contractual Duties

In health care professional continuing education settings,[10] breach of contract liability issues can arise in at least three ways:

1. Involving continuing education course presenters and sponsors, based on either compensation or presentation performance disputes. This type of contract legal action typically involves straightforward interpretation of express contractual language.

2. Involving continuing education course presenters or sponsors, and participants, based on the content or perceived value of particular presentations or courses. This type of contract legal action is often complex and may require that a court examine the language in course brochures, announcements, and other correspondence. To prevent these kinds of disputes from arising, continuing education course sponsors and presenters are urged to carefully review the language in their marketing materials—particularly course objectives—to ensure that what is promised to participants is substantially delivered.

3. Involving continuing education course presenters and demonstration subjects (patients), based on the scope and duration of professional (treatment) intervention. This type of contract legal action may involve the issue of patient abandonment by the presenter, i.e., did the termination of professional care comport with the parties' understandings? Another question may be whether treatment by a presenter meets licensure and practice standards.

It is strongly advised that continuing education presenters who treat patients at courses always consider the following recommendations:

- Clearly define the scope and duration of treatment in a written agreement signed by presenter and patient(s) to prevent misunderstandings and patient dissatisfaction.

- Determine the legal requirements regarding practice and continuation of care in the state where the treatment takes place.

Chapter Summary

The majority of civil litigation cases involve, not allegations of tortious conduct, but contractual and other business disputes. The beauty of contract law is that parties to contracts are largely free to create their own enforceable "private law," consistent with legal, business, and professional ethical considerations, as well as public policy considerations.

The four basic required elements common to all contracts are (1) contractual *agreement* between or among the parties, (2) mutual *consideration* in support of parties' contractual promises, (3) recognized legal *capacity* on the part of the parties to enter into a binding contract, and (4) *legality* of the subject matter of the agreement.

Most contracts are not written and are not required by law to be in writing. Prudence in business affairs, however, mandates that health care professionals and other businesspeople always reduce their contractual agreements to writing.

In contractual litigation cases, courts may remedy breach of contract through the award of monetary damages or through imposition of equitable remedies, such as the issuance of an injunction or an order for specific performance. An order for specific performance of a personal services contract, such as a health services contract, is inappropriate, because it violates the constitutional prohibition against involuntary servitude.

All health care professionals, from all practice settings, are strongly advised to review their business contracts with their personal legal counsel before signing them.

Cases and Questions

1. *A*, a physical therapist in private practice, is approached by *B*, another physical therapist and lifelong friend of *A*, who proposes that they form a professional partnership for practice. What initial advice would you offer to *A* and *B*?

2. *C*, an occupational therapist in private practice, treats *D*, a 17-year-old male patient and an emancipated minor, for right wrist movement dysfunction secondary to a fall onto his outstretched hand while skateboarding. *D* is being treated pursuant to a proper physician referral. *C*'s normal billing charge is $25 per hour. Can *C* legally enforce her normal billing charges if *D* refuses to pay?

3. *E*, a certified prosthetist, evaluates *F*, a 32-year-old male patient and professional golfer, who sustained a traumatic left below-knee (B-K) amputation, for an appropriate B-K prosthesis. *F* concedes during the course of the evaluation that he does not know anything about prostheses and is putting his full confidence in *E* to select the most appropriate prosthesis to enable him to return to professional play. Money is no object for *F*. *E* has a specific computer-designed prosthesis in mind for *F*, and warrants that it will be the best one for him. Several months later, *F* is experiencing difficulty controlling his prosthesis. On what basis might *F* have a contractual cause of action against *E*?

Suggested Answers to Cases and Questions

1. The first thing that *A* and *B* should do is to consult with their respective personal legal advisors before coming to any enforceable agreement. It is imperative that a professional partnership contract be negotiated and reduced to a signed writing. Legal counsel can help initially by apprising their clients of the legalities concerning forms of business organization and the particulars of the law of partnership for the parties' state(s).

2. *C* may not be able to enforce her normal fee for services in court. *C* has contracted with a minor and, even though the services are necessary, *C* may be limited to recovering what a court determines to be the reasonable value of her services (which may be less than her normal fee). (In most states, the fact that *D* is an emancipated minor does not prevent him from disaffirming his contract with *C*.)

3. *E* may face breach of (product) warranty liability. *E* has made an express warranty to *F* concerning the quality of the prosthesis *E* has selected for *F*. *E* also knows that *F* is relying on *E*'s special knowledge and expertise to choose the best limb for him. *E* may be liable in contract for breach of an express warranty and breach of an implied warranty of fitness for a particular purpose regarding *F*'s B-K prosthesis.

References

1. U.S. Constitution, Article I, Section 10.
2. Restatement (Second) of Contracts, Section 1.
3. Calamari, J.D., Perillo, J.M. *Contracts*, 2nd ed. St. Paul, MN: West Publishing Company, 1977, Chs. 2, 4, 8, and 22.
4. Restatement (Second) of Contracts, Section 22.
5. See *Tunkl* v. *Regents of the University of California*, 60 Cal. 2d 92 (1963).
6. Calamari, J.D., Perillo, J.M. *Contracts*, 2nd ed. St. Paul, MN: West Publishing Company, 1977, p. 134.
7. Uniform Commercial Code, Section 2-201.
8. *Sullivan* v. *O'Connor*, 296 N.E. 2d 183 (Mass.1973).
9. U.S. Constitution, Amendment Thirteen.
10. Scott, R.W. "Liability Considerations in Continuing Education." *PT Magazine,* May 1994, pp. 54–57.

Suggested Readings

1. Calamari, J.D., Perillo, J.M. *Contracts*, 2nd ed. St. Paul, MN: West Publishing Company, 1977.
2. Lewis, K. "Part 2: Physical Therapy Contracts." *Clinical Management*, 1992; 12(5):15–20.
3. Rasmussen, B. "Contracts and Fees: Part 2." *Clinical Management*, 1992; 12(3):24–27.
4. Restatement (Second) of Contracts.
5. Scott, R.W. *Health Care Malpractice: A Primer on legal Issues*. Thorofare, NJ: Slack, Inc., 1990.
6. Scott, R.W. "Liability Considerations in Continuing Education." *PT Magazine*, May 1994, pp. 54–57.

Chapter 6

Criminal Law

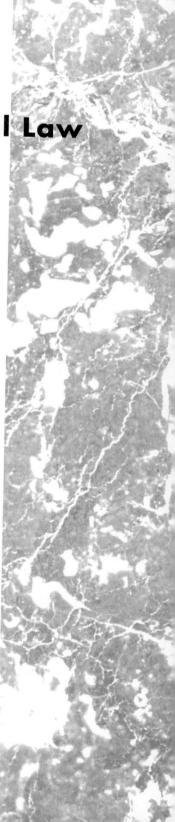

This chapter defines basic criminal law concepts and explores offenses commonly charged against health care professionals. Many criminal offenses bear the same names and elements of proof as their intentional tort counterparts, including assault and battery, sexual assault and battery, and fraud.

The successful prosecution of most crimes by the state requires proof of two elements: culpable conduct (actus reus) and a culpable state of mind (mens rea). The burden of proof on the state in a criminal case is proof of guilt beyond a reasonable doubt.

Defenses to most crimes include consent by the victim (not normally applicable in the health care setting), defense of others and self-defense, infancy, insanity, intoxication, and the statute of limitations, among others. Avoidance of allegations of health care clinical misconduct that can give rise to criminal and civil liability is the formidable responsibility of all health care practitioners and administrators.

The Nature of Criminal Law

A licensed or certified health care provider confronted with an allegation of professional misconduct may face legal action in one or more of the following venues, based on a single incident: (1) in civil court, for health care malpractice; (2) in adverse administrative proceedings affecting licensure; (3) before a judicial committee of a professional association of which the respondent is a member, for a violation of professionals ethics; and (4) in criminal court. All of these judicial and administrative legal actions may take place simultaneously, but more probably will be conducted at different times, because of docketing, evidentiary, and other considerations.

Health care professionals, like other business professionals and citizens in general, are directly affected as potential victims by the rampant violent crime wave sweeping the United States and by so-called nonviolent, "white-collar" crime, while at work,[1] home, or elsewhere. Reported criminal legal case files also reveal that health care professionals are no less subject to being charged as perpetrators of crime than other similarly-situated professionals. The primary purpose for the material presented in this chapter is to familiarize health care professionals with basic criminal law and procedure, so that they both understand it better and have a healthy respect for its power.

Classifications and Types of Criminal Actions

Unlike morals and ethics, which govern the conduct of select individuals or groups of people, the law compels all persons within its reach (jurisdiction) to comply with its mandates. The purpose of law, then, is to delineate what constitutes socially unacceptable conduct and to impose sanctions for noncompliance. A crime may be generally defined as:

> conduct which violates a recognized duty owed to society as a whole, for which, society will demand satisfaction.[2]

With very few exceptions,[3] conviction for all crimes requires a bifurcated form of proof of culpability: (1) proof of commission of a criminal act (the *actus reus*, Latin for "guilty act") and (2) proof of a wrongful state of mind (*mens rea*). Criminal law recognizes varying degrees of *mens rea* along a continuum, ranging from *specific*, malicious criminal intent at one extreme, to *criminal negligence* (gross negligence or recklessness) at the other extreme.

There are many ways to classify crimes. For instance, crimes are classified according to whether they affect people or property interests and whether they involve, or do not involve, allegations of *moral turpitude*.[4] As alluded to in an earlier paragraph, crimes may also be classified as either violent or nonviolent offenses.

Criminal activity is also classified as either *mala in se* (Latin for "wrongs in themselves") or *mala prohibita* (Latin for "prohibited acts"). *Mala in se* crimes include wrongful acts that are clearly criminal in nature, such as the wrongful use of violence against another person (e.g., robbery) and fraud offenses. *Mala in se* crimes are often also labeled as "substantive" offenses.

Mala prohibita crimes, on the other hand, consist of "petty" offenses that are only criminal law violations because society says that they are so. *Mala prohibita* crimes are not inherently wrongful. Offenses such as speeding while driving a motor vehicle and minor building code and Occupational Safety and Health Administration (OSHA) workplace violations are examples of *mala prohibita* "criminal" offenses.

There are two basic types of crimes: misdemeanor offenses and felony crimes. *Misdemeanor* offenses include crimes of relatively minor importance, such as moving traffic violations, which generally are punishable by incarceration for less than one year and/or fines of less than $1,000. Jurisdictions may subdivide misdemeanor offenses into categories, or classes, ranging from A (most serious) to C (least serious).

Crime: any social harm defined and made punishable by law.[5]

Felony crimes include all of the classic serious offenses, such as felonious homicide, robbery, burglary, rape, and fraud. Felonies are generally punishable by imprisonment for greater than one year, and in some cases even by death. Like misdemeanors, felonies are often subdivided into categories, or degrees, ranging from capital offenses (punishable by death) to third degree (punishable by a maximum of five years imprisonment).[6]

Public Interest

Unlike tort (civil) legal actions, which involve disputes between private parties over "private wrongs," criminal legal actions involve disputes between the state and a private defendant over "public wrongs." The term "the state" is intended to be inclusive of all governmental prosecutorial entities, at the city, county or parish, state, and federal levels.

Crimes, then, are wrongs against society and social order. It is society that exclusively circumscribes what conduct is and is not criminal (by statute), and it is societal interests that are satisfied through *sentencing* when an alleged criminal offender is convicted of a crime. An individual crime victim does not have an absolute right to have a criminal case prosecuted. Criminal prosecution is largely discretionary to public prosecutors.

Criminal legal cases differ, then, in many respects from civil (tort) cases that may emanate from the same wrongful conduct. Criminal wrongs are public wrongs against society as a whole, while torts (e.g., health care professional intentional [mis]conduct malpractice) are private wrongs against the personal interests of private victims. Criminal cases are prosecuted at the discretion of public officials, while private parties prosecute civil tort cases. Also, criminal law is largely statutory law, while tort law may be statute-based, but largely is common (judge-made) law.

Parties

In tort cases and other forms of civil litigation, the parties to the cases are private parties—individuals, business entities, and even governmental entities. Civil cases are *captioned* ("titled") with the private litigants' names. For example, a physical therapy malpractice case might be captioned, *Smith by Smith*[7] v. *Doe, P.T.*

In criminal cases, however, cases are captioned with the title of the governmental entity as plaintiff and the name of the private defendant. A criminal case against a physical therapist might be captioned, *People (or State, Commonwealth, or United States)* v. *Doe, P.T.* The victim of a crime is not a party in a criminal case.

Hint *The victim of a crime is not a party in a criminal case.*

Elements and Burdens of Proof in Criminal Cases

In tort cases, civil plaintiffs must fulfill their evidentiary burden of proving specific elements of the torts in issue in order to prevail. For example, in a health care (professional negligence) malpractice case brought by a patient against an occupational therapist, the patient must specifically prove each of the following elements:

1. the defendant-occupational therapist owed a duty of special care to the plaintiff-patient
2. the occupational therapist somehow breached the duty owed in the course of professional care delivery
3. the occupational therapist's breach of professional duty caused the patient to sustain injury
4. the injuries sustained by the patient warrant the payment of monetary damages in order to make the patient "whole"

The civil plaintiff must prove all of the required elements of his or her case by a *preponderance* (or greater weight) *of evidence* to the satisfaction of a civil jury or a judge.

In a criminal prosecution, the state's attorney-plaintiff also bears the entire legal burden to prove the state's case against a criminal defendant. Each and every statutory element of a crime must be proved in order to prevail. Failure of proof of any material element of a criminal case results in *acquittal* (a finding of "not guilty").

In part because of the relative potential severity of criminal sanctions (compared to civil sanctions), and in part because of constitutional, statutory, and judicially-imposed safeguards designed to protect the rights of criminal defendants, the quantum of proof required for a criminal conviction is much greater than that required to prevail in a civil case. The state's representative in a criminal case must convince a trier-of-fact of a criminal defendant's culpability *beyond a reasonable doubt* in order to merit a *guilty* verdict. This lofty standard of proof requires that the criminal defendant's guilt be proven to a "moral certainty," so that there is no legitimate, lingering question concerning the defendant's culpability in the minds of any jurors or in that of the judge.

Why is such a high burden of proof required of government prosecutors in criminal cases? The adage goes, "Society would rather free a truly guilty defendant than to wrongfully convict an innocent one." The adverse consequences to a criminal defendant's life, liberty, and property interests are potentially so severe that the strongest proof of culpability under the law is required for a conviction.

A verdict of "not guilty" in a criminal case does not equate to a lack of culpability on the part of the defendant. It simply stands for the proposition that a unanimous finding of guilty beyond a reasonable doubt could not legitimately be reached by the fact-finders in the case. As O. J. Simpson (and interested parties following his very public legal cases) discovered in 1995, a finding of not guilty in a criminal case does not preclude the institution of a civil case based on the exact same facts that formed the basis for criminal prosecution. The "not guilty" finding in the criminal case only precludes retrial in the same jurisdiction (i.e., state or federal system) of the defendant for the same offense. This Fifth Amendment constitutional protection against criminal retrial is called *double jeopardy*.

Defenses to Criminal Actions

Like the civil law system, the criminal legal system recognizes a number of defenses to criminal charges that defendants can attempt to take advantage of in order to escape liability. Some of these defenses operate as *complete defenses* to exonerate defendants from any criminal liability, while others are *incomplete defenses* that may serve to exonerate criminal defendants of some, but not all, offenses. Normally, the burden of establishing (proving) affirmative defenses is incumbent upon criminal defendants, not the state.

Examples of legitimate defenses to criminal charges include alibi, automatism (a state of unconsciousness), coercion, consent (of the victim), defense of others, duress, entrapment, immunity from prosecution, infancy, intoxication, insanity, mistake of fact or (sometimes) of law, self-defense, and expiration of the statute of limitations. The following comments are intended only to introduce some key concepts about selected defenses to criminal liability, not to be an exhaustive overview of this area of law.

In the health care delivery setting, public policy considerations do not permit the use of the defense of patient consent (in either civil or criminal litigation) to wrongful conduct on the part of a defendant-health care provider. Self-defense and defense of others (including of staff, patients, and visitors in health care environments) allows for the use of anticipatory or reciprocal force to prevent or to repel the imminent application of criminal force. The *objective entrapment* defense normally requires that a criminal defendant not be predisposed to commit a crime in the absence of an unlawful inducement by law enforcement officials or agents. Mistake of law is normally a tenuous defense, unless a criminal defendant can prove justifiable reliance on an official, erroneous pronouncement of law. Generally, though, the adage, "ignorance of the law is no excuse," applies.

The fact that a criminal defendant is a minor may operate as a defense to successful prosecution. This defense is known as the "infancy" defense. At early common law, minors seven years of age or younger could not be held to account for criminal conduct at all. For minors between the ages of seven and fourteen, there was, at common law, a *rebuttable presumption* that the minor was incapable of forming the *mens rea* to commit a criminal act, which the state could try to rebut, in order to try the minor as an adult for the offense. Between ages 14 and the age of legal majority, the rebuttable presumption at common law was that the minor could form the requisite criminal intent to commit any crime, and the legal burden to rebut that presumption rested with the minor's criminal defense attorney. Most states have retained this approach to holding minors responsible for criminal acts, while other states have enacted other systems for liability-determination.

The defense of intoxication may relieve a criminal defendant of legal responsibility for criminal conduct, particularly if the actor's intoxication was involuntary, i.e., he or she was drugged or forced to imbibe alcohol. Even voluntary intoxication may operate as a complete defense to crimes that require a specific criminal intent, such as murder, sexual battery, and fraud. Voluntary intoxication cannot successfully be proffered as a defense to crimes where the required culpable mental state is recklessness or criminal negligence, as in most crimes arising from driving while intoxicated or, in the case of health care providers, treating patients while impaired.

There are two principal tests that courts use to adjudge whether a criminal defendant is insane. In some states (and throughout the federal system), the Model Penal Code definition of *insanity* is used, which reads:

A person is not responsible for criminal conduct if at the time of such conduct as a result of mental disease or defect the person lacks substantial capacity either to appreciate the wrongfulness of his conduct or to conform his [or her] conduct to the requirements of the law.[8]

Other jurisdictions use a more traditional rule of decision, the M'Naghten test, which excuses criminal behavior under the defense of insanity if the defendant is incapable, because of a substantial mental defect, from distinguishing right from wrong.[9] Courts differ on whether a criminal defendant bears the burden of proving insanity (by a preponderance of, or clear and convincing, evidence), or whether the state bears the legal burden of establishing a criminal defendant's sanity (beyond a reasonable doubt).

Anticipatory or reciprocal deadly force may legitimately be employed in order to prevent or repel *deadly force* (i.e., force reasonably likely to cause imminent serious bodily harm or death). The statute of limitations defense is similar to the civil health care malpractice statute of limitations defense. It is a time bar to initiation of legal action. While some defenses, such as the failure of police to comply with Miranda rights warnings,[10] are Constitution-based, the defense of statute of limitations is purely a technical defense. This means that a criminal defendant who successfully invokes it literally "gets off on a technicality." (The statute of limitations does not apply to murder or treason charges.)

Criminal Procedure

Unlike the civil legal system, in which both parties to a lawsuit are simultaneously aided and impeded by the same procedural rules regarding evidence, testimony, and burdens of proof, in criminal procedure, a criminal defendant enjoys substantially greater protection than the state. This is so primarily because of the dire potential consequences to the defendant of a conviction, including imprisonment, loss of reputation and citizen privileges, and even imposition of the death penalty.

Special federal constitutional rights operate in favor of criminal defendants. These include:

- the Fourth Amendment protection against (most) warrantless searches and seizures of property and against unreasonable searches and seizures of property and the person of the defendant

- the Fifth Amendment requirement for fundamental fairness in judicial proceedings—"due process of law," prevention of involuntary self-incrimination by the defendant, and protection against retrial, after acquittal, for the same charges (double jeopardy)
- the Sixth Amendment rights to have the assistance of personal legal counsel, to have a speedy and public trial, to confront adverse witnesses before and at trial, and to have one's criminal action heard before a jury of one's peers (i.e., citizens drawn from the local community)
- the Eight Amendment rights not to be subjected to cruel or unusual punishment nor to have excessive bail or criminal fines imposed before or at trial

Statutes, case law, and state constitutions may afford criminal defendants even greater rights than those enumerated in the federal Constitution. These sources of law, however, may not limit or take away the basic federal constitutional rights of criminal defendants. The following section describes basic criminal procedures common to all jurisdictions: arrest, indictment or information, arraignment, pre-trial (discovery) processes, trial, and appeal.

Arrest

In the United States, unlike in many other countries, people generally enjoy the right to be free from unreasonable intrusion on their privacy and freedom of movement from the police and the state. While police may temporarily detain anyone based on reasonable suspicion of criminal activity, they may not arrest a person without *probable cause*, i.e., evidence of a substantial likelihood that (1) a crime has been committed, and (2) the person to be arrested committed the crime.

Before questioning an arrestee about criminal activity, police officials must apprise the person being subjected to custodial interrogation of his or her Miranda rights, which are based on the Fifth Amendment right against self-incrimination. The Miranda warnings consist of the following points:

- the right not to speak to police about any offense
- the fact that anything said might be used by police and, by the state, against the person
- the right to have an attorney present during questioning and to have the government provide an attorney, if the arrestee cannot afford to retain one[11]

Without proof that these rights were explained to a criminal defendant and proof that the defendant waived, or gave up, the right to not to speak, no evidence obtained from any subsequent interrogation (either directly or indirectly) may be used against the defendant in a criminal trial. The severity of the consequences of this exclusionary rule starkly demonstrates the preeminent value that the United States places on fundamental human rights.

Indictment or Information

After arrest and processing, a grand jury, a magistrate, or another judicial official determines anew whether probable cause exists to bind the suspect over for criminal trial. The formal complaint that results is either called an *indictment* (if issued by a grand jury) or an *information* (if issued by a public official).

Arraignment

After the issuance of a formal indictment or information, the criminal suspect is arraigned, i.e., brought before a trial judge to be apprised of the formal charges against him or her and to be required to enter a plea (answer) to the charges. Most criminal cases are disposed of without resort to a full trial by *plea bargaining*, in which criminal defendants and prosecutors bargain over specific offenses to be pleaded guilty to, sentencing limitations, and conditions to be imposed on the parties. Conditions include cooperation and assistance by the defendant in other prosecutions and recommendations of the prosecutor regarding sentencing, among others. A plea bargain is an express business contract between a criminal defendant and a criminal prosecutor and a necessary instrument for any semblance of efficiency in the operation of a very busy legal system.

Pre-trial (Discovery) Processes

Pre-trial discovery in criminal cases is very similar to discovery processes in civil cases. During this period, both the prosecution and the defense interview witnesses and prospective witnesses, locate and examine evidence, and formulate trial strategies and tactics. Plea bargaining often continues during pre-trial discovery. The state has the affirmative legal duty to expeditiously turn over to the defense exoneration and exculpatory evidence. Judges order the parties to appear in court for pre-trial conferences and hearings (especially in the federal court system) to monitor processes and to narrow issues.

Trial

As described earlier in this chapter, at trial a criminal defendant nominally has no legal burdens. He or she is presumed innocent until proven guilty by the state, beyond any legitimate, reasonable doubt. Even in the face of seemingly overwhelming physical and testimonial evidence against a criminal defendant, a "not guilty" verdict can result. This is what happened in 1995 in the celebrated California case of *People* v. *O.J. Simpson*. Despite substantial public dissatisfaction with the decision, it must fairly be conceded that the jury could have legitimately found reasonable doubt, based on alleged racism and evidence tampering on the part of former Los Angeles Police Detective Mark Fuhrman.

Appeal

Whenever a guilty verdict results in a criminal case, the defendant has an absolute right to appeal the case for a review of legal and factual issues by an appellate court.

At the appellate level, the case is largely a "paper case," without live witnesses or the presence of another jury.

Although it is often said that a defendant enjoys the right to appeal his or her case to the U.S. Supreme Court, such is not the case. The U.S. Supreme Court reviews selected criminal cases as a matter of judicial discretion and normally hears only those cases presenting important constitutional issues.

State and Federal Jurisdiction and Interests

The overwhelming majority of criminal cases are tried in state courts, because such cases exclusively affect intrastate interests. The Tenth Amendment to the U.S. Constitution reserves the general "police power" to the states as follows:

The powers not delegated to the United States by the Constitution, nor prohibited by it to the States, are reserved to the States respectively, or to the people.[12]

Federal criminal courts try cases involving criminal activity having interstate, national, or international effects, such as drug and mail fraud cases, crimes committed on federal installations and against federal officials, and immigration cases, among others. Federal criminal and civil procedure may differ greatly from that of state court systems.

Remedies and Sentencing Principles

In civil tort legal system, the principal purpose of a liability award in a given case is to make a tort victim "whole." Remedies in tort are relatively flexible and are largely based on judicial precedent guided by the principle of *stare decisis*.[13] In the criminal legal system, however, remedies are primarily based on statute and are more formalized for specific offenses. In fact, criminal court judges may be required to comply with relatively rigid sentencing guidelines (as in the federal system) when sentencing criminal defendants.

In a criminal case, the remedy awarded reflects societal needs and concerns, as well as any impact on individual victims of crime. The criminal law equivalent to the civil remedy of monetary damages is incarceration, or the threat of incarceration (probation) of a criminal defendant. A criminal sentence serves to make society whole, in a sense, by punishing the criminal wrongdoer.

The factors that are considered in arriving at a criminal sentence, referred to as *sentencing principles*, reflect societal needs for:

- retribution, or punishment of an offender, i.e., "just desserts"
- isolation of a dangerous offender from members of society
- specific deterrence of further criminal activity by a convicted criminal

- general deterrence of others who know of a criminal's conduct and might otherwise be tempted to emulate it
- rehabilitation of an offender to make him or her a productive member of society

A specific sentence in a given case reflects how a sentencing authority (judge or jury) weighs and prioritizes these sentencing principles. In addition to incarceration or probation, a criminal defendant may be ordered to make monetary restitution to a crime victim or to multiple victims. A convicted criminal may also face a criminal monetary fine as part of sentencing and risk the forfeiture of personal property and assets, either those used in the commission of a crime or those obtained with illicit assets as "fruits" of the crime.

Crimes in the Health Care Environment

Crimes of Violence

Assault and Battery

Criminal *assault and battery* are essentially the same under criminal law as under civil law. Assault involves the apprehension or fear, on the part of a victim, of impending unlawful harmful or offensive contact. Battery involves the unlawful application of harmful or offensive force, by a perpetrator, to the person of a victim.

A subclassification of criminal battery that too frequently arises as an allegation in the health care environment is criminal sexual battery. It may be defined as:

> any nonconsensual touching of a patient's or a health care provider's sexual or other body parts (or clothing) by the other party, for the purpose of arousing or gratifying the sexual desires of either party, or for the purpose of sexually abusing a patient.[14]

A health care provider facing an allegation, or multiple allegations, of sexual assault or battery incident to patient care may be required to defend him- or herself in criminal court, as well as in civil court, and before licensure boards and professional association ethics committees. Conviction of a health care professional of sexual assault or battery of a patient in a criminal trial provides overwhelming evidence that can be introduced against the provider in civil and administrative proceedings.

Robbery

Robbery may be defined as the unlawful, forcible taking of a victim's property from the person of the victim. Robbery is distinguished from other unlawful seizures of property, such as larceny and burglary, in that (1) the property seized is taken directly from the person of the victim (as in a mugging), and (2) there is involved the use or threat of force. Thus, theft of property that occurs while a victim is asleep—a hospital patient, for example—would not constitute robbery, since no force is used or threatened. Similarly, when a pickpocket lifts a victim's wallet—in the hospital or in any other setting—the crime committed is larceny, but not robbery. A criminal charge of robbery may be elevated from simple to aggravated robbery if a deadly weapon is brandished during the crime or if the victim suffers serious injury during the unlawful taking of the victim's property.

Homicide

Homicide literally means the killing of one human being by another. Many patient deaths occur in health care settings. Most patient deaths, however, do not give rise to criminal charges against health care professionals. Some patient deaths facilitated by health care professionals, however, such as through the unlawful practice of *active euthanasia*, may give rise to criminal prosecution. There have been many publicized criminal cases against physicians[15] and other providers in recent years, the most notorious being the ongoing Michigan state court prosecutions against Dr. Jack Kevorkian, a pathologist, for alleged physician-assisted suicide. (As of the time this book was written, Kevorkian has yet to be convicted by a jury of unlawful homicide in the deaths of any of his terminally ill patients.) Health care providers responsible for the deaths of patients under their care may be charged criminally with any of the homicide offenses described below.

Murder *Murder* is the unlawful killing of a person (or of a fetus, in some states) with *malice aforethought* (i.e., with a predetermined, unlawful intent to kill). The Model Penal Code defines murder in the following way:

Criminal homicide constitutes murder when: (a) it is committed purposely or knowingly, or (b) it is committed recklessly under circumstances manifesting extreme indifference to the value of human life. Such recklessness and indifference are presumed if the actor is engaged or is an accomplice in the commission of, or is attempting to commit: robbery, rape or deviate sexual intercourse by force or threat of force, arson, burglary, kidnapping or felonious escape.[16]

In addition to a specific intent to murder, the state of mind of extreme criminal negligence constituting a "depraved heart" can be a basis for conviction for murder.

Manslaughter *Manslaughter* involves a less culpable state of mind than murder and can be defined as an unlawful homicide without *malice*, or the specific intent to kill the victim. This crime can be subdivided into voluntary and involuntary manslaughter.

Voluntary Voluntary manslaughter involves a victim's death that occurs during the commission of some unlawful act, such as during a fight arising from the "heat of passion."[17] The death of a patient during an illegal abortion would probably give rise to a charge of voluntary manslaughter against a physician performing the abortion.

Involuntary Involuntary manslaughter occurs when a victim dies during the (reckless) commission of a lawful act.[18] Consider the following hypothetical example.

A patient with extensive third-degree burns is being treated by a physical therapist in a whirlpool tub. A radio is positioned by the therapist on the edge of the tub to distract the patient's attention during debridement. If the radio falls into the water, causing the electrocution death of the patient, the most likely unlawful homicide charge against the physical therapist would be involuntary manslaughter, since the patient's death arguably occurred during the (reckless) commission of an otherwise lawful act.

Negligent Homicide *Negligent homicide* involves the death of victim caused by another person, where the latter's conduct constitutes gross negligence. Gross negligence is conduct that falls well below the standards established by law for the reasonable protection of others. As with involuntary manslaughter, in criminally negligent homicide, the perpetrator displays neither wanton depravity nor any specific intent to kill another human being. Most homicide charges lodged against health care professionals for patient deaths are labeled as criminally negligent homicide.

Nonviolent Crimes

Fortunately for patient safety and the safety of others, most criminal activity that occurs in health care settings involves the commission of nonviolent, or so-called "white-collar" offenses. However, nonviolent crime arguably has an equally devastating impact as violent crime does on society in general and on business in particular. The following are selected examples of nonviolent crimes that affect business (including the business of health care delivery).

Burglary

Burglary is now defined as the unlawful breaking and entry (trespass) onto another person's property with the specific intent to commit a felony crime on the victim's premises. While the felony crime intended to be committed may be a violent offense, most often the intended felony is larceny. An example of burglary is where a thief breaks into a health care clinic at night to steal a computer that is visible through a closed window. As with robbery, a burglary charge can be elevated to *aggravated burglary* if a deadly weapon is used in commission of the crime.

Larceny

Larceny is defined as the unlawful taking of another person's property with the intent to permanently deprive the true owner of its use. Threshold amounts for the value of property taken determine whether the crime to be charged is a misdemeanor (*petit larceny*) or a felony (*grand larceny*). Shoplifting is a form of larceny, as is stealing a vehicle (*grand theft auto*).

Embezzlement

Embezzlement is theft of money or other property by someone in a *fiduciary* (special trust) relationship with the victim. Unlike in larceny, the embezzler is in lawful possession or engaged in lawful use of the victim's property at some point. While the eventual return of the victim's property may operate in *extenuation and mitigation* to reduce the severity of a criminal sentence, the crime of embezzlement is complete once the wrongful misappropriation occurs.

Employment and Reimbursement Fraud

Fraud in any setting involves the unlawful misrepresentation of a material fact, specifically intended to deceive a victim and cause him or her to act to the victim's detriment. The U.S. General Accounting Office (GAO) estimates that the health care system loses ten percent of gross revenues (or $100 billion annually) to fraud.[19] Since 1992, the federal Department of Justice has reported a 76-percent increase in the number of criminal health care fraud cases filed and a 76-percent increase in the conviction rate. On the civil side of the ledger, fraud settlements and judgments garnered by federal litigators have increased 140 percent since 1992.[20]

While most health care fraud involves active misrepresentation to third-party payers of health care (non)delivery, passive fraud is of growing concern, especially under managed care models. Passive managed care health fraud (more accurately "abuse") involves deliberate underprovision of health care to plan beneficiaries to prop up profits. This area of fraud and abuse is more difficult to investigate, ferret out, and eliminate. However, state and federal agencies are making slow, incremental progress against it.

An interesting example of (pre)employment fraud involved Eugene Roscoe, who purportedly was a physical therapist. Mr. Roscoe reportedly "earned" over $100,000 per year from job interviews. He allegedly undertook job interviews in 38 states before his arrest in Houston, Texas. Reportedly, Roscoe, age 55, was never licensed.[21]

Corporate Crime

Perhaps the fiercest weapon that federal law enforcement authorities have in the fight against corporate crime—violent and nonviolent—is RICO, or the Racketeer Influenced and Corrupt Organizations Act,[22] which Congress enacted as part of the Organized Crime Control Act of 1970. Although authorities reasonably debate the intended scope for RICO, it has been used successfully to curb organized crime's encroachment into legitimate business—including health care delivery. RICO makes interstate "racketeering" activity a federal felony crime that may be prosecuted anyplace along the trail of criminal activity. "Racketeering" includes the unlawful commission (or *conspiracy* [unlawful agreement] to commit) of two or more of 26 enumerated federal felonies or nine specified state-law offenses.[23] In addition to criminal prosecution under RICO, the government and private individuals may sue defendants civilly for monetary damages.

Chapter Summary

The application of criminal law to health care has received ever-increasing attention in recent years. Out of a single act or omission—such as the wrongful injury to or death of a patient, a health care professional can face legal action in civil and criminal court, as well as adverse administrative action before licensure boards and professional associations.

A criminal act almost always requires culpable conduct (*actus reus*) and a culpable state of mind (*mens rea*) to subject a defendant to possible criminal liability. Both violent (e.g., sexual battery) and nonviolent (e.g., reimbursement fraud) criminal offenses are on the rise in the health care environment, as are federal and state investigatory and prosecutorial efforts. The RICO (Racketeer Influenced and Corrupt Organizations) federal statute has given criminal prosecutors a most formidable weapon to brandish and use in the fight against health care fraud and other related racketeering activities.

Cases and Questions

1. *A*, a physical therapist in one state, is solicited by *B*, a physician practicing nearby in an adjacent state, to defraud Medicare and Medicaid through phony billing for patient services. *A* agrees to take part in the plan. What are the consequences when *A* is caught?

2. *C*, an occupational therapy aide, is working on a neurosurgical ward, when suddenly *D*, a closed-head injury patient, begins to physically attack *E*, a licensed practical nurse. *C* screams for help, but no one is nearby. *C* then tries to forcibly remove *D* from his position on top of *E*, but to no avail. Finally, sensing that *E* is in imminent danger of losing her life, *C* breaks a chair over *D*'s head, killing *D*. Is *C* liable for murder?

Suggested Answers to Cases and Questions

1. *A* has committed two offenses: conspiracy (unlawful agreement) to defraud Medicare and fraud. Because these are interstate crimes, prosecutors may be aided by the federal RICO statute in prosecuting *A* under a racketeering, or "criminal enterprise," theory. If convicted, *A* also faces adverse licensure administrative action and adverse action by *A*'s professional association for ethics violations, as well as mandatory exclusion from participation as a provider in federal health programs (assuming that *A* still has a professional license).

2. *C* is not guilty of murder or of any crime involving unlawful homicide. *C* acted lawfully in defending *E* against deadly force. *D*'s death was justifiable homicide. No criminal or adverse administrative action should result. *C* should also prevail if charged civilly with wrongful death on the same grounds.

References

1. Violence in the American workplace is a most serious human resources management problem. Since 1980, an average of 750 people per year have been victims of homicide in work settings, making homicide the third leading cause of occupational deaths. Seventy-five percent of workplace homicides are committed with firearms. Solomon, J., King, P. "Waging War in the Workplace." *Newsweek*, July 19, 1993, pp. 30–34. Perhaps the most infamous workplace crime in U.S. history (at the time of the writing of this book) was the suspected domestic terrorist bombing of the Alfred P. Murrah Federal Building, Oklahoma City, Oklahoma, in April 1995, that resulted in 169 deaths and more than 500 injuries. Two defendants, Timothy J. McVeigh and Terry Lynn Nichols, await trial on murder and terrorism charges stemming from this incident. Gerlin, A. "The Oklahoma City Bombing: Did They Kill 169 People? The Accused Terrorists Come to Trial." *Wall Street Journal*, February 1, 1996, p. B1.

2. Adapted from *Black's Law Dictionary*, 5th ed. St. Paul, MN: West Publishing Company, 1979, p. 334.

3. For example, the crime of *statutory rape*, or carnal knowledge of a (usually female) child (consensual sex with a legal minor) is punishable (in most states) even if the adult party made a legitimate and reasonable mistake as to the minor's status as a minor. Valid and reasonable mistake of age eliminates *mens rea*. However, conviction under such circumstances is justified by basing it on social policy disfavoring sexual relations between adults and minors.

4. *Moral turpitude* describes intentionally wrongful *mala in se* criminal conduct that violates public standards of moral decency. Crimes of moral turpitude evince heinousness, vileness, and depravity. These crimes include offenses such as nonconsensual sexual relations (ranging from intercourse to lewd and lascivious behavior) between health care professionals and patients and consensual or nonconsensual sexual activity between adults and young children. Traditionally, conviction of crimes of moral turpitude was alone a legitimate basis for adverse action affecting professional licensure and health professional association membership. Now, though, the precise definition of "moral turpitude" is so difficult to articulate that it may be successfully challenged as unconstitutionally "vague" when it is invoked as a basis for adverse professional actions.

5. Perkins, R. *Perkins on Criminal Law*, 2nd ed. Mineola, NY: Foundation Press, 1969, p. 9.

6. See generally Model Penal Code, American Law Institute, 1962.

7. The malpractice plaintiff's name in the case caption, *Smith by Smith*, indicates that Smith, a legal representative (e.g., parent or guardian) is bringing suit on behalf of Smith, the *real party in interest*.

8. Model Penal Code, American Law Institute, Section 4:01.

9. See *M'Naghten's Case*, 8 Eng. Rep. 718 (1843).

10. See *Miranda v. Arizona*, 384 U.S. 436 (U.S. Supreme Court, Chief Justice Earl Warren, 1966).

11. Baird, P.D. "Critics Must Confess, Miranda Was the Right Decision." *Wall Street Journal,* June 13, 1991, p. A19.

12. U.S. Constitution, Tenth Amendment, 1791.

13. *Stare decisis* is Latin for "the decision stands," and, as a legal principle, requires lower courts within a jurisdiction to abide by the prior judicial pronouncements of

higher-level courts within the jurisdiction, applicable to the same or similar facts. Only where constitutional or statutory law, or public policy considerations, require it, will case precedent normally be overturned.

14. Adapted from Model Penal Code Section and Colorado Revised Statutes, Section 18-3-401(4).
15. See, e.g., Kuriansky, E.J. (In Letters to the Editor). "The Doctor as Criminal." *Wall Street Journal,* March 13, 1995, p. A19; Crane, M. "Practice Medicine, Land in Jail." *Wall Street Journal*, February 21, 1995, p. A24 (describing the conviction of internist Dr. Gerald Einaugler of New York City for criminally negligent homicide, for the negligent delay in admitting a patient to the hospital with end-stage renal disease. Dr. Einaugler was sentenced to serve 52 consecutive weekends in confinement at Riker's Island State Prison. His conviction is on appeal.)
16. Model Penal Code, American Law Institute, Section 210.2.
17. Model Penal Code, American Law Institute, Section 210.3(1)(b).
18. Model Penal Code, American Law Institute, Section 210.3(1)(a).
19. "Legislation and Regulations: Fraud Crackdown in Health Care." *Advance for Physical Therapists,* July 17, 1995, pp. 4, 17.
20. *Ibid.* at 17.
21. Harlan, C. "He Apparently Succeeded Better Than Most of Us at Avoiding Work." *Wall Street Journal*, March 14, 1991, p. B1.
22. See Title 18, United States Code Sections 1961 *et. seq.*
23. *Ibid.* at Section (1)(A).

Suggested Readings

1. Harlan, C. "He Apparently Succeeded Better Than Most of Us at Avoiding Work." *Wall Street Journal*, March 14, 1991, p. B1.
2. "Health Care Fraud Convictions Up 73 Percent." *Advance for Physical Therapists*, March 27, 1995, p. 20.
3. "Legislation and Regulations: Fraud Crackdown in Health Care." *Advance for Physical Therapists*, July 17, 1995, pp. 4, 17.
4. Model Penal Code, American Law Institute, 1962.
5. Perkins, R. *Perkins on Criminal Law*, 2nd ed. Mineola, NY: Foundation Press, 1969.
6. Pozgar, G.D. *Legal Aspects of Health Care Administration*, 5th ed. Gaithersburg, MD: Aspen Publishers, Inc., 1993, Ch. 3.
7. Scott, R.W. *Health Care Malpractice: A Primer on Legal Issues for Professionals.* Thorofare, NJ: Slack, Inc., 1990, pp. 9–11.
8. Scott, R.W. *Legal Aspects of Documenting Patient Care.* Gaithersburg, MD: Aspen Publishers, Inc., 1994, pp. 17–18.
9. Title 18, United States Code Sections 1961 *et. seq.*
10. U.S. Constitution.

Chapter 7

Education Law

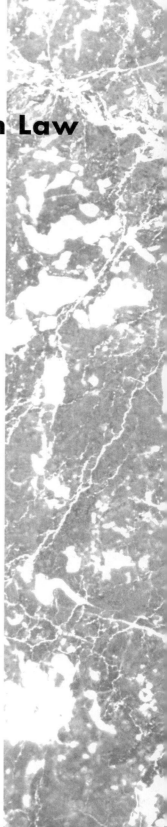

Τhis chapter introduces basic concepts related to legal aspects of educational processes. Important federal statutory law, including Title IX of the 1972 Educational Amendments, Title VI of the Civil Rights Act of 1964, the Buckley Amendment, the Individuals with Disabilities Education Act (IDEA), and the Americans with Disabilities Act (ADA, Titles II and III) are discussed. Legal and ethical issues associated with academic discipline and dismissal are explored, as are such issues as they relate to the admissions process. The chapter concludes with a discussion of legal responsibility for health professional student conduct in the clinic.

Introduction

Education, training, and development are related concepts that, in health care education and delivery systems, affect the conduct of academicians, professional students, clinical and administrative professionals, and support personnel. The process of "education" involves the acquisition of general or specific knowledge with or without specific learning goals. "Training," on the other hand, encompasses the acquisition of job-specific or other ADL-related proficiency skills. "Development" embraces the furtherance of knowledge or skill either under education or training.

It is commonly believed that there is a constitutional right to public education in the United States. While there may be such a right under selected state constitutions, there is no express right to public education in the federal Constitution. Under federal law, educational rights largely fall under limited federal statutes addressing educational issues within the restricted domain of federal jurisdiction (interests). Other federal educational rights derive from case law based on interpretation of federal constitutional provisions such as equal protection, privacy, and due process.

Education law is comprised of both federal and state laws. Education law may be grounded in federal and/or state constitutions, statutes, case law, and administrative rules and regulations.

Selected Federal Statutes Impacting Education

Congress has enacted a number of statutes designed to assist state and local government educational agencies to meet the many special needs of students at all levels in the education process—preschool, elementary, secondary, collegiate, graduate, and professional. For example, the Elementary and Secondary Education Act of 1965[1] (as amended) addresses bilingual and drug education, high school completion, and other issues within the purview of interests of the federal government.

Other federal statutes place specific mandates on the states, based on federal constitutional authority, including equal protection, privacy, due process, and Congress's plenary power to regulate interstate commerce. Title VI of the Civil Rights Act of 1964,[2] for example, prohibits discrimination against students by schools receiving federal financial assistance (i.e., almost all schools) on the basis of race or national origin. The statute reads:

> No person in the United States shall, on the ground of race, color, or national origin, be excluded from participation in, be denied the benefits of, or be subjected to discrimination under any program or activity receiving Federal financial assistance.

Title IX of the Educational Amendments of 1972,[3] patterned after Title VI of the Civil Rights Act of 1964, prohibits gender discrimination in educational programs and activities that receive federal funds. This law, enacted in the same year that gender was added as a protected class to the Civil Rights Act of 1964, was intended to "round out" federal educational antidiscrimination policy by including as prohibited conduct gender discrimination in educational programs and activities receiving federal dollars. The statute reads in pertinent part:

> Section 1681(a). No person in the United States shall, on the basis of sex, be excluded from participation in, be denied the benefits of, or be subjected to discrimination under any education program or activity receiving Federal financial assistance, except that:
> (1) in regards to admissions to educational institutions, this section shall apply only to institutions of vocational education, professional education, and graduate higher education, and to public institutions of undergraduate higher education;
> (2) in regards to admissions to educational institutions, this section shall not apply . . . (B) for seven years from the date an educational institution begins the process of changing from being an institution which admits only students of one sex to being an institution which admits students of both sexes. . . .

(3) this section shall not apply to an educational institution which is controlled by a religious organization if the application of this subsection would not be consistent with the religious tenets of such organization;

(4) this section shall not apply to an educational institution whose primary purpose is the training of individuals for the military service of the United States, or the merchant marine;

. . .

(h) this section shall not apply to membership practices—(A) of a social fraternity or social sorority which is exempt from taxation under section 501(a) of Title 26, the active membership of which consists primarily of students in attendance at an institution of higher education, or (B) of the Young Men's Christian Association, Young Women's Christian Association, Girl Scouts, Boy Scouts, Camp Fire Girls, and voluntary youth service organizations which are so exempt, the membership of which has traditionally been limited to persons of one sex and principally to persons of less than nineteen years of age. . . .

While there was initially some ambiguity over whether only specific programs receiving federal funds or entire educational institutions were bound not to discriminate on the basis of gender, this issue was resolved in 1987 when Congress enacted the Civil Rights Restoration Act,[4] which applied Title IX to entire institutions, not just to specific programs or activities receiving federal funds. Subsequent federal case law applied Title IX protections not just to female students, but to female faculty and staff as well.

The Family Educational Rights and Privacy Act of 1974,[5] popularly known as the Buckley Amendment, established uniform standards for educational institutions concerning the privacy of student records. This federal statute was enacted contemporaneously with the federal Privacy and the Freedom of Information Acts[6] which regulate the confidentiality of and access to information about individuals in the possession of the federal government. The Buckley Amendment gave students and their parents access to official school records and the right to challenge the accuracy of information contained in them. It also required that student records be kept confidential and that they be released only with the written consent of students over age 18 or of parents of students under age 18.

This law also established a five-year retention requirement for official student records. Clinical affiliation reports on health professional students are official student records for purposes of the Buckley Amendment.

Under case law interpreting the Buckley Amendment, personal notes made by teachers about students are not considered to be official education records and are exempt from maintenance and disclosure requirements. Case law also established as permissible practice the posting of student grades on examinations, so long as students cannot be individually identified in such postings.

The Education for All Handicapped Children Act of 1975 (EHA)[7] was one of the first federal statutes to address the educational needs of disabled children. Signed into law by President Ford, EHA mandated equal educational opportunity for disabled children between the ages of three and 21. This statute was subsequently amended and eventually incorporated into a successor federal statute entitled the Individuals with Disabilities Education Act of 1990 (IDEA).[8]

The Individuals with Disabilities Education Act of 1990 built upon the Rehabilitation Act of 1973, Section 504[9] and EHA by specifically enumerating qualifying disabilities in children. IDEA clearly established the right of disabled children to free public education without any legal burden on their parents to show demonstrable benefit from it.

IDEA established the concept of inclusion ("mainstreaming") of physically and mentally challenged students into regular classes and other educational experiences to the extent feasible, in order to optimally normalize the education of disabled students. Under the law, individualized student educational program plans must be developed. School districts are also required to provide supportive "related services" to disabled students including transportation services; assistive technology devices; medical, psychological, physical, and occupational therapy; and audiology and speech-language evaluative services required to assist disabled students to benefit from special education.[10]

IDEA is pending reauthorization before the 104th Congress. In an era of cost containment, possible looming cuts in IDEA's budget include overall funding cuts and reduction or elimination of funding for "related services," including evaluative therapy services.[11]

The Equal Access Act of 1984,[12] enacted into law by Congress during President Ronald Reagan's first term, made public (secondary) schools into limited public fora by requiring that schools that receive federal funds allow use of their facilities for religious extracurricular clubs and activities, if they allow them for nonreligious extracurricular clubs and activities. The statute reads in pertinent part:

It shall be unlawful for any public secondary school which receives Federal financial assistance and which has a limited open forum to deny equal access or a fair opportunity to, or [to] discriminate against, *any* students who wish to conduct a meeting within that limited open forum on the basis of *religious, political, philosophical, or other content of the speech* at such meetings. [emphasis added]

The Americans with Disabilities Act of 1990 (ADA)[13] (discussed in greater detail in Chapter 8) was a landmark federal civil rights statute which empowered 43 million disabled Americans. It mandated equality in opportunity for them in employment

(Title I), and access to public services (including education) and public transportation services (Title II), public accommodations and services operated by private entities (Title III), and telecommunications services (Title IV). The ADA expanded the scope of the Rehabilitation Act of 1973 to include under its jurisdiction all business entities, in the public and private sectors, having 15 or more employees.

The ADA expressly excluded from protection the following classes of individuals: current users of illegal drugs[14] (except under supervision of a licensed health care professional) and/or alcohol, compulsive gamblers, klepto- and pyromaniacs, homosexuals, bisexuals, transvestites, transsexuals, exhibitionists, voyeurs, pedophiles, and those persons affected by other gender identity or sexual behavioral disorders.[15] The Rehabilitation Act of 1973 was similarly amended to exclude these conditions from the definition of "handicap."[16]

There have been a number of reported judicial ADA higher education cases.[17] Issues addressed include accommodation of testees in admissions tests, student disabilities unknown to school officials, requirements for sign language interpreters for deaf students, and the nature of "undue (financial) hardship" regarding modifications to school sites for disabled students. In general, if educational institutions take reasonable measures to accommodate known student disabilities so as to give qualified disabled students and applicants equal opportunity vis-a-vis nondisabled students and applicants, then they are complying with both the letter and spirit of Titles II and III of the ADA, as applicable.

> **Hint** *Under the ADA, educational institutions are required to take reasonable measures to accommodate known student disabilities, so as to give qualified disabled students and applicants equal opportunity in admissions, education, and services vis-a-vis nondisabled students and applicants.*

Federal Education Law Premised on Federal Constitutional Protections

Federal and applicable state constitutional protections apply to people and actions in school settings with equal force as to any other place or circumstances. *Due process* of law, applicable to the states under the Fourteenth Amendment and to the federal government under the Fifth Amendment, requires that school officials treat students with substantive fairness in all aspects of educational processes, and particularly, that they procedurally give adequate notice to students and their parents or guardians of potential adverse administrative actions (such as suspension or expulsion) and afford students an opportunity to be heard on such issues before final decisions are made. The amount of "process" that is "due" turns on the severity of the disciplinary action in issue.

Equal protection under law, also applicable to the states under the Fourteenth Amendment and to the federal government under the Fifth Amendment, requires (at least) that school officials treat similarly-situated students in a similar way. The Equal Protection Clause of the Fourteenth Amendment was a post-Civil War federal constitutional amendment designed to eliminate government-endorsed racial discrimination in the United States.

While the "similarly situated" standard applies to treatment of students generally by school officials, school actions or policies that intentionally discriminate against, or even have a disparate adverse impact upon protected minorities—including women and racial or ethnic minorities—are judged by courts under higher standards of review. Actions that adversely impact women, for example, such as the creation or maintenance of all-male schools or programs, must be proven to be substantially related to important governmental interests in order to survive judicial scrutiny. In recent times, all-male educational institutions of higher learning have become all but nonexistent, because they cannot meet this intermediate-tier legal standard of scrutiny.

School actions or policies that discriminate against students on the basis of race/ethnicity or religion are judged under the highest judicial standard of review. In order to be upheld, such actions or policies must directly advance compelling state interests, such as the preservation of life, health, or public safety. Because no school policy conceivably is justifiable under this highest-tier judicial standard of review, public school-based racial and religious discrimination, such as the maintenance of racially segregated schools,[18] is prohibited.

The constitutional right of (student) *privacy* applies with nearly equal force in the school setting as in other settings. The courts have ruled that the right of privacy under the Fourth Amendment applies in school settings. However, they have also held that, in order to conduct searches of students or their property, school officials need have only *reasonable* ("common sense") *suspicion* of wrongdoing, not *probable cause* (i.e., substantial, objective, credible evidence that a particular suspect committed a specific offense), which is the higher standard of justification required for searches by police.

The First Amendment to the Constitution simultaneously requires the official separation of church and state and governmental tolerance of the free exercise of individual and group religious beliefs. The balance struck between these two dichotomous mandates is that no religious instruction (of any faith) may be included in official public educational curricula, yet to the extent that secular extracurricular activities are supported by schools, religious activities must be supported as well.

Academic Disciplinary Issues Involving Health Professional Students

Official conduct on the part of public university faculty and administration are considered "state action," triggering the protections of individual liberty and property interests under the federal Constitution. Constitutional safeguards entitle public university students facing academic disciplinary action to both substantive and procedural due process protection in adjudication of their cases. Under substantive due process, the key question is, "Does the student facing discipline have a protected property or liberty interest in continued, unconditional enrollment in the institution of higher learning?" The procedural due process question is, "Was the student given clear notice of specific academic or disciplinary noted deficiencies and a reasonable opportunity to respond to charges?" An additional procedural due process question for courts on reviews may be, "Was the deficient student afforded a reasonable opportunity to improve his or her performance prior to execution of adverse administrative action?"

Disciplinary actions taken by private universities against students are subject to less judicial scrutiny than in public settings. Because there is no "state action" with private university actions, the questions to be answered on judicial review of private university disciplinary actions against students are, "Did the private university have reasonable academic disciplinary rules in place and well-publicized? Did the university follow its own procedures in deciding whether to discipline or dismiss a student for academic or disciplinary reasons?

There have been several noted legal cases concerning the propriety of academic dismissal by colleges and universities. In all of the following cases, courts displayed substantial deference to the professional judgments of school administrators and faculty.

In *Board of Curators of the University of Missouri* v. *Horowitz*,[19] the U.S. Supreme Court reviewed an academic dismissal decision involving a medical student from a state university. The student in question failed a major examination and reportedly had a poor overall academic record. In finding in favor of the university on both procedural and substantive due process grounds, the court found that the student had adequate notice of poor academic performance and reasonable opportunities for improvement, and that the school's decision to dismiss the student was careful, deliberate, and fair. The opinion held that:

> *Like the decision of an individual professor as to the proper grade for a student in his course, the determination whether to dismiss a student for academic reasons requires an expert evaluation of cumulative information as is not readily adapted to the procedural tools of judicial or administrative decisionmaking. . . . Courts are particularly ill-equipped to evaluate academic performance.*[20]

In a concurring opinion, Justice Powell added that "university faculty must have the widest range of discretion in making judgments as to the academic performance of students."[21]

In *Regents of the University of Michigan* v. *Ewing*,[22] the U.S. Supreme Court again deferred to academicians in affirming the academic dismissal of a medical student attending a state university Inteflex (combined undergraduate and medical education) program. In this case, the student was dismissed after failing an NBME (National Board of Medical Examiners) qualifying examination for clinical rotations after his fourth year of study. Because the dismissal was based on the student's overall academic record, it was deemed to be fair and not arbitrary and capricious, as the student had claimed.

In *Tobias* v. *University of Texas*,[23] the Texas Court of Appeals reviewed the case of a nursing student who was dismissed for academic deficiency after twice failing a required course entitled "Nursing During the Childbearing Experience." The student appealed his failing grades through academic channels, invoking the university's grievance procedure outlined in its catalog. When he was not permitted to take the course for a third time, the former student sued the university (and three professors individually, as state officials, under 42 U.S.C. Section 1983, for violation of his civil rights), claiming due process and equal protection violations under the federal and Texas constitutions and breach of contract. The appellate court affirmed the lower court decision of summary judgment in favor of the university, rejecting all of the former student's claims. In his opinion, Justice Lattimore held that:

> *Substantive due process protection in the academic arena protects an individual from actions that are arbitrary and capricious. A judge may not override the faculty's professional judgment in academic affairs unless [their judgment] is such a substantial departure from accepted academic norms as to demonstrate that the person or committee responsible did not actually exercise professional judgment. Where a reviewing court has found* minimal *[emphasis added] evidence of professional judgment, such evidence has been considered sufficient to justify judgment against a student as a matter of law.*

Based on the case decisions cited above, the following risk management measures are recommended for health care professional collegiate programs, in order to protect student, faculty, and administration rights and to minimize litigation exposure incident to student disciplinary actions.

- Identify deficient academic performance by a student as early as possible, and promptly notify the affected student.

- Afford reasonable opportunity for the student to be heard on the matter. (These first two elements together constitute "procedural due process.")

- Offer the deficient student specific recommendations for improvement. Explain the adverse consequences of continued unsatisfactory performance. Allow adequate time for remediation and improvement.

- Have in place in the institution, clear, well-disseminated standards for minimally acceptable academic and clinical performance on the part of students. Have in place grievance and appeals processes for student use. Always follow these processes when adjudicating cases. Post procedures for filing grievances and appeals of adverse actions in institutional catalogs and/or student handbooks.

- Consider (after consulting with institutional legal counsel) including a disclaimer in catalogs and handbooks that no contractual agreement concerning student continuation in, or graduation from, the institution exists as a result of catalog or handbook information or language.

- Document student counseling sessions. Maintain documentation in a secure location.

- Involve institutional legal counsel in student disciplinary matters *ab initio.*

Academic Admissions Issues

The same considerations concerning student constitutional and common law rights that apply to academic disciplinary processes also apply to admissions decisions in public institutions, including substantive and procedural due process, equal protection, and antidiscrimination considerations. Because admissions to public colleges and universities constitute "state action," admissions committees, their staff, and institutional administration must ensure that processes are fundamentally fair to all applicants.

Under Title VI of the Civil Rights Act of 1964,[24] certain questions on applications and in interviews are prohibited, including questions about:

- race or ethnicity
- religious affiliation or beliefs
- nationality
- marital status
- existence of dependent family members
- perceived disabilities
- military discharge classification
- economic status

In addition to inquiries prohibited by law, certain questions and comments should not be asked or made, because they can reasonably be misconstrued as discriminatory. For example, avoid:

- offering compliments, criticism, or suggestions about personal appearance

- questions concerning foreign language ability or region of the state or country in which an applicant grew up

- inquiring about social organizations that the applicant may belong to, unless directly related to the applicant's abilities as a health professional

During interviews of multiple applicants, remember to ask each applicant questions from the same basic shell of questions, allowing some latitude for specific inquiries to individual applicants. This promotes uniform treatment of applicants and should meet the equal protection requirement to treat similarly situated people similarly.

Liability for Student Conduct in Clinical Settings

An important consideration for academic and clinical faculty who supervise health professional students is who bears legal responsibility for liability-generating conduct on the part of students. Faculty and clinical supervisors may incur primary liability for their own liability-generating conduct that results in patient injury. One or more of them may also be vicariously, or indirectly, liable for student liability-generating conduct, even when faculty and supervisors themselves do not directly cause patient injury.

Any licensed or certified health care professional who has the legal duty to care for a patient may be primarily liable for physical and mental injury incurred by a patient as a result of (1) professional negligence (substandard care delivery), (2) intentional (mis)conduct, (3) breach of a contractual therapeutic promise made to a patient, and (4) patient injury that results from the use of a dangerously defective modality or product. A clinical faculty member who supervises the official activities of students, assistants, aids, and others, may be vicariously, or indirectly, liable for patient injury resulting from the liability-generating conduct of these persons when it occurs within the scope of their employment or affiliation.

The party vicariously liable for health professional student conduct usually is the party who has accepted such legal responsibility under a clinical affiliation agreement, or contract. The clinical affiliation contract should clearly delineate the scope of vicarious liability for both the clinical site and the academic institution and should only be created in close consultation with both parties' legal counsel. As an additional protective measure for both clinical site and school, such a contract may also include express language that memorializes the mutual understanding of the parties that the academic institution will send to the clinical site only those students who are adequately prepared to participate in clinical experiences.

In the absence of clear contractual language spelling out who (or rather whose liability insurer) is responsible for student conduct, a court may invoke a common-law doctrine called the "borrowed servant rule" to assign liability, based on whose interests (the school or site) the student was primarily serving at the time of an adverse patient incident.

In addition to vicarious liability, clinical sites and academic institutions may incur primary liability for their own negligence in supervising and preparing students who injure patients, respectively. An academic institution, for example, may incur primary liability for the negligent instruction or academic preparation of a student and/or for the negligent or intentional misrepresentation of a student's competency or status.

A clinical instructor (CI) or site may incur primary liability for the negligent failure to review a referral order, a patient's treatment records, or a student's evaluation note before allowing the student to treat a patient. CIs and sites may also be primarily liable for the negligent failure to provide on-site and, when appropriate, direct supervision of a student during patient intake, evaluation, and treatment. State practice acts usually define the degree of supervision of students required of CIs.

Failure to supervise primary liability is often couched in legal terms of art, such as patient or student abandonment. A CI who permits a health professional student to evaluate and/or care for patients without the degree of supervision required by law may face, in addition to civil malpractice liability, a criminal legal action for the aiding and abetting of physical therapy by an unlicensed practitioner, as well as possible adverse administrative action affecting professional licensure and professional association action for ethics violations.

Malpractice exposure may also occur when a CI imparts negligent instruction or guidance to a student that results in patient injury, or when there is a negligent or intentional failure to include students in systematic quality oversight activities, such as peer review of patient care activities carried out in the clinic.

Center coordinators for clinical education (CCCEs) and clinic managers must ensure that CIs thoroughly understand the rules of appropriate supervision of students. CIs must also exercise sound professional judgment when assigning patients to students, based on factors such as student competence and special considerations associated with particular patients.

It is essential that CIs review all student evaluations and countersign their notes (as required) before allowing students to carry out initial treatment of patients. This precaution helps to protect all participants in the treatment process—the patient, the student, the CI, and the clinical site. Because health professional students are not licensed providers, the "student note" is not valid without CI review and approval. The CI adopts, or is deemed legally to have adopted, all evaluation and treatment notes written by students under his or her supervision as his or her own notes. Whenever a health care malpractice case from an intervention involving a health professional student results in the payment of a monetary settlement or judgment, it is normally the supervising CI's name—and not the student's name—that is reported for permanent inclusion in the National Practitioner Data Bank.

CIs have not only the ethical responsibility, but also a legal duty to honestly and accurately evaluate and report on a health professional student's clinical performance to academic coordinators of clinical education (ACCEs). Any critical, candid comments about a student should be accurate, fair, objective, and well-supported by prior written counseling statements, in which the student was given clear notice of deficient performance, an opportunity to respond to the allegation(s), and the opportunity to remedy any deficiencies. A CI who misrepresents a student's level of competence may be held legally accountable for directly-related patient injury when that student enters professional practice.

Remember that federal and state statutory law and common law and customary practice require that clinical site personnel, as well as academicians, treat official information concerning health professional students as confidential. Everyone who has official knowledge about students and their performance must understand the gravity of this reponsibility and not disseminate confidential student information outside of the chain of those who have an official need to know, and the legal right to receive, the information.

Special Informed Consent Considerations When Students Are Involved in Patient Care

The basic legal and ethical rule is that all health care professionals have the duty to make sufficient disclosure of treatment-related information to patients so as to enable them to make informed choices about care. Informed consent to treatment is premised on respect for the patient rights of autonomy and self-determination.

The disclosure elements for legally sufficient patient informed consent to evaluation and treatment when students are involved in patient care include:

- the type of treatment recommended or ordered

- any material (decisional) risks of serious harm or complication associated with the proposed treatment

- the expected benefits of the proposed treatment, i.e., patient goals

- information about any reasonable alternatives to the proposed treatment, including their relative material risks and benefits

- the identification and role of a student or students in the patient's evaluation and treatment

In addition to the above disclosure elements, the health professional clinician must solicit and satisfactorily answer all patient questions about the treatment process. CIs should remember that it is their personal legal responsibility—not the student's—to obtain patient informed consent to treatment. (Similarly, this professional responsibility cannot legally be delegated to assistants, aids, or others.)

Student Responsibility

A student is always personally legally responsible for his or her own negligence or wrongdoing in the clinic. A student may be singularly responsible for patient injury when the student fails to comply with clear and reasonable instructions given by his or her CI. A student also may be held singularly liable when the student engages in reckless or malicious injurious conduct.

Just as with licensed health care professionals, students may be (and have been) charged with committing, against patients, intentional liability-generating misconduct. For example, a student may commit or be accused of battery (inappropriate or offensive touching of a patient), defamation (false assertions about a patient that harm the patient's good personal reputation), invasion of patient privacy, breach of patient confidentiality, or sexual harassment and misconduct.

Liability Risk Management Strategies for Clinical Instructors and Affiliation Sites

The following clinical risk management strategies represent a basic framework of ideas, to which other strategies and practices may be added to form a comprehensive clinical risk management program.

Center coordinators of clinical education should consider implementing a policy that requires student affiliates to wear name badges that clearly identify them as health care professional students. Similarly, student-generated evaluation and treatment notation should bear, after the student's name, an identifier such as "SPT," "SOT," "PTA(S)," "COTA(S)," or whatever is appropriate.

Clinical site managers should also have a policy in place that assigns only seasoned clinicians as CCCEs and CIs. Information about the selection process and copies of documentation concerning specific selection of CCCE and CI personnel should be generated and retained as legal documents.

Upon their arrival to the clinic, CCCEs and/or CIs should thoroughly orient all students to the physical facility and its written policies, protocols, treatment guidelines, and other standardized operating procedures, before students are asked to commence even supervised patient evaluation and treatment. Similarly, students should be thoroughly oriented to clinic equipment and supplies that they may use in their patient care duties during their affiliations. The student orientation process itself should be documented in a procedures manual, and CCCEs should consider having students sign off that they have read and understand all applicable clinic policies and procedures and are familiar with clinic equipment.

Taking these minimally burdensome steps is not practicing defensive health care clinical education. These measures are established for the protection of all participants in the health care professional student clinical education process—students, clinical site, CCCE, CI, and, most importantly, patients.

Chapter Summary

As with professional health care clinical practice, the academic and clinical components of health care professional student education are governed by legal and ethical rules of conduct, with which academicians and clinical faculty and managers are bound to comply. This chapter overviews important federal statutes, case law, and risk management strategies for minimizing liability exposure in academic and clinical education settings.

Governmental influence over public education (at all levels) resides primarily with state governments, but with strong federal influence. Significant federal educational statutes have been enacted in recent decades. The Civil Rights Act of 1964, Title VI, mandates nondiscrimination on the basis of race or national origin in educational programs and activities that received federal funds. Title IX of the 1972 Educational Amendments added gender nondiscrimination to existing protections. The

Individuals with Disabilities Education Act of 1990 (IDEA) replaced the Education for All Handicapped Children Act of 1975, and established as national policy that students with disabilities are entitled to free, mainstreamed (whenever possible) public education. The Americans with Disabilities Act of 1990 (ADA) further codified the rights of the disabled in educational and all other public and private settings.

The Family Educational Rights and Privacy Act of 1974,[5] popularly known as the Buckley Amendment, established uniform standards for educational institutions concerning the privacy and maintenance of official student records. The Equal Access Act of 1984 made public educational institutions into limited public fora for purposes of access to its facilities by religious, political, and other extracurricular special-interest groups.

In addition to federal statutes, federal constitutional protections apply to governmental actions in educational settings. These rights include the right to due process of law (fairness, notice and opportunity to be heard), equal protection under the law, and the right to privacy.

Regarding academic discipline, educators and administrators must take reasonable steps to ensure that their reasonable disciplinary processes are disseminated to all those who potentially might be adversely affected by them, and, in particular, must abide by their own rules and policies when disciplining students. Before adverse administrative action against a student may be taken in public educational institutions, the student is entitled to due notice of an infraction and the opportunity to state his or her side of the case.

Responsibility for health care professional student liability-generating conduct in clinical settings is normally pre-established in clinical affiliation agreements or contracts. Students are always personally legally responsible for their own conduct. In addition to vicarious, or indirect, liability, academic faculty and institutions may be primarily liable for failing to adequately prepare students for clinical experiences. Clinical instructors and sites may incur primary liability for failing to or for negligently supervising students placed in their facilities.

Cases and Questions

1. *Z*, a CI at XYZ Community Hospital, conducts a cursory review of an evaluation note for a patient with a diagnosis of herniated lumbar disc lesion, L4-5, written by *X*, a student physical therapist. *X*'s proposed treatment plan includes the administration of Williams' flexion exercises, not the prone-lying extension exercises that were ordered by the referring neurosurgeon. *Z* countersigns *X*'s note. The treatment is carried out, resulting in acute exacerbation of the patient's right lower limb radicular signs and symptoms. As a result of the worsening of the patient's condition, the neurosurgeon performs a laminectomy-discectomy the next day. What are the liability issues in this scenario?

2. *A* is a physical therapy student on affiliation at ABC HealthCare, Inc., a one-therapist hand clinic. Her CI, *B*, wants to leave the clinic early today, to begin an overnight drive to a nearby city for a continuing education course that starts tomorrow. Can *B* legally leave *A* alone for two hours in the afternoon to treat only *A*'s existing patients, with instructions not to evaluate new ones? (Note: *A* is a senior student physical therapist, and functions virtually independently.)

3. *D*, an occupational therapy student on an internship at X-O Hospital, is not progressing well, in the viewpoint of his CI. The CI shares her concerns about *D*'s affective conduct with the school's ACCE, and indicates that she plans to fail the student for the affiliation, based primarily on his spotty attendance and poor attitude. The CI ends up passing *D*, without making any adverse comments on his evaluation sheet. The CI does, however, inform *C*'s future employer, with whom *D* is contractually bound to work after graduation, of her concerns about this student's affect. What are the liability issues in this scenario?

Suggested Answers to Cases and Questions

1. While *X* is personally legally responsible for his or her own negligence, *Z* also faces probable liability in this scenario. *Z* is primarily responsible for negligent supervision of *X*'s evaluation and negligent failure to check the referral order for specific instructions. Once *Z* countersigned *X*'s evaluation note, it became *Z*'s note for legal purposes.

2. *B* is legally and ethically obligated to supervise *A*. Failure to comply with these requirements may subject *B* to primary civil liability for professional negligence or intentional misconduct, criminal liability for aiding and abetting unlicensed professional practice, adverse administrative action affecting licensure, and professional association action for ethical misconduct. The last three types of actions may take place even if no patient injury resulted from *B*'s lack of supervision of *A*.

3. *D*'s CI had the legal and ethical duty to accurately report *D*'s performance during *D*'s affiliation. The CI violated this duty. The CI, however, had no right to discuss *D*'s alleged poor performance with *D*'s prospective employer. This breach of confidentiality violates the federal Buckley Amendment and constitutes a common law invasion of privacy (public disclosure of private facts).

References

1. The Elementary and Secondary Education Act of 1965, 20 United States Code Section 2701 *et. seq.*

2. The Civil Rights Act of 1964, Title VI, 42 United States Code Section 2000d-1.

3. Title IX of the Educational Amendments of 1972, 20 United States Code Sections 1681–1683.

4. The Civil Rights Restoration Act of 1987, 20 United States Code Section 1687.

5. The Family Educational Rights and Privacy Act of 1974, 20 United States Code Section 1232g.

6. 5 United States Code Section 552.

7. The Education for All Handicapped Children Act of 1975, 20 United States Code Section 1401.

8. The Individuals with Disabilities Education Act of 1990, 20 United States Code Sections 1400–1485.

9. The Vocational Rehabilitation Act of 1973, 29 United States Code Section 706(8), Section 504, which prohibits discrimination against qualified "handicapped" persons by federal executive agencies and by the approximately 50 percent of American businesses that contract with the federal government, reads in pertinent part:

   "Qualified handicapped person" means. . .with respect to. . .elementary and secondary. . .education services, a handicapped person (i) of an age during which nonhandicapped persons are provided such services, (ii) of any age during which it is mandatory under state law to provide such services to handicapped persons, or (iii) to whom a state is required to provide a free appropriate public education under Section 612 of the Education of the Handicapped Act. 34 Code of Federal Regulations Section 104.3(k)(2), 1988.

10. The Individuals with Disabilities Education Act of 1990, 20 United States Code Section 1401(17).

11. Phillips, P. "IDEA Legislation—A Positive for PT and Children with Disabilities." *PT: Magazine of Physical Therapy*, 1996; 4:(1):20, 22.

12. The Equal Access Act of 1984, 20 United States Code Section 4071.

13. The Americans with Disabilities Act of 1990, Public Law 101-336, codified at 42 United States Code Section 12101–12213.

14. For a listing of illegal drugs covered by the ADA, see Controlled Substances Act, 21 United States Code Section 812.

15. 42 United States Code Section 12211.

16. For example, the new subsection 7(8)(C)(i) reads:

    For purposes of programs and activities providing educational services, local educational agencies may take disciplinary action pertaining to the use or possession of illegal drugs or alcohol against any handicapped student who currently is engaging in the illegal use of drugs or in the use of alcohol to the same extent that such disciplinary action is taken against nonhandicapped students. Furthermore, the due process procedures at 34 C.F.R. 104.36 shall not apply to such disciplinary actions.

17. Mirone, J. "ADA Case Law: Cases in Higher Education." *PT: Magazine of Physical Therapy*, 1994; 2:(6):33.

18. It was only just over 40 years ago, in *Brown v. Board of Education* of Topeka, Kansas, 347 U.S. 483 (1954), that the U.S. Supreme Court ruled that separate-but-equal public schools constituted unconstitutionally illegal, intentional racial discrimination.

19. *Board of Curators of the University of Missouri* v. *Horowitz*, 435 U.S. 78 (1978).

20. *Ibid.* at 89–90.

21. *Ibid.* at 96, note 6.

22. *Regents of the University of Michigan* v. *Ewing*, 474 U.S. 214 (1985).

23. *Tobias* v. *University of Texas*, 824 S.W. 2d 201 (Tex. App. Ft. Worth 1991).

24. The Civil Rights Act of 1964, Title VI, 42 United States Code Section 2000d-1.

Suggested Readings

1. "Adverse Academic, Disciplinary and Licensing Decisions." *Journal of College and University Law*, 1993; 20(2):198–201.

2. Cherrington, D.J. *The Management of Human Resources*, 4th ed. Englewood Cliffs, NJ: Prentice Hall, 1995, p. 319.

3. *Clinical Education Guidelines and Self-Assessment.* Alexandria, VA: American Physical Therapy Association, 1994.

4. Gordon, D.J. "The Duties of a Clinical Instructor." *Clinical Management*, 1989; 9(5): 39–41.

5. Gostin, L.O., Beyer, H.A. *Implementing the Americans with Disabilities Act: Rights and Responsibilities of All Americans.* Baltimore, MD: Brooks Publishing Company, 1993.

6. Mirone, J. "ADA Case Law: Cases in Higher Education." *PT: Magazine of Physical Therapy*, 1994; 2:(6):33.

7. Phillips, P. "IDEA Legislation—A Positive for PT and Children with Disabilities." *PT: Magazine of Physical Therapy*, 1996; 4:(1):20, 22.

8. Scott, R.W. "CIs and Liability." *PT: Magazine of Physical Therapy*, 1995; 3:(2):30–31.

9. Smith, H.G. "Introduction to Legal Risks Associated with Clinical Education." *Journal of Physical Therapy Education*, 1994: 8(2):67–70.

10. The Americans with Disabilities Act of 1990, Public Law 101-336, codified at 42 United States Code Section 12101–12213.

11. The Civil Rights Act of 1964, Title VI, 42 United States Code Section 2000d-1.

12. The Family Educational Rights and Privacy Act of 1974, 20 United States Code Section 1232 *et. seq.*

13. The Individuals with Disabilities Education Act of 1990, 20 United States Code Section 1400–1485.

14. Title IX of the Educational Amendments of 1972, 20 United States Code Sections 1681–1683.

Chapter 8

Employment Law

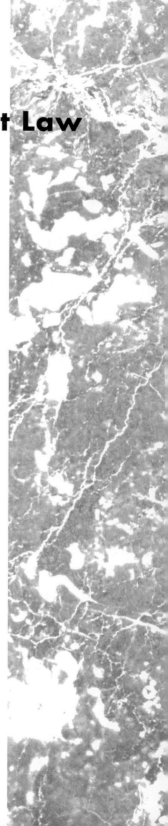

This chapter overviews key employment law issues. The principle federal statute governing employment discrimination is Title VII of the
Civil Rights Act of 1964, which prohibits discrimination in all aspects
of employment on the basis of race/ethnicity, gender, religion, and
national origin. Augmenting Title VII are the Americans with Disabilities
Act of 1990 and the Age Discrimination in Employment Act of 1967,
which prohibit employment discrimination against disabled and older
workers, respectively.

The vast majority of employment in the United States is "at will,
"meaning that either the employee or employer can terminate the relationship without notice or penalty. Employment at will creates a significant job-security problem for health care professionals under managed
care. Health care human resource managers have the formidable task
of recruiting and managing scarce health care workers in this unpre-
dictable environment.

The Importance of Human Resource Management in Business

With one of the highest standards (and costs) of living in the world and
123,060,000 citizens and legal aliens[1] working full-time in order to enjoy the
fruits of that standard, employment in the United States is probably *the* central socioeconomic issue facing individuals, families, and businesses today.
Recent phenomena, such as corporate downsizing and managed health care
delivery, add significant stress to employees (and managers) who understand
all too well that there is a very fine balance between optimal efficiency and
productivity on one hand and employment stability and quality of work life
on the other hand.

It is the herculean responsibility of human resource managers to oversee
and manage the work lives of the people that make America work.
According to Shortell and Kaluzny,[2] human resource management is the most
important managerial function in any business organization, including health
care service organizations. Cherrington[3] identifies seven classic functions of

human resource managers: staffing (recruitment, selection, and retention), compensation (wages/salary, benefits, and incentives), training and development, labor-management relations, performance assessment, safety and health, and human resource management research.

The term *human resource management* is relatively new to American business. Traditionally, people management in business and government was referred to as *personnel management.* (It still is so labeled in the Federal Civil Service system and in many state and local governmental agencies.) Personnel management was a philosophy of people management that worked fairly well into the mid-1900s, when the roles of personnel managers were largely limited to employee selection, recordkeeping, and overseeing early union-management relations. Since the end of World War II, however, the responsibility of managing human resources has become very complex.

Human resource managers today must also know how to accommodate employees' sophisticated personal and family needs; manage elaborate benefits programs (which were virtually nonexistent pre-World War II); implement often esoteric legislative, judicial, and administrative legal mandates that never affected their predecessors; and contribute coequally with the "line" to the corporate "bottom line," among other considerations. In fact, human resource management is now a distinct profession with all of the requisite characteristics common to other traditional professions: a defined body of knowledge, a code of ethics and self-governance, a professional organization (the Society for Human Resource Management[4]), and practice specialization and certification.

Employment at Will vs. Employment Under Contract

Traditionally, all employees were employed "at will." The vast majority of employees are still employed at will. Under the common law concept of employment at will, an employee is free at any time to terminate his or her employment with an employer, with or without justification. The reciprocal right rests also with the employer under employment at will. Absent some legally recognized exceptions, an employer is free, under employment at will, to discharge an employee at any time, with or without just cause.

Employment at will is generally mutually advantageous to employees and employers. Whenever a better employment opportunity arises, an employee knows, under employment at will, that he or she can terminate an existing employment relationship (with reasonable advance notice) and take advantage of the new opportunity without stigma. Similarly, in a time of corporate downsizing, employers can generally adjust the size and composition of their workforces without adverse legal consequences (with due regard to their social responsibility[5]).

There are several recognized exceptions to the concept of employment at will. Obviously, a valid employment contract for a specific term of days, weeks, months, or years, is an exception to employment at will. Such a contract must comply with all of the legal requisites for a valid contract, including a valid offer and acceptance (mutuality of assent), consideration (mutuality of obligation), legal capacity of the parties to contract, legality of the subject matter, and compliance with the statute of frauds, as applicable.

Some courts have found language in employee handbooks, such as a promise not to discharge an employee except for just cause or the promise of "steady employment," to be implied contractual promises that modify the common law doctrine of employment at will. An employer may be able to disclaim an implied employment contract in an employee handbook by prominently featuring the express disclaimer in the handbook and phrasing it clearly in simple English.[6] Many other employers have chosen to do away with employee handbooks to avoid altogether the possible declaration of an implied employment contract incident to language in the handbook.

Courts have also declared illegal employee discharges based on protected conduct under federal or state statutes. Examples of such wrongful discharges include discharges for *whistleblowing* (making a good faith report of a suspected violation of law to appropriate authorities); union activities permitted by law; illegal discrimination against racial and ethnic minorities, women, and disabled workers; and the proper filing of workers' compensation and disability claims. Rarely, courts have also declared illegal, as violative of public policy, employee discharges that are deemed fraudulent, malicious, or abusive, such as when a supervisor conspires with coworkers to create a case for discharge against an employee.

Similarly, it would constitute wrongful discharge for an employer to fire an employee who refuses to commit an illegal act. In physical and occupational therapy, an example of such a wrongful discharge might be the situation in a managed care setting in which a clinical therapist is fired for refusing to allow unlicensed support personnel to carry out clinical duties that cannot legally be delegated to them.

Labor-Management Relations

Before 1926, organized labor activity in the United States was significantly impeded by industry, state and federal government, and public opinion. At various points in time, organized labor was viewed either as a criminal or communist conspiracy, or both. As a result of this unfair and distorted view of organized labor, ordinary employees existed largely at the mercy of their employers, and arbitrary wage cuts and terminations without cause were commonplace.

In 1926, Congress enacted the Railway Labor Act,[7] which permitted, for the first time, collective bargaining over compensation, benefits, and conditions of employment between railroad (and later airline) employees and their employers. In 1935, Congress expanded the scope of workers' rights granted under the Railway Labor Act to nearly all of the private sector when it enacted the National Labor Relations Act (NLRA), or "Wagner Act."[8] The NLRA specifically sanctioned as legitimate organized union activity on behalf of private sector employees and bargaining units and declared collective bargaining to be public policy. The NLRA also defined certain employer misconduct as "unfair labor practices" and created the administrative agency, the National Labor Relations Board, to oversee collective bargaining activities in the private sector.

Unfair labor practices were later extended to unions by the Labor-Management Relations Act of 1947,[9] or "Taft-Hartley Act." Federal public sector employees were first given the right to organize and bargain collectively over conditions of employment by an executive order signed by President Kennedy in 1962.[10]

It was not until 1974 that Congress authorized employees of nonprofit hospitals to engage in union activity by amending the NLRA. Health care unions are required by statute to give advance notice of an impending strike to the Federal Mediation and Conciliation Service, which then will attempt to avert the strike through mediation.[11] Except where restricted by law (e.g., by federal employees, or during a national emergency), the exercise by unionized employees of the strike option is recognized by law as a legitimate, last-resort option under collective bargaining, just as the lock out is for employers.

Under administrative rules established by the National Labor Relations Board, hospital-based employees can only form into eight bargaining units (with a minimum of six employees in each) representing physicians, registered nurses, other health care professionals (including physical and occupational therapists), technicians, skilled maintenance workers, other non-health professional employees, clerical employees, and guards. Implementation of the NLRB's plan was delayed until the U.S. Supreme Court approved it in a case decision in 1991, after it was challenged in the courts by the American Hospital Association.[12]

For a variety of reasons, the percentage of the total workforce represented by unions has decreased dramatically since its high point of about one-third of the workforce in the mid-1950s.[13] However, with the ongoing drastic restructuring of health care delivery under managed care and the resultant actual and perceived loss of job security and erosion of benefits for health care employees, unions may begin to attract health professional members in very large numbers if they carefully analyze and target this population and meet its special needs.

Selected Federal and State Laws and Agencies

Age Discrimination in Employment Act of 1967; Older Workers Benefit Protection Act of 1990

The Age Discrimination in Employment Act of 1967 (ADEA),[14] as amended, prohibits employment-related discrimination by private- and public-sector employers of workers age 40 or older (except executives and top policy-making officials). The legal analysis used to process and adjudicate age discrimination cases under federal law parallels that used in Title VII, Civil Rights Act of 1964 cases. Therefore, employment discrimination against older workers is prohibited in recruitment, selection, training, promotion, and conditions of employment.

The ADEA was augmented in 1990 by the Older Workers Benefit Protection Act,[15] which clarified Congress's intent that benefits protection was included in age-related federal antidiscrimination statutory law. The amendment also permits employers to ask dismissed older workers to waive their rights to sue for age discrimination under the ADEA in exchange for compensation.

The Equal Employment Opportunity Commission (EEOC) is the federal agency that administers and enforces the ADEA (and several other federal antidiscrimination laws discussed below). State statutes and judicial law may afford additional protection to older workers. In 1991, the EEOC and state agencies responsible for protecting older workers' rights processed 27,748 age discrimination claims.[16]

Americans with Disabilities Act of 1990

The Americans with Disabilities Act of 1990 (ADA)[17] was enacted by Congress on July 26, 1990, for the express purpose of "establish[ing] a clear and comprehensive prohibition of discrimination on the basis of disability."[18] This federal statute completed the decades-long effort of Congress, under the Fourteenth Amendment (Due Process and Equal Protection) and under its plenary power to regulate interstate commerce, to prohibit employment discrimination in both the public and private sectors. For the approximately 43,000,000 Americans with physical or mental disabilities, the ADA ensures equal access to public accommodations and services and equal opportunities in employment.

Before the ADA was signed into law, 34 states had already enacted legislation protecting disabled workers against employment-related discrimination. The ADA was modeled after the Rehabilitation Act of 1973,[19] which prohibits disability-related employment discrimination in federal executive agencies and by the approximately 50 percent of private sector businesses that contract with the federal government.

The ADA has five sections, or "titles," that protect the rights of people with disabilities. Title I (discussed in greater detail below) protects against disability-related employment discrimination. Title II ensures equal access for the disabled to public services (i.e., all activities of state and local governments), including public transportation services. Title III ensures equal access for the disabled to public accommodations, including all private businesses and services (except for some private clubs and all religious organizations and places of worship[20]). This title includes private health care facilities under its jurisdiction. Title IV provides for equal access by disabled patrons to telecommunications services. Title V is a miscellaneous section addressing, among other considerations, the relationship of the ADA to other federal statutes, key definitions, and an affirmation that the states cannot claim immunity (Eleventh Amendment) from the requirements of the ADA.

Title I became effective for businesses employing 25 or more people on July 26, 1992, and for businesses with 15 or more employees on July 26, 1994. Title I covers private and public employers, employment agencies, and labor union organizations.

Title I of the ADA prohibits employment discrimination by employers against employees and job applicants who are qualified to perform the essential functions of their jobs. This prohibition against employment discrimination is all-encompassing, applying to recruitment, selection, training, benefits, promotion, discipline, and retention. The ADA does not, however, establish a quota system for hiring or retaining disabled workers.

If a job candidate with a disability is legitimately found to be unable to perform the essential functions of a position, then that person may be rejected as a candidate for employment for that position. The legal burden of challenging such a decision rests with the rejected candidate, who must prove that he or she is the best qualified person for the position. Qualification standards also require that a candidate not pose a "direct threat" to others in the workplace, i.e., "a significant risk to the health or safety of others that cannot be eliminated by reasonable accommodation."[21]

Title I includes several key definitions. *Disability* is defined in one of three ways.[22] An employee or job applicant has a disibility if one or more of the following are true:

- The person has a physical or mental impairment that substantially limits one or more major life activities.

- The person has a record of such an impairment.

- The person is regarded as having such an impairment.

"Major life activities" include all of the important activities of daily living already well-known to rehabilitation professionals, including the ability to see and hear, speech, cardiorespiratory functions, ambulation, self-care, the performance of manual tasks, and formal and informal learning activities, among others.[23]

Precisely which functions are "essential" for any given job is a matter of business judgment for employers.[24] Prudent liability risk management and fundamental fairness require, however, that standards in job descriptions and delineation of essential functions for positions be clear, justifiable, and in writing. Business decisions regarding the labeling of job tasks as "essential functions" should be reviewed by legal counsel before implementation.

A "qualified individual with a disability" means a job applicant or employee who can perform essential job functions, with or without reasonable accommodation.[25] "Reasonable accommodation" is defined by the EEOC[26] as:

any change or adjustment to a job or work environment that permits a qualified applicant or employee with a disability to participate in the job application process, to perform the essential functions of a job, or to enjoy benefits and privileges of employment equal to those enjoyed by employees without disabilities . . . and may include:

- acquiring or modifying equipment or devices
- job restructuring
- part-time or modified work schedules
- reassignment to a vacant position
- adjusting or modifying examinations, training materials or policies
- providing readers and interpreters, and
- making the workplace readily accessible to and usable by people with disabilities.

Reasonable accommodation must be carried out upon request of an applicant or employee (or if a disability is obvious to the employer), unless the employer can prove that to do so would amount to an "undue hardship." *Undue hardship* is defined as a situation in which accommodation is excused because to do so would be unduly burdensome (excessively disruptive, costly, or difficult to implement) or would fundamentally alter the very nature of the employer's business operations.[27] The accommodation provided need not be one specifically requested by a disabled applicant or employee, just one that enables the applicant or employee to perform the essential functions of his or her job. The applicant or employee can be asked to contribute to funding the accommodation if its cost amounts to an undue hardship for the employer.[28]

The ADA does not require that employers hire or promote anyone but the "best qualified," however, the law mandates that disabled applicants and employees be afforded equal consideration in the selection process. Excluded from the statutory definition of "disabled" are:

- current illegal drug users and abusers of alcohol

- compulsive gamblers, klepto- and pyromaniacs

- pedophiles, exhibitionists, and voyeurs

- homosexuals and bisexuals
- persons with gender identification and miscellaneous sexual behavior disorders (including transsexualism and transvestism).[29]

Employers must continuously review their hiring, promotion, training, and benefits programs to ensure compliance with the ADA. They must especially ensure that, during the hiring process, prospective employees are judged on their abilities, not disabilities, and that candidates and current employees are made aware of their ADA rights (through posting of federal anti-employment-discrimination requirements in a prominent place[30]).

Regarding pre-employment inquiries and screening tests, the following rules apply. It is unlawful to inquire about applicants' disabilities and to require pre-offer medical examinations. Pre-offer drug screening tests, however, are permissible by management, as are non-medically-related physical agility and psychological tests.

Once a conditional offer has been extended to an applicant, it is permissible to carry out a job-related medical examination, if such an examination is universally given to all similarly-situated conditional offerees. A final offer of employment may lawfully be conditioned on the results of such an examination.

According to final EEOC regulations on pre-employment questions released in October 1995, it is permissible for an employer to inquire about an applicant's ability to perform specific tasks, including requiring a demonstration of job skills, as long as such an inquiry is made of all applicants. Although it is generally unlawful to inquire about reasonable accommodation(s) during pre-offer interviews, the EEOC sanctions such inquiries when one of the following occurs:

- The employer reasonably believes that reasonable accommodation might be required for a job, because the applicant displays an obvious disability, such as blindness or paralysis.
- The applicant voluntarily discloses an unidentified disability, and the employer reasonably believes that accommodation might be required.
- The applicant requests accommodation.

The EEOC establishes rules and regulations interpreting, and enforcing, the ADA. Although there were a relatively small number of claims of disability-related job discrimination lodged by complainants with the EEOC during 1992 (approximately 400 per month), the number of complaints grew to 1,600 per month by March, 1993.[31] By the end of 1994, the EEOC had processed over 30,000 claims. The specific impairment most often cited in complaints was back pain syndrome (20 percent), followed by neurological impairment (12 percent) and emotional and psychiatric impairment (11 percent).[32] Fully a quarter of all ADA complaints lodged with the EEOC relate to the alleged failure on the part of employers to provide appropriate reasonable accommodation for disabled applicants and employees.[33]

Litigation over the scope of duty on the part of employers to provide reasonable accommodation to disabled workers has helped to clarify the mandates of the ADA. For example, courts have ruled in favor of employees, requiring a teacher's aide for a teacher with physical and mental limitations post-automobile accident,[34] reasonable alternatives for an employee unable to drive (an "essential function") because of terminal cancer,[35] lifting restrictions for a nurse with low back dysfunction,[36] and home-based work for a clerical employee with multiple sclerosis,[37] among other required accommodations. Courts have also ruled in favor of employers, holding that extensive workplace redesign required to accommodate a paraplegic employee constitutes excessive cost and therefore undue hardship[38] and accommodation short of a total workplace smoking ban for an asthmatic employee is acceptable,[39] among other pro-employer decisions.

Courts are divided, in reasonable accommodation ADA litigation cases, over whether the employee or the employer bears the legal burden of proof in the case. Some courts take a middle ground, first requiring a disabled employee to establish that he or she can perform the essential functions of a particular job (with or without accommodation), and then shifting the burden of proof to the employer to establish why the employer should be excused from providing accommodation.[40]

Despite the substantial number of administrative and litigation cases involving the ADA, employers should not be fearful of the ADA. In addition to reinforcing a business's social responsibility to recruit, hire, train and develop, retain, and promote workers with disabilities, the ADA makes good business sense. Total public support of a person who has a disability averages one million dollars over the person's lifetime, whereas employment of that person results in a net gain to public coffers of

$65,000 in taxes paid. Studies and experience show that people with disabilities want to work and perform their work very well, relative to the total workforce. One recent study concluded that persons with severe physical or mental disabilities or both can be successful in the workplace through supported employment.[41]

Employers who are strongly committed to the principles of the ADA also benefit from an enhanced public image and increased goodwill. Employers should not take a defensive approach to compliance with the ADA because, as has been the case with health care malpractice prevention, a defensive posture only serves to increase the likelihood of litigation.

Despite the call from some legislators in the current highly politicized Congress for ADA reform, based in part on the financial burden of compliance,[42] the ADA remains a linchpin for employment and civil rights, crucial to the prestige and maintenance of the United States as a world leader. Rehabilitation professionals have a unique opportunity to serve as consultants to both employers (to meet their legal responsibilities) and to employees (to exercise their rights and rehabilitation and vocational potential).

Civil Rights Act of 1964, Title VII

The most important (or at least most pervasive) federal statute addressing employment discrimination and civil rights is Title VII of the Civil Rights Act of 1964.[43] This law was critically important for the full integration of racial and other minorities into the American workforce, yet its passage was stalled for years in the U.S. Senate by repeated filibusters.

President John Kennedy, Attorney General Robert Kennedy, and congressional Democratic leaders grounded the statute in Congress's plenary power to regulate interstate commerce,[44] rather than in constitutional due process or equal protection under law, believing that this was the only way that the law could survive a legal challenge by noncompliant private sector businesses. The legal premise justifying enactment of the Civil Rights Act of 1964 was that discrimination of minorities—especially of African-Americans—by business had an immeasurable adverse impact on interstate commerce, and that Congress was empowered to remedy this by means of a federal nondiscrimination mandate to all public and private business entities.

Title VII specifically prohibits discrimination against job applicants and employees on the basis of race/ethnicity, gender (as of 1972), religion, and national origin, at all stages along the continuum of employment processes. The groups enumerated in Title VII are referred to in case and administrative law as "protected classes." Specifically, Title VII states in pertinent part that:

It shall be an unlawful employment practice for an employer:

1. to fail or refuse to hire or to discharge any individual, or otherwise to discriminate against any individual with respect to his compensation, terms, conditions, or privileges of employment, because of such individual's race, color, religion, sex, or national origin, or

2. to limit, segregate, or classify his employees or applicants for employment in any way which would deprive any individual of employment opportunities or otherwise adversely affect his status as an employee, because of such individual's race, color, religion, sex, or national origin.[45]

_ .. _ . _ .. _ . _ .. _ . _ .. _ . _ .. _ . _ .. _ . _ .. _ . _ .. _ . _ .. _ . _ .. _ . _

Title VII applies to all private sector businesses with 15 or more employees; labor unions; and federal, state, and local governmental entities. Title VII is administered and enforced by the EEOC. States are free to provide additional constitutional, statutory, judicial, and administrative protections to their citizens over and above that provided by federal law. Forty-one states, the District of Columbia, and Puerto Rico all have statutes similar to Title VII.[46]

Employers are required by EEOC regulations to create, submit for review, and maintain records that evidence compliance with Title VII. For reporting purposes, race/ethnicity is divided into five classifications: white (non-Hispanic), black, Hispanic, Asian/Pacific Islander, and American Indian/Alaskan native.[47]

Title VII expressly permits employment discrimination against protected classes of persons on the basis of bona fide occupational qualifications, or BFOQs.[48] A BFOQ must be based on business necessity, i.e., reasonably necessary for the normal operation of a particular business. BFOQs are allowed for gender, religion, and national origin (and age under the ADEA) classifications, provided that employers can establish business necessity. (BFOQs based on race violate public policy and are generally disallowed.) An example of a legitimate gender-based BFOQ is the requirement, based on social mores, that dressing room attendants be of the same gender as patrons. An example of a legitimate religion-based BFOQ is the requirement that a parish priest be Catholic.

Title VII prohibits both intentional and unintentional employment discrimination. Intentional wrongful employment discrimination is referred to as "disparate treatment," while other employment practices, though they appear to be protected class-neutral on their face, have a particular adverse "disparate impact" on the employment rights of protected class members.

Pending before the U.S. Supreme Court is a legal case involving the interpretation of whether "15 or more workers on the job" (triggering Title VII jurisdiction over private businesses) means on payroll or physically present at work. The Census Bureau reported in 1991 that there were 550,000 businesses that employed between ten and 19 employees, accounting for 7.4 million workers.[49]

Civil Rights Act of 1991

The Civil Rights Act of 1991[50] was enacted to clarify congressional intent regarding employment discrimination, after the U.S. Supreme Court reportedly "weakened the scope and effectiveness of federal civil rights protections"[51] in its 1989 decision in *Wards Cove Packing Co. v. Atonio.*[52] The provisions of this federal statute affect the Civil Rights Act of 1964 and the Rehabilitation Act of 1973.

The Civil Rights Act of 1991 invalidates the Supreme Court's holding in *Wards Cove*, in part, by reshifting part of the burden of proof in disparate impact employment discrimination cases from plaintiffs to employers, to prove business necessity for any business practice that is proven (by a plaintiff) to have a disparate impact on a Title VII-protected class.

The Civil Rights Act of 1991 also permits, for the first time, not only the equitable remedies of reinstatement, back pay (with interest), and restoration of seniority for proven employment discrimination, but also compensatory and punitive damages for intentional discrimination under Title VII or the ADA. Title VII and ADA plaintiffs have the right, for the first time, to request a jury trial for determination of monetary damages. Monetary damages are graduated according to company size and are capped at $300,000.[53]

Prohibited for the first time under the Civil Rights Act of 1991 is the process of "race norming," under which raw scores on pre-employment tests were sometimes scaled differently for racial and ethnic minority applicants as a form of affirmative action. The law also protects U.S. citizens from employment discrimination who are employed outside of the United States by U.S. firms. (An exception to this extraterritorial application of Title VII is that firms are allowed to comply with local foreign customs in their employment practices.)

Drug-Free Workplace Act of 1988

The Drug-Free Workplace Act of 1988[54] requires that companies and individuals who enter into contracts with the federal government, valued at $25,000 or more, certify that their facilities are drug-free workplaces. Federal contractors are required, at least, to:

- have in place an effective workplace drug education program

- post and give to each employee a copy of the prohibition against the "unlawful manufacture, distribution, [use], or [possession] of controlled substances. . . in the workplace,"[55] specifying potential disciplinary actions for violation of the prohibition

- notify the federal contracting agency, within ten days, of any drug-related criminal convictions of its employees

The Drug-Free Workplace Act of 1988 does not specifically mandate that employers carry out workplace drug testing; however, neither are they prohibited by the statute from doing so. Workplace drug testing is of relatively recent vintage. It first began in the military during the 1970s. By 1983, three percent of companies in the United States carried out workplace drug testing. Currently, about one-third of

Fortune 500 corporations test their employees for illicit drug use.[56]

Employee drug testing includes the following tests[57]:

- *Pre-employment* drug screening, the most commonly used employee drug test type. Pre-employment drug testing is recognized as a common law management right to promote an employer's legitimate business interests.

- *Reasonable suspicion* drug testing, done when a supervisor of an employee reasonably believes that the employee may be under the influence of mind-altering drugs. Legal bases for reasonable suspicion drug testing include the fact that employers are vicariously liable for the conduct of employees acting within the scope of employment and the statutory requirement under the Occupational Safety and Health Act of 1970 for employers to maintain a workplace free of serious safety hazards.

- *Periodic* drug testing of employees, such as during a periodic physical examination, or as part of a promotion into a position that requires the employee to handle classified documents or carry a firearm.

- *Post-accident* drug testing, after serious accidents, with or without suspicion of employee misconduct.

- *Random* drug testing, the least often used and most effective and controversial form of employee drug testing.

- *Exculpatory* drug testing,[58] designed to exculpate an employee who erroneously tests positive for illicit drug use, by comparing the blood types of the suspect and blood group substances found in the positive urine sample. Approximately 80 percent of the population are "secretors" of such substances, for whom exculpatory testing, based on ABO blood groups, is feasible.

Case law to date addressing the constitutionality and propriety of employee drug testing has generally upheld the practice, with one proviso. Except for military service members and prisoners, direct observation of a subject rendering a urine sample is universally considered to be repugnant and an unconscionably impermissible violation of personal human dignity and privacy. In business settings, therefore, only indirect observation of subjects rendering urine samples is permitted, such as the posting of a guard outside of a lavatory so that extraneous paraphernalia is not carried in by testees.

Effective January 1, 1996, all transit employers regulated by the U.S. Department of Transportation (DOT) were required to have, in addition to drug awareness programs, alcohol abuse prevention programs that comply with DOT's specific regulations. These federal regulations preempt any conflicting state laws concerning alcohol misuse. Safety-sensitive employees, including truck and bus drivers, are prohibited from imbibing alcohol four hours prior to driving and are subject to testing to confirm that they are alcohol-free and (other) drug-free on the job.[59]

Employee Polygraph Protection Act of 1988

The Employee Polygraph Protection Act of 1988 (EPPA)[60] severely curtailed the use of polygraph examinations in the workplace. This federal statute, based on respect for individual privacy, prohibits the use of "lie detector" examinations of any kind by private sector employers, except for:

- job applicants in the security industry

- job applicants in companies that manufacture or market controlled drugs

- current employees, as part of an investigation concerning a specific economic loss, such as theft from, or sabotage of, a firm

The polygraph is an instrument that measures the physiologic responses of heart rate, respiration, and perspiration through a galvanic skin response. Physiologic responses to "control" or background lies are compared to those of "relevant" lies to determine whether a polygrapher believes that a subject is truthful or deceptive. If no determination as to truthfulness can be made, the test is reported as inconclusive.

The congressional Office of Technological Assessment has concluded that a polygraph only has validity when the control question technique is used in the area of specific criminal investigations.[61] The EPPA correctly reflects the widely held belief that the use of polygraphs for other purposes constitutes an unwarranted invasion of individual privacy.

Results of private sector employment-related polygraph examinations may not be released to anyone except the employee tested and appropriate governmental agencies (such as the police), but only with a court order. Employers are required to conspicuously post a notice of employee rights under the EPPA. The law is administered by the Employment Standards Division of the U.S. Department of Labor.

Employee Retirement Income Security Act of 1974

The Employee Retirement Income Security Act of 1974 (ERISA)[62] was enacted by Congress to regulate private pension and benefit plans. A key original intent behind the legislation was the desire to ensure that pensioners receive what is due them at the end of a working career. ERISA preempts all conflicting state laws (except for state insurance laws) concerning employee benefits and pensions.

Regarding employee health benefit plans, the employer self-insured plan and risk retention plan fall outside of state jurisdiction, because they are not legally considered to be "insurance." This means that state law mandates of nondiscrimination and minimum coverage do not apply to such plans, which include two-thirds of current employee health benefit plans. ERISA itself fails to address such issues, creating what has been called "the ERISA vacuum."[63]

Under ERISA, employer contributions to pension plans fully vest after five years of employment. The portability option is a voluntary option under ERISA under which employees can roll over vested pension benefits when they leave their current place of employment. Pensions are of two types: the traditional (and more costly) defined benefit plan and the defined contribution plan, including the popular 401(k) plan.

Companies and their pension insurers and trustees are legal *fiduciaries* to pension beneficiaries, meaning that they stand in a legal position of trust toward beneficiaries and must act prudently to safeguard the assets of the pension fund. Companies also have substantial disclosure (to beneficiaries) and reporting (to the federal government) requirements concerning employee pension plans. ERISA is co-administered by the Department of Labor and the Internal Revenue Service.

Equal Employment Opportunity Commission

The Equal Employment Opportunity Commission (EEOC) is a federal administrative agency created by Congress in the Civil Rights Act of 1964 to administer and enforce Title VII of that statute. The EEOC also administers and enforces the ADA, ADEA, and the Equal Pay Act of 1963,[64] and provides oversight and coordination of all federal regulations, policies, and practices affecting equal employment opportunity.

The EEOC consists of five commissioners and a general counsel, all appointed by the president and confirmed by the Senate. The president designates the chairman, who acts as chief executive officer of the commission. All commissioners serve for five-year, staggered terms. The commissioners make EEOC policy, while the general counsel supervises equal employment opportunity litigation brought on behalf of complainants.

EEOC staff process and investigate complaints of employment discrimination against private and public entities. In most instances, charges must be filed with the EEOC within 180 days of the alleged employment discrimination. If the EEOC's investigation of a charge concludes that there is reasonable cause that actionable employment discrimination occurred, it will initiate conciliation procedures to try to resolve the charge to the reasonable satisfaction of the complainant at this lowest level of adjudication. That failing, the EEOC may sue the respondent in federal court on the alleged victim's behalf. (Only the Justice Department may bring suit against a state or local governmental entity, however.) If the EEOC declines to litigate a case, a notice of right to sue will be issued to a complainant 180 days after a charge is filed.[65]

The EEOC currently has a backlog of over 100,000 cases and is capable of litigating only about 500 cases per year. In the face of ongoing budget cuts and freezes, the situation is likely to get worse. As a result, the EEOC now utilizes contract mediation services to help resolve many disputes.[66]

Family and Medical Leave Act of 1993

The Family and Medical Leave Act of 1993 (FMLA)[67] was signed into law by President Clinton just after his inauguration and became effective on February 5, 1993. The

FMLA requires covered employers to provide up to 12 weeks of unpaid, job- and benefit-protected leave per year to eligible employees for childbirth, adoption, and personal and family medical illnesses. About 45 million workers in the United States are eligible to take advantage of the FMLA.[68]

Employees eligible for FMLA protection are those who have worked for at least 1,250 hours during the previous 12 months at a location in which their employer has 50 or more employees located within a 75-mile radius. Under Department of Labor administrative rules, which became effective in April 1995, covered illnesses under the FMLA include those conditions which incapacitate an employee or family member (spouse, child, or parent) for at least three days, require consultation with a health care professional, and are treated with prescription medications.[69]

Under the administrative rules implementing the FMLA, an employee on FMLA leave of absence for personal illness is not required to accept an employer's offer of "light duty" or other reasonable accommodation.[70] This rule is seemingly inconsistent with the ADA, and probably results in significant confusion on the part of human resource managers who must co-administer the FMLA and the ADA for their companies. Interagency coordination and reconciliation of this inconsistency is needed on the part of the Department of Labor and EEOC.

Although eligible employees must provide 30-day advance notices of covered leave whenever feasible, employers fear abuses and an adverse effect on productivity.[71] Employers may require the production of a medical certificate of illness and even a second opinion regarding a claimed covered illness (at the employer's expense). Employer retaliation against an employee invoking the protection of the FMLA is prohibited. The law is enforced by the U.S. Department of Labor.

Occupational Safety and Health Act of 1970; Occupational Safety and Health Administration

The Occupational Safety and Health Act of 1970 (OSHA)[72] was enacted to establish and enforce workplace safety and health standards. The Occupational Safety and Health Administration (also called OSHA) is the federal administrative agency which promulgates rules and enforces OSHA. Its rules, covering workplace issues from universal precautions to standards for the minimization of cumulative trauma disorders in industry, apply to almost all private sector employers, except family farmers and self-employed persons.

OSHA is enforced by the U.S. Department of Labor, and compliance is monitored through mandatory reporting and scheduled and surprise (but pursuant to a warrant) administrative inspections. Employers with more than ten employees must make and maintain detailed occupational injury and illness records for their employees. Like the EEOC, OSHA is facing ongoing budgetary reductions.

Pregnancy Discrimination Act of 1978

The Pregnancy Discrimination Act of 1978[73] is a codicil statute amending Title VII of the Civil Rights Act of 1964. Under the Pregnancy Discrimination Act, the definition of unlawful gender-based employment discrimination is expanded to include discrimination based on pregnancy, childbirth, and related medical conditions (including complications of pregnancy and therapeutic abortions). The law does not mandate that employers covered by Title VII provide pregnancy-related medical benefits (or any benefits), however, if medical benefits are provided to employees, pregnancy must be treated in the same manner as any other covered disability. If reasonable job accommodation is provided by an employer for other disabilities, it must also be provided for (temporary) disability related to pregnancy. Under the Pregnancy Discrimination Act, employers are also prohibited from mandating a specific numbers of days after which pregnant employees must return to work after childbirth.

Workers' Compensation Statutes

State workers' compensation statutes were first introduced on a voluntary basis in five states in 1911[74] to provide some degree of protection to industrial workers injured while on the job. Before that time, workers who were injured on the job, who almost universally had neither health nor disability insurance, were normally summarily discharged from their employment since they could no longer work. As a result, many industrial worker injury cases became the subject of lawsuits, most of which were won by employers, on theories ranging from the "fellow servant rule" (another worker, not the employer, was at fault) and "contributory negligence" on the part of the injured worker. This social injustice led to the enactment of mandatory workers' compensation statutes in all 50 states by 1948.[75]

Workers' compensation statutes provide for income continuation and payment of related medical and rehabilitation expenses for covered workers injured on the job. The sole issues to be adjudicated by state workers' compensation administrative agencies are (1) whether the employee was injured while functioning within the scope of employment, and (2) the degree of resultant disability. Workers' compensation laws generally do not consider who was at fault for a covered incident resulting in employee injury. In that sense, workers' compensation laws are no-fault laws.

Because of a sense that workers' compensation laws are subject to abuse (despite the fact that few, if any, injured employees reap a financial windfall from workers' compensation benefits), many state legislatures recently have enacted workers' compensation reform measures. Some of the reform measures include reducing the roles of personal injury attorneys in the administrative process, risk-shifting for minor job-related injuries, and case management of individual workers and their rehabilitation.

Sexual Harassment in the Workplace

Even though sexual harassment has long been a widespread problem affecting productivity, morale, and every other aspect of interpersonal relations in the workplace, only recently have allegations of sexual harassment lodged against prominent public officials brought this problem "out of the closet" and into every board room, work setting, and living room in the United States and elsewhere.

The EEOC defines[76] sexual harassment as:

> Unwelcome sexual advances, requests for sexual favors, and other verbal or physical conduct of a sexual nature, when (1) submission to such conduct is made either explicitly or implicitly a term or condition of employment, (2) submission to or rejection of such conduct by an individual is used as a basis for employment decisions affecting such individual, or (3) such conduct has the purpose or effect of unreasonably interfering with an individual's work performance or creating an intimidating, hostile, or offensive work environment.

The EEOC definition of sexual harassment has a dual focus on (1) the types of inappropriate conduct that constitutes sexual harassment and (2) the possible adverse employment consequences for victims of sexual harassment and for others in the workplace. Conduct that constitutes sexual harassment could include:

- unwelcome comments of a sexual nature about a victim's person or body parts

- solicitation of others for sexual relations

- inappropriate touching of another person on a private area of his or her body with the intent to arouse or gratify sexual desires (i.e., commission of sexual battery)

Employment consequences fall into two categories: adverse employment decisions resulting from *quid pro quo* situations and hostile work environments. *Quid pro quo* describes a situation in which a victim's response to sexual harassment is the basis for employment-related decisions involving the victim or other workers. A *quid pro quo* complaint typically is lodged either by an employee who has been denied opportunities because he or she refused a perpetrator's sexual advances or by an employee who has been denied opportunities because another employee obtained those opportunities by submitting to a perpetrator's sexual advances. An example of a *quid pro quo* sexual harassment situation would be the case in which an employer's decision to fund a staff occupational therapist's attendance at a professional conference turned on whether the occupational therapist submitted to the employer's sexual advances.

In a hostile work environment scenario, sexual harassment unreasonably interferes with either the target victim's or another person's work performance. Complaints related to hostile work environments can be made by any person in the workplace who is reasonably offended by a perpetrator's sexual harassment (of the complainant or of another person in the work setting) and whose work is impeded by that harassment. An example of a hostile work environment sexual harassment situation would be the case in which a physical therapy aide is unable to concentrate on patient care activities because of the misconduct of a physical therapist who is making sexual advances toward a patient.

The EEOC and the courts adjudicating sexual harassment cases traditionally have utilized the "ordinary reasonable person" standard to assess whether an individual's conduct constitutes sexual harassment. This is the same standard commonly used to determine whether a defendant in a civil tort (e.g., health care malpractice) case violated a duty owed to a plaintiff. Under this standard, as applied in a sexual harassment case, a trier of fact (judge or jury) puts him- or herself into the shoes of an ethereal "person of ordinary care and diligence"[77] and determines how such a person would be likely to perceive the conduct in issue and decides the case accordingly.

The problem with the traditional "ordinary reasonable person" standard is that it frequently is translated into a "reasonable man" standard, with the result that the trier of fact assesses interpersonal conduct exclusively from a male point of view. To ensure that a gender-neutral standard is applied in administrative and legal sexual harassment cases, some federal courts have established a modified standard that eventually may supplant the traditional standard of review. Under this modified standard, the trier of fact still puts him- or herself into the shoes of an "ordinary reasonable person" when determining whether specific conduct constitutes sexual harassment, but that ordinary reasonable person must be of the same gender as the alleged victim of sexual harassment or misconduct.

Expert testimony has been presented in sexual harassment cases to support the notion that men and women view sexually-oriented conduct—in the workplace and elsewhere—very differently. In testifying in *Robinson* v. *Jacksonville Shipyards*,[78] Alison Wetherfield of the National Organization for Women's Legal Defense and Education Fund cited a study in which 75 percent of men polled said that they were flattered by sexual advances by women in the workplace; only 15 percent claimed that they would be offended by such conduct. Of women surveyed, however, 75 percent stated that they would be offended by sexually-oriented conduct in the workplace.[79] In *Robinson*, the court employed an "ordinary reasonable woman" standard to hold an employer responsible for the sexually harassing conduct of male employees toward a female co-worker.

Supporting Alison Wetherfield's assertion that men and women view sexually-oriented conduct differently is a recently-reported study done by the spousal research team of Struckman-Johnson and Struckman-Johnson, reported in 1994 in the journal *Sex Roles*.[80] In a study of 277 college men, subjects were asked to imagine that they were the target of unsolicited sexual advances from casual female acquaintances. Conduct to be imagined ranged from a gentle touch on the genitals, to a push, to coercion with and without a deadly weapon. Nearly 25 percent of the men stated that they would willingly continue sexual activity with an "attractive" female aggressor, even if coerced by the assailant with a deadly weapon.

In another legal case, *Ellison* v. *Brady*,[81] a federal appeals court evaluated what were described as "bizarre," repetitive, unwelcome love letters written by a male co-worker to a woman in a federal government office. The lower court had found that the man's conduct did not constitute sexual harassment. In reversing that decision, the appellate court adopted an "an ordinary reasonable woman" standard to assess whether the letters constituted sexual harassment.

Another model for assessing interpersonal conduct was developed by the U.S. Navy[82] after the Tailhook convention in which a number of male officers were accused of sexually harassing female colleagues. This model categorizes conduct as either:

- "green light," i.e., interpersonal conduct that is clearly acceptable behavior in the eyes of an ordinary reasonable person of either gender

- "yellow light," i.e., conduct that may be unacceptable in the eyes of some reasonable persons of the same gender as the target of the conduct

- "red light," i.e., conduct that is always unacceptable in the eyes of an ordinary reasonable person of the same gender as the target of the conduct

Green light conduct might include such things as complimenting a colleague about his or her dress in an inoffensive and nondiscriminatory manner. Yellow light behavior might include soliciting a date with a co-worker for the first time. Red light behavior includes such conduct as repeated solicitations for a date after rejection, indecent exposure, and sexual assault or battery.

In the workplace, managers bear the formidable responsibility of ferreting out, eliminating, and preventing sexual harassment. Managers may even be held liable for sexual harassment of which they are unaware, especially if the organization or work unit does not have in place a reporting or grievance mechanism for receiving and investigating complaints of sexual harassment. Management also is liable when it fails to take appropriate action on a complaint found to be valid at the conclusion of an investigation.[83] Managers are not free to assume an "ostrich defense." They will be held responsible for what they should have observed and corrected.[84]

Specific management responsibilities regarding sexual harassment include:

- *Sensitizing and educating employees about what constitutes sexual harassment, how men and women may differ in their attitudes toward sexual conduct, and the types of conduct that reasonable persons might find offensive.* This process not only should be a part of new employee orientations, but also should be regularly reinforced as continuing education for all employees. Managers might wish to consult with human resource management specialists to lead sessions at which employees are given information about current administrative and legal sexual harassment cases and are asked to participate in group cooperative learning processes, such as brainstorming about what interpersonal conduct constitutes permissible and impermissible behavior in the workplace.[85]

- *Expressing strong disapproval of sexual harassment and developing and enforcing appropriate sanctions to stop sexual harassment whenever it is found to exist.* Managers are responsible for taking immediate action to stop known sexual harassment, regardless of who the perpetrator[86] or the victim might be. Reporting, investigation, and grievance procedures for internal resolution of sexual harassment complaints should be in place. Managers must be fair and impartial in their investigations of such complaints, respecting the rights of all parties involved to the maximum extent possible.[87] If employees and others view management's commitment as strong, the investigatory process as equitable, and the awarding of sanctions as appropriate, then minor complaints stand a better chance of being resolved at the organizational level instead of through the EEOC or the courts.

- *Alerting employees, as required by federal law, of their right to initiate formal charges with the EEOC.* Although victims of sexual harassment should be encouraged to resolve grievances at the lowest appropriate level, under the EEOC sex discrimination guidelines, managers are responsible for making their employees aware of

Hint *Although managers have the primary responsibility for preventing and eliminating sexual harassment, responsibility is ultimately shared by everyone in an organization.*

their right to pursue unresolved complaints at higher administrative or legal levels. Making employees aware of their rights could be done as part of the sensitization process (discussed above). In addition, managers should ensure that both a statement of employees' rights and the organization's policy statement on sexual harassment, with a clear description of the internal grievance process, is posted in a prominent place.

Human Resource Management Issues

Recruitment and Selection

The same equal employment opportunity legal considerations that govern employment discrimination generally apply specifically to employee recruitment and selection procedures in both the private and public sectors. Job applicants, like current employees, are protected from employment discrimination by federal statutes, including the Civil Rights Act of 1964, the Equal Pay Act of 1963, the Age Discrimination in Employment Act of 1967, and the Americans with Disabilities Act of 1990, among others. Federal constitutional, case law, and administrative law protections augment federal statutory protections. State anti-employment-discrimination statutes and case and administrative law provide additional protection to job applicants.

Administrative guidelines promulgated by the EEOC offer employers specific guidance concerning prohibited and precautionary pre-employment inquiries.[88] Prohibited inquiries generally include questions concerning:

- race, ethnicity, national origin (Note that every employer has the right and legal duty to inquire about an applicant's legal right to work in the United States. This should be done for every job applicant.)
- marital status, number of children, child care arrangements, existence of an opposite- or same-gender "domestic partner"
- religious beliefs and practices
- disabilities, whether obvious or perceived
- age

Precautionary inquiries, i.e., ones that must pass the threshold test of being specifically job-related in order to be legitimate, generally include questions concerning:

- height, weight
- educational level
- criminal convictions
- military discharge classification (if less than honorable)
- financial status

Most or all of the precautionary inquiries listed above have been found, in administrative and judicial cases, to have a disparate impact on federally-protected classes of people. Employers may legally inquire about the existence of an applicant's criminal convictions, but should include a disclaimer in the job application that an affirmative response will not necessarily preclude selection of the applicant, but that the conviction will be considered in light of the totality of circumstances, including the nature of the offense, the applicant's age at the time the offense occurred, and indices of post-conviction rehabilitation. Most of the prohibited and precautionary pre-employment inquiries above become legitimate areas of inquiry, i.e., for activation of benefits,[89] EEOC reporting requirements, and other legitimate business and legal requirements, once an applicant is selected for employment.

Under what is known as the "four-fifths rule," the EEOC attributes as possible evidence of disparate discriminatory impact employee selection rates for protected classes that are less than 80 percent of the rate of the group with the highest selection rate. Consider the following example:

Thirty applicants are hired as home health aides for a managed care organization (MCO). Forty white males applied for employment with the MCO, as did 40 females (ten of whom are African-Americans). Twenty successful applicants are white males and ten are females, three of whom are African-Americans. Is the EEOC's four-fifths rule violated? Yes. The selection rate for the group with the highest selection (white males) is 50 percent. To avoid closer scrutiny by the EEOC, the selection rates for females generally, and African-American specifically, must be at least 40 percent (80 percent of 50 percent). Here, only 25 percent of females (30 percent of African-American females) were selected.

Employers, especially in occupations where employees are in close contact with clients (e.g., the health professions), need to be concerned about liability exposure for *negligent hiring*, a claim that may arise when a client or other person is injured by an employee. Negligent hiring means that the employer may be liable for injury to others when the employer fails to take reasonable steps to ascertain that a job applicant poses a danger to others and, once employed, that employee causes harm to the person or property of another in the course of employment.

Employers should take appropriate steps to screen for dangerousness through pre-employment inquiries about criminal convictions and gaps in employment or education and by conducting appropriate background investigations, pursuant to signed releases by applicants[90] (including inquiries to the National Practitioner Data Bank for licensed/certified health care professionals). In addition, employers should check as many employment references as is feasible and document the process and reference responses.

Employees vs. Independent Contractors

The distinction between employees and contract workers has enormous consequences for both employers and workers. By definition, an independent contractor is a person who works independently of detailed control of an employer. The employer is not normally vicariously liable for the contractor's work-related conduct. Employers, however, may be vicariously liable for the conduct of contractors under ostensible agency, when contractors are indistinguishable from employees in the eyes of the public.

Employers are primarily liable for the negligent selection and retention of contractors, areas over which employers do have control. Health care employers are additionally subject to primary liability for the negligent failure to monitor the quality of health care delivery throughout their organizations, irrespective of whether the care is delivered by employees, contractors, or others.

There are also tax consequences for employers, employees, and independent contractors for labeling workers as either employees or contractors. Employers are required by law to withhold federal income tax and social security contributions from employees, but not from contract workers, who are responsible for their own withholding. The complex and admittedly (by the Internal Revenue Service) ambiguous set of criteria for distinguishing employees and contractors, based on common law, classifies workers based on the nature, duration, and location of their work, and on the degree of permissible supervision of their work product by employers, among other factors.[91]

Employee Discipline and Termination

There are two basic approaches to employee discipline: a punitive, negative approach and a constructive, positive approach.[92] The constructive approach is always preferred when an employer wants to retain his or her employees because it promotes personal responsibility and self-correction by employees and a positive attitude and work ethic, which leads to enhanced productivity. Under either approach, employees are entitled to administrative due process, consisting of:

- procedural due process, i.e., notice of an infraction and an opportunity to be heard on the matter before disciplinary action is taken
- substantive due process, i.e., fundamental fairness. Under this prong of due process, the sanction(s) awarded for an offense must be reasonable in light of the totality of the circumstances. By analogy to criminal law, the punishment must fit the "crime."

In addition to being constructive and in compliance with due process standards, employee discipline should be progressive in nature. This means that discipline takes place along a continuum of possible actions, ranging at one extreme from no action, to discharge from employment at the other extreme. In between are progressive disciplinary steps, including a verbal warning, a written reprimand, a disciplinary transfer, and suspension from employment. For some offenses, the appropriate first step (after investigation) is discharge. Such offenses might include violent behavior causing injury to others and sex offenses committed on the job.

Scenarios that may lead to disciplinary action against employees have recently been augmented by newly publicized ones, including resume fraud[93] and office romances.[94] While employers are urged to have written policies making resume fraud grounds for dismissal from employment, the actual dismissal of an employee for resume fraud must be assessed on a case-by-case basis, taking into account the employee's whole record and the employer's financial and time investments in that employee. A 1993 survey conducted by the Society for Human Resource Management of its 65,000 members revealed that 90 percent of human resource professionals believe that, unless a superior-subordinate relationship exists, dating among employees should not be prohibited.[95]

Discharge from employment has been labeled as the "key employment rights issue of the 1990s."[96] The following procedural steps are recommended before executing disciplinary terminations of employees:

- Do not discharge an employee "on the spot" for any offense.
- Conduct a prompt and complete investigation of an alleged offense, affording all relevant parties (including the subject of the investigation) the opportunity to be heard.
- Consult with human resource management specialists and legal counsel for advice *ab initio* and throughout the process.
- If disciplinary termination is found to be warranted, ground it on a specific reason or reasons, and notify the employee in person, if feasible.
- Carefully and thoroughly document the investigatory process and retain it for at least the period of the legal statute of limitations for *wrongful discharge*,[97] along with all supporting documentation.

Health Professional Student Pre-Employment Contracts

The successful negotiation of pre-employment contracts permit many health professional students to contribute meaningfully toward self-funding their education, without being saddled with excessive loans upon entering the workforce. Employers also benefit from pre-employment contracting with health professional students, in that their staffing processes are made more predictable, with relatively firm work commitments on the part of prospective scarce health care professionals.

There are also several important potential disadvantages to pre-employment contracting. The process of seeking out and negotiating pre-employment contracts may foster excessive competition among students in selected job markets and practice settings. Employment contracts are formal legal instruments—just like any other business contract—with obligations incumbent on both parties, including penalties for breach of respective promises. Such contracts are often very complex, containing elements such as conditions precedent to the receipt of employment bonuses and liquidated (pre-established) monetary damages provisions for non-performance. There also are tax consequences for students who receive monetary bonuses from employers. Health professional program directors and student advisors should counsel students to have all pre-employment agreements reviewed by legal counsel before signing them.

Students also should be counseled concerning potential ethical dilemmas associated with pre-employment contracting. Potential issues include the issue involving the hypothetical student who "shops" for other employment after having signed a contractual agreement with another entity from whom the student has received money. Students under contract to an employer may also be subject to preferential treatment in clinical affiliations and internship experiences vis-a-vis those not under contract by clinical faculty having undisclosed conflicts of interest.

The professions of physical[98] and occupational[99] therapy have proposed guidelines for student pre-employment contracts. Professional students, academicians, employers, and legal counsel for students, employers, and educators should review these guidelines before entering into, or educating or advising on, such agreements.

Letters of Recommendation: To Write or Not to Write?

Employers, professors, clinical educators and managers, and other professionals are frequently asked to write letters of recommendation for employees, students, volunteers, and others. Prospective writers of recommendations may be torn ethically between the conflicting duties of helping someone whom they may like personally and conveying accurate information about the person. Human resource management scholars are of the opinion that letters of recommendation are biased and of little value, holding that "employers usually disregard such letters unless they contain negative information."[100]

Writers of letters of recommendation often are constrained from making candid comments about candidates because of a fear of liability exposure. The legal morass surrounding letters of recommendation is indeed complex. Potential litigation over recommendations may include:

- *Defamation* of character, i.e., the communication of false information injurious to a person's good reputation in the community. *Slander* is defamation communicated orally, and *libel* encompasses all other forms of defamation, including that conveyed in letters of recommendation.

- *Invasion of privacy*, i.e., the public disclosure of private facts about a person, such as arrests, drug use, and sexual orientation. Courts have found liable and imposed punitive damages against employers who unlawfully release confidential employee information, such as a credit history, drug test results, and human immunodeficiency virus (HIV) status.

- *Intentional infliction of emotional distress*, i.e., unreasonable conduct (including the communication of information about a person) that results in severe physical and psychological injury.

At the opposite end of the legal spectrum, individuals may also face liability exposure for failing to provide a reference when they have agreed to do so, as may be spelled out in an employment contract or employee handbook. Litigation might also result if one candidate learns that an employer, or other official, has written a favorable reference for one candidate, but has declined to do so for the litigant.

The growing concern over potential litigation over letters of recommendation has prompted many employers and individuals to change their policies on references. Many employers limit the information they convey to basic employment and salary data, even though, in some states, recommenders enjoy qualified immunity from liability as long as they act in good faith. Even with such protection, the burden of litigation over whether the writer is protected by qualified immunity is enough to prevent many individuals and companies from giving out information about others.

As rehabilitation "helping professionals," physical and occupational therapists are altruistic, and it runs counter to their nature to refuse to provide references to prospective candidates for employment, schooling, or other opportunities. With that in mind, the following risk management suggestions are recommended for writers of letters of recommendation.

- Require a written request for information from a prospective employer or other requestor and a written release from the candidate (especially when the recommendation will be anything less than sterling) before releasing any information.

- Respond to requests for information about employees, students, or others only in writing, so that your words will not be misconstrued. Maintain file copies of correspondence for at least the length of time of the state statute of limitations on legal actions. (Check with your legal advisor regarding the length of the tort statute of limitations for your state.)

- If possible, centralize formal responses to reference requests. Have your human resource manager and/or legal advisor review and send out any responses to requests for information about current or former employees, students, volunteers, or others.

Restrictive Covenants in Employment Contracts

Restrictive *covenants* in employment contracts limit the ability of parties to act without restraint in specified ways. In health care contracts, the principal types of restrictive covenants affecting employees are the non-solicitation provision and the covenant not to compete. A non-solicitation clause in an employment contract prevents a former professional employee from marketing his or her professional services to the employer's existing clients after termination of the employment relationship. A covenant not to compete is a contractual general promise made by an employee not to compete directly with a former employer.

A covenant not to compete is, in essence, a restraint on trade, which is generally considered to be against public policy. For that reason, a few states prohibit it altogether in employment contracts.[101] Most states, however, allow the covenant not to compete in employment contracts as a means to protect an employers' legitimate business interests.[102]

A covenant not to compete in an employment contract must meet four criteria in order to be valid and enforceable:

- It must be supported by consideration, that is, the covenant not to compete must have been made as part of a bargained-for exchange, and value must have been given by the employer in exchange for the employee's promise not to compete.

- A covenant not to compete must be reasonable in three areas[103] in terms of:

  — the geographic area of practice restriction

  — specific practice restrictions

  — time

Chapter Summary

Employment law is governed primarily by common and statutory law. The common law principle of employment at will governs most employment relationships and permits either an employee or employer to terminate the business relationship at will without penalty. Exceptions to employment at will include employment under contract for a specific term and employment treated as contractual, because of considerations such as language contained in employee handbooks and public policy considerations. The principle federal statute governing employment discrimination is Title VII of the Civil Rights Act of 1964, which prohibits employment discrimination against protected classes of workers, based on race/ethnicity, gender, religion, and national origin. Supplementing Title VII, among other federal and state statutes, are the Americans with Disabilities Act of 1990 and the Age Discrimination in Employment Act of 1967, protecting disabled and older workers from discrimination in employment.

The current complex work environment—especially under managed care—requires careful professional management of human resources. Human resource managers and legal counsel are key consultants to both employers and employees.

Cases and Questions

1. Develop five legitimate bona fide occupational qualifications that justify employment discrimination.

2. How might physical and occupational therapists serve as ADA consultants to employees and to industry?

3. Name five risk management measures, specific to your practice setting, that can be implemented to minimize the occurrence of sexual harassment of co-workers by employees.

Suggested Answers to Cases and Questions

1. The following are examples of legitimate bona fide occupational qualifications that justify employment discrimination:
   a. Requirement that a religious minister be credentialed by the same denomination as the congregation.
   b. Requirement that a wet nurse be female.
   c. Requirement for male-only applicants for the position of attendant for a men's dressing room at a public swimming pool.
   d. Requirement for female-only applicants to play the role of Selena in the upcoming movie based on her life.
   e. FAA regulations requiring airline pilots to retire at age 60.

2. As rehabilitation professionals, physical and occupational therapists possess unique understanding of the special needs of disabled workers, and can advise employers on how best (and at least expense) to meet their legal duty to accommodate them in the workplace. Physical and occupational therapists can also serve as consultants to disabled employees and job applicants concerning suggested requests for accommodations.

3. The following are examples of risk management measures that can be implemented to minimize the occurrence of sexual harassment of co-workers by employees:

a. Clinic policy recognizing sexual harassment as prohibited behavior.

b. Strong managerial commitment to preventing, investigating, and (where established) punishing sexual harassment.

c. Effective complaint and investigatory processes that are fair to all parties.

d. Orientation and ongoing training of the workforce concerning sexual harassment.

e. Regular consultation and coordination with legal and human resource management specialists.

References

1. *The World Almanac and Book of Facts 1996*. Mahwah, NJ: World Almanac Books, Inc., 1995, p. 146.
2. Shortell, S.M., Kaluzny, A.D. *Health Care Management: Organization Design and Behavior*, 3rd ed. Albany, NY: Delmar Publishers, 1994, p. 87.
3. Cherrington, D.J. *The Management of Human Resources*, 4th ed. Englewood Cliffs, NJ: Prentice Hall, 1995, pp. 11–15.
4. The Society for Human Resource Management, 606 North Washington Street, Alexandria, VA 22314-1997, telephone 1-800-283-SHRM.
5. "Companies Told They Have Duty to Workers." *San Antonio Express News*, March 24, 1995, p. 30A.
6. Furey, M.K., Ohnegian, S.A. "Employee Handbooks May Be Implied Contracts." *The National Law Journal*, October 24, 1994, p. B12.
7. The Railway Labor Act of 1926, 45 United States Code Sections 151 *et. seq.*
8. The National Labor Relations Act of 1935 (Wagner Act), 29 United States Code Sections 151–187.
9. The Labor-Management Relations Act of 1947 (Taft-Hartley Act), 29 United States Code Sections 141 *et. seq.*
10. See Executive Order No. 10988, 1962.
11. 29 United States Code Sections 158, 183.
12. *American Hospital Association* v. *National Labor Relations Board*, 499 U.S. 606 (1991).
13. "33.2 percent of the total work force in the United States was unionized in 1955; 15.5 percent in 1994." *The World Almanac and Book of Facts 1996*. Mahwah, NJ: World Almanac Books, Inc., 1995, p. 157, citing Bureau of Labor Statistics, U.S. Department of Labor, 1995.
14. The Age Discrimination in Employment Act of 1967, 29 United States Code Sections 621–634.
15. The Older Workers Benefit Protection Act of 1990, 29 United States Code Section 623.
16. Perry, P.M. "Don't Get Sued for Age Discrimination." *Law Practice Management*, May/June 1995, pp. 36–39.

17. The Americans with Disabilities Act of 1990, 42 United States Code Section 12101–12213.

18. Preamble, The Americans with Disabilities Act of 1990, Public Law 101-336, 104 Stat. 327, July 26, 1990.

19. The Rehabilitation Act of 1973, 29 United States Code Section 794a.

20. 42 United States Code Section 12187.

21. 42 United States Code Section 12111.

22. 42 United States Code Section 12102.

23. *The Americans With Disabilities Act: Your Responsibilities as an Employer.* Washington, DC: Equal Employment Opportunity Commission, Publication No. EEOC-BK-17, 1991, p. 2.

24. 42 United States Code Section 12111.

25. *Ibid.*

26. *The Americans With Disabilities Act: Your Responsibilities as an Employer.* Washington, DC: Equal Employment Opportunity Commission, Publication No. EEOC-BK-17, 1991, p. 4.

27. *Ibid.*, pp. 5–6; 42 United States Code Section 12111.

28. *The Americans With Disabilities Act: Your Responsibilities as an Employer.* Washington, DC: Equal Employment Opportunity Commission, Publication No. EEOC-BK-17, 1991, p. 6.

29. 42 United States Code Sections 12114, 12211.

30. *The Americans With Disabilities Act: Your Responsibilities as an Employer.* Washington, DC: Equal Employment Opportunity Commission, Publication No. EEOC-BK-17, 1991, p. 15.

31. "Disability Cases Rise." *Wall Street Journal*, May 6, 1993, p. B10.

32. "Backlash With ADA Emerging, Education Needed." *PT Bulletin*, February 24, 1995, p. 15.

33. Mirone, J.A. "Reasonable Accommodation in Disability Law." *PT: The Magazine of Physical Therapy*, 1995; 3(3):68–69.

34. *Borkowski* v. *Valley Central District*, 63 F.2d 131 (2d Cir. 1995).

35. *EEOC* v. *AIC Security Investigations, Ltd.*, 820 F. Supp. 1060 (N.D. Ill. 1993).

36. *Tuck* v. *HCA Health Services of Tennessee, Inc.*, 7 F.3d 465 (6th Cir. 1993).

37. *Langan* v. *Department of Health and Human Services*, 959 F.2d 1053 (D.C. Cir. 1992).

38. *Vande Zande* v. *Wisconsin Department of Administration*, 44 F.3d 538 (7th Cir. 1995).

39. *Harmer* v. *Virginia Electric & Power Company*, 831 F. Supp. 1300 (E.D. Va. 1993).

40. Phelan, G. "Reasonable Accommodation: Linchpin of ADA Liability." *Trial*, February 1996, pp. 40–44, at 44. In this excellent overview article, the author describes many additional reasonable accommodation ADA cases. For additional reasonable accommodation ADA cases, see Mirone, J.A., note 32.

41. Wehman, P., Revell, W., Kregel, J., *et. al.* "Supported Employment: An Alternative Model for Vocational Rehabilitation of Persons with Severe Neurological, Psychiatric, or Physical Disability." *Archives of Physical Medicine and Rehabilitation*, 1991; 72(2):101–105.

42. "States, Cities Stagger Under Financial Burden of Disabilities Law." *PT Bulletin*, December 15, 1993, pp. 36–37.

43. Civil Rights Act of 1964, Title VII, 42 United States Code Section 2000e - 2000e-17.

44. U.S. Constitution, Article I, Section 8.

45. Civil Rights Act of 1964, Title VII, Section 703(a).

46. Cherrington, D.J. *The Management of Human Resources*, 4th ed. Englewood Cliffs, NJ: Prentice Hall, 1995, p. 95.

47. 29 Code of Federal Regulations Sections 1602.20(b), 1607.4(B), 1993.

48. Civil Rights Act of 1964, Title VII, Section 703(e).

49. Barrett, P.M. "Job Bias Law to Be Clarified by High Court." *Wall Street Journal*, March 19, 1996, p. B9.

50. The Civil Rights Act of 1991, Public Law 102–166, 105 Stat. 071, 42 United States Code Sections 1981a and 2000e.

51. 42 United States Code 1981 note.

52. *Wards Cove Packing Co.* v. *Atonio*, 490 U.S. 642 (1989).

53. Davidson, M.J. "The Civil Rights Act of 1991." *Army Lawyer*, March 1992, pp. 3–11, at 3–4.

54. The Drug-Free Workplace Act of 1988, 41 United States Code Section 701–707.

55. *Ibid.*, Section 701(a)(1)(A).

56. Cherrington, D.J. *The Management of Human Resources*, 4th ed. Englewood Cliffs, NJ: Prentice Hall, 1995, p. 601.

57. Aalberts, R.J., Rubin, H.W. "A Risk Management Analysis of Employee Drug Abuse and Testing." *Chartered Property and Casualty Underwriters Journal*, 1988; 41(2):105–111.

58. Scott, R.W. "Defending the Apparently Indefensible Urinalysis Client in Nonjudicial Proceedings." *Army Lawyer*, November 1986, pp. 55–60.

59. Allen, T.Y. "DOT Drug-Testing Rules Require Detailed Plans." *HR News*, March 1996, pp. 3, 9.

60. The Employee Polygraph Protection Act of 1988, 29 United States Code Section 2001–2009.

61. Scott, R.W. "Defending the Apparently Indefensible Urinalysis Client in Nonjudicial Proceedings." *Army Lawyer*, November 1986, pp. 55–60, at 56, note 8.

62. The Employee Retirement Income Security Act of 1974, 29 United States Code Section 1001 *et. seq.*

63. Gostin, L.O., Widiss, A.I. "What's Wrong with the ERISA Vacuum? Employers' Freedom to Limit Health Care Coverage Provided by Risk Retention Plans." *Journal of the American Medical Association*, 1993; 269:2527–2532.

64. The Equal Pay Act of 1963, 29 United States Code Section 206, an amendment to the Fair Labor Standards Act, provides in pertinent part that:

   No employer shall discriminate between employees on the basis of sex by paying wages to employees less than the rate at which he pays wages to employees of the opposite sex for equal work on jobs which require equal skill, effort, and responsibility, and similar working conditions. (29 U.S.C. Section 206d[1])

65. *EEOC: Information for the Private Sector and State and Local Governments*. Washington, DC, EEOC-BRP-E (undated).

66. "EEOC and OSHA Prepare to Make Better Use of Limited Resources." *Issues in HR*, May/June 1995, pp. 2–3.

67. The Family and Medical Leave Act of 1993, 29 United States Code Section 2601–2654.

68. Lublin, J.S. "Family-Leave Law Can Be Excuse for a Day Off." *Wall Street Journal*, July 7, 1995, pp. B1, B10.

69. *Ibid.*, at B1.

70. Young, R.S. "Managing Medical Leaves of Absence." *HR Magazine*, August 1995, pp. 23–30.

71. *Ibid.*, citing Survey of 123 Fortune 500 companies by Labor Policy Association, Washington, DC.

72. The Occupational Safety and Health Act of 1970, 29 United States Code Section 651–678.

73. The Pregnancy Discrimination Act of 1978, 42 United States Code Section 2000e(k).

74. White, B. "Workers' Compensation Rates Drop as Reform Legislation Takes Hold." *Houston Business Journal*, November 29, 1993, p. 30.

75. Cherrington, D.J. *The Management of Human Resources*, 4th ed. Englewood Cliffs, NJ: Prentice Hall, 1995, p. 509. Three states—Texas, New Jersey, and South Carolina—permit employers to opt out of coverage under state-sponsored workers' compensation insurance plans. Those employers who exercise this option lose most of the common law defenses that so often shielded them from liability in the past and are held liable for employee injuries for which they are in any way at fault. Merlo, C. "Texas Non-Subscribers Still Have Protections." *Risk Management*, June 1992, p. 7.

76. Sex Discrimination Guidelines, Equal Employment Opportunity Commission, 29 Code of Federal Regulations 1604.11, *Federal Register*, November 10, 1980; 45:74677.

77. *Black's Law Dictionary*, 3rd ed. St. Paul, MN: West Publishing Company, 1979, p. 990.

78. *Robinson v. Jacksonville Shipyards*, 760 F. Supp. 1486 (Middle District of Florida 1991).

79. Hays, A.S. "Courts Concede That the Sexes Think in Unlike Ways." *Wall Street Journal*, May 28, 1991, pp. B1, B5.

80. Struckman-Johnson, C.S., Struckman-Johnson, D. "Men's Reactions to Hypothetical Female Sexual Advances." *Sex Roles*, 1994; 1:387–405.

81. *Ellison v. Brady*, 924 F.2d 871 (9th Circuit 1991).

82. *Resolving Conflict: Following the Light of Personal Behavior*. Washington, DC: U.S. Government Printing Office, Naval Personnel Bulletin 15620, 1993.

83. Plevan, B.B., Borg, J.A. "Expanded Employer Liability for Supervisors' Conduct in Hostile Work Environments." *The National Law Journal*, August 8, 1994, pp. B5–B10.

84. Kruger, P. "See No Evil." *Working Woman*, June 1995, pp. 32–35, 64, 77.

85. Graf, L.A., Hemmasi, M. "Risque Humor: How It Really Affects the Workplace." *HR Magazine*, November 1995, pp. 64–69.

86. Niven, D. "The Case of Hidden Harassment." *Harvard Business Review*, March/April 1992, pp. 12–27. The scenario presented in this case study involves a female office worker who is sexually harassed by her supervisor's superior. The victim's supervisor learns of the sexual harassment by chance and, when questioned about it, the victim does not want it to be reported. The case analysis offers the opinions of several human resource management and legal experts on how the victim's immediate supervisor should proceed.

87. Lopez, J.A. "Control the Damage of a False Accusation of Sexual Harassment." *Wall Street Journal*, January 12, 1994, p. B1.

88. *Preemployment Inquiries*. Washington, DC: Equal Employment Opportunity Commission, 1991.

89. Only about 150 of the 6,000,000 employers in the United States have expanded the benefits penumbra to include "domestic partners" of employees. Employers who offer this extended benefit to employees do so for one or more of the following reasons: to right perceived inequity in benefits protections; to proactively accommodate an increasingly diverse workforce; to attract select employees; and for business goodwill. Only a small percentage (2 to 3 percent) of eligible employees accept domestic partner benefits, and two-thirds of those have opposite-sex domestic partners. Swoboda, F. "Extending the Benefits Umbrella to a Wider World." *The Washington Post*, June 4, 1995, p. H5.

90. Jackson, S., Loftin, A. "Proactive Practices Avoid Negligent Hiring Claims." *HR News*, September 1995, p. 9.

91. Selz, M., Mehta, S.N. "Small Businesses Get Big Bills as IRS Targets Free-Lancers." *Wall Street Journal*, August 24, 1995, pp. B1–B2.

92. Cherrington, D.J. *The Management of Human Resources*, 4th ed. Englewood Cliffs, NJ: Prentice Hall, 1995, p. 594.

93. O'Neal, L.L., Loftin, A.T. "Consider Context Before Firing for Resume Fraud." *HR News*, February 1996, p. 13.

94. Hicks, M. "Love Amid the Cubicles." *San Francisco Examiner*, February 12, 1995, pp. D1, D6.

95. *Ibid*.

96. *Legal Report: Cardinal Rules for Disciplinary Terminations*. Alexandria, VA: Society for Human Resource Management, 1995, p. 1.

97. Korotkin, M.I. "Damages in Wrongful Termination Cases." *American Bar Association Journal*, May 1989, pp. 84–87.

98. Winter, K. "APTA House Members Prepare to Discuss Proposed Guidelines for Fairness in Student Pre-Employment Contracts." *PT Bulletin*, June 17, 1992, pp. 8–9, pp. 107–108.

99. Perry, R., Crist, P. "Strategies for Negotiating Preemployment Agreements." *The American Journal of Occupational Therapy*, 1994; 48:824–831.

100. Cherrington, D.J. *The Management of Human Resources*, 4th ed. Englewood Cliffs, NJ: Prentice Hall, 1995, p. 228.

101. Lewis, K. "Physical Therapy Contracts." *Clinical Management*, 1992; 12(6):14–18. Most states that prohibit employment-related covenants not to compete permit such contractual provisions involving the sale of an ongoing business to another professional in order to protect the "goodwill" value of the business being sold.

102. Wallen, E. "A Restrictive Covenant Can Lessen Practice's Risk of Losing Patients." *Physicians Financial News*, May 1991, p. 26.

103. Freed, C., Martinez, W.L. "Non-Compete Covenant Has to Be Reasonable." *San Antonio Medical Gazette*, June 9–15, 1993, p. 8.

Suggested Readings

1. Aalberts, R.J., Rubin, H.W. "A Risk Management Analysis of Employee Drug Abuse and Testing." *Chartered Property and Casualty Underwriters Journal*, 1988; 41(2):105–111.

2. Armbruster, K.R., Ellard, W.M., Holtzclaw, S.R. "ERISA Preemption: State-Law Claims by Health-Care Providers." *The Health Lawyer*, 1995; 8(2):12–14.

3. *A Short History of the American Labor Movement*. Washington, DC: American Federation of Labor-Congress of Industrial Organizations, 1981.

4. "Backlash With ADA Emerging, Education Needed." *PT Bulletin*, February 24, 1995, pp. 15, 32.

5. Cherrington, D.J. *The Management of Human Resources*, 4th ed. Englewood Cliffs, NJ: Prentice Hall, 1995.

6. Colan, B.J. "Five Years Later: Is ADA Meeting Needs?" *Advance for Physical Therapists*, June 19, 1995, pp. 5, 24.

7. "Companies Told They Have Duty to Workers." *San Antonio Express News*, March 24, 1995, p. 30A.

8. Davidson, M. J. "The Civil Rights Act of 1991." *Army Lawer*, March 1992, pp. 3–11.

9. "Employers Face a Difficult Burden of Proof When Attempting to Enforce a Disability-Based Distinction in Employee Benefits." *The Health Lawyer*, 1993; 7(1):2, 15.

10. Ensman, R.G. "Don't Ask! Twenty Questions to Avoid During Employment Interviews." *Advance for Health Information Professionals*, December 13, 1993, p. 15.

11. Freed, C., Martinez, W.L. "Non-Compete Covenant Has to Be Reasonable." San *Antonio Medical Gazette*, June 9–15, 1993, p. 8.

12. Fishman, R.H. "Where Silence Is Golden." *Nation's Business*, July 1991, pp. 48–49.

13. Furey, M.K., Ohnegian, S.A. "Employee Handbooks May Be Implied Contracts." *The National Law Journal*, October 24, 1994, p. B12.

14. Gostin, L.O., Widiss, A.I. "What's Wrong with the ERISA Vacuum? Employers' Freedom to Limit Health Care Coverage Provided by Risk Retention Plans." *Journal of the American Medical Association*, 1993; 269:2527–2532.

15. Graf, L.A., Hemmasi, M. "Risque Humor: How It Really Affects the Workplace." *HR Magazine*, November 1995, pp. 64–69.

16. Hays, A.S. "Courts Concede That the Sexes Think in Unlike Ways." *Wall Street Journal*, May 28, 1991, pp. B1, B5.

17. Hicks, M. "Love Amid the Cubicles." *San Francisco Examiner*, February 12, 1995, pp. D1, D6.

18. Jackson, S., Loftin, A. "Proactive Practices Avoid Negligent Hiring Claims." *HR News*, September 1995, p. 9.

19. Jones, D.L., Watzlaf, V.J.M., Hobson, D., Mazzoni, J. "Responses Within Nonfederal Hospitals in Pennsylvania to the Americans with Disabilities Act of 1990." *Journal of the American Physical Therapy Association*, 1996; 76:49–60.

20. King, B. "ADA Update: Making Room, Title III: Accessibility to Programs and Services." *Advance for Directors in Rehabilitation*, May/June 1993, pp. 47–52.

21. Korotkin, M.I. "Damages in Wrongful Termination Cases." *American Bar Association Journal*, May 1989, pp. 84–87.

22. Kruger, P. "See No Evil." *Working Woman*, June 1995, pp. 32–35, 64, 77.

23. *Legal Report: Cardinal Rules for Disciplinary Terminations*. Alexandria, VA: Society for Human Resource Management, 1995, p. 1.

24. Lewis, K. "Physical Therapy Contracts." *Clinical Management*, 1992; 12(6):14–18.

25. Lopez, J.A. "Control the Damage of a False Accusation of Sexual Harassment." *Wall Street Journal*, January 12, 1994, p. B1.

26. Lublin, J.S. "Family-Leave Law Can Be Excuse for a Day Off." *Wall Street Journal*, July 7, 1995, pp. B1, B10.

27. Miller, G. "At-Will Employment Doctrine—Are Patient Care Employers Vulnerable?" *Hospital & Health Services Administration*, 1991; 36(2):257–270.

28. Niven, D. "The Case of Hidden Harassment." *Harvard Business Review*, March/April 1992, pp. 12–27.

29. O'Neal, L.L., Loftin, A.T. "Consider Context Before Firing for Resume Fraud." *HR News*, February 1996, p. 13.

30. Perry, P.M. "Don't Get Sued for Age Discrimination." *Law Practice Management*, May/June 1995, pp. 36–39.

31. Perry, R., Crist, P. "Strategies for Negotiating Preemployment Agreements." *The American Journal of Occupational Therapy*, 1994; 48:824–831.

32. Phelan, G. "Reasonable Accommodation: Linchpin of ADA Liability." *Trial*, February 1996, pp. 40–44.

33. Plevan, B.B., Borg, J.A. "Expanded Employer Liability for Supervisors' Conduct in Hostile Work Environments." *The National Law Journal*, August 8, 1994, pp. B5–B10.

34. *Preemployment Inquiries*. Washington, DC: Equal Employment Opportunity Commission, 1991.

35. Reichley, M.L. "ADA Update: Titles II and III, Lesser Known, Just as Important." *Advance for Physical Therapists*, March 13, 1995, pp. 10, 24.

36. *Resolving Conflict: Following the Light of Personal Behavior*. Washington, DC: U.S. Government Printing Office, Naval Personnel Bulletin 15620, 1993.

37 Rybski, D. "A Quality Implementation of Title I of the Americans with Disabilities Act of 1990." *The American Journal of Occupational Therapy*, 1992; 46:409–418.

38. Scott, R.W. "Defending the Apparently Indefensible Urinalysis Client in Nonjudicial Proceedings." *Army Lawyer*, November 1986, 55–60.

39. Scott, R.W. "The ADA and You." *Clinical Management*, 1992; 12(1):16–17.

40. Shortell, S.M., Kaluzny, A.D. *Health Care Management: Organization Design and Behavior*, 3rd ed. Albany, NY: Delmar Publishers, 1994.

41. Struckman-Johnson, C.S., Struckman-Johnson, D. "Men's Reactions to Hypothetical Female Sexual Advances." *Sex Roles*, 1994; 1:387–405.

42. Swoboda, F. "Extending the Benefits Umbrella to a Wider World." *The Washington Post*, June 4, 1995, p. H5.

43. The Americans with Disabilities Act of 1990, 42 United States Code Section 12101 *et. seq.*

44. *The Americans With Disabilities Act: Your Responsibilities as an Employer*. Washington, DC: Equal Employment Opportunity Commission, Publication No. EEOC-BK–17, 1991.

45. *Understanding the ADA*. New York: Atlantic Mutual Insurance Company, 1992.

46. Wallen, E. "A Restrictive Covenant Can Lessen Practice's Risk of Losing Patients." *Physicians Financial News*, May 1991, p. 26.

47. Winter, K. "APTA House Members Prepare to Discuss Proposed Guidelines for Fairness in Student Pre-Employment Contracts." *PT Bulletin*, June 17, 1992, pp. 8–9, 107–108.

48. Young, R.S. "Managing Medical Leaves of Absence." *HR Magazine*, August 1995, pp. 23–30.

49. Youngberg, B.J. "The Americans with Disabilities Act: Meeting the Challenge in the Health Care Arena." *Quality & Risk Management in Health Care*, 1991; 1(6):1–8.

Chapter 9

Insurance Law

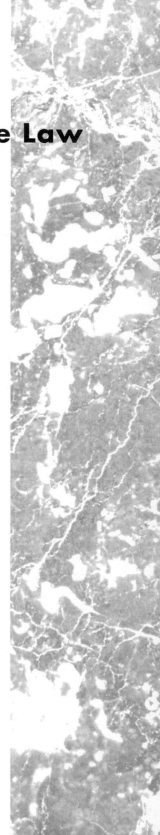

T his chapter introduces basic insurance law concepts. The chapter begins with a discussion of the nature of business financial risk and the need to minimize personal risk through the purchase of insurance. Insurance law is described as being largely under state vs. federal control, evidenced by the fact that the insurance industry enjoys a statutory exemption from compliance with federal antitrust law under the McCarran-Ferguson Act of 1945.

Insurance contracts have characteristics common to all legal contractual instruments and impose mutual legal duties on the insured and his or her insurer. As a result of the insurance crisis of the 1970s and 1980s, health care professional liability insurance companies began to write claims-made policies, instead of the traditional occurrence-coverage policies, which are described in detail in the chapter. The chapter concludes with a discussion about who needs professional liability insurance coverage (almost everyone).

The Nature of Insurance

Virtually every business undertaking—including the rendition of health care delivery services—carries with it a degree of risk of financial loss. Such is the nature of business. Financial losses may be incurred by business owners, investors, and professionals from fire damage and other natural disasters, spoilage of goods, theft of goods and services, and claims and litigation. The purchase of insurance is one of the most important ways that professionals can minimize their business-related financial losses, by transferring the legal responsibility to pay for covered outlays to third-party insurance professionals.

Several of the common types of insurance are very familiar to health care professionals. As part of their employee benefits programs, most health care professionals enjoy employer-paid or subsidized health and life insurance. Many professional employees also have employer-paid or subsidized employment-related short- or long-term disability insurance coverage. Those who own homes and are encumbered with mortgages are required by their mortgagees (and by good business sense) to take out homeowner's insurance for the mutual protection of mortgagees and mortgagors (homeowners). Personal property insurance protects the insurable interests of persons and businesses in *chattels*, or moveable items of personal property.

General liability insurance covers insured persons and businesses against losses from claims and litigation brought by parties against policyholders for monetary damages incident to personal injury or property damage for which the policyholders are legally responsible to pay. Automobile liability insurance is a special form of liability insurance with which most drivers are familiar.

While the remainder of this chapter is devoted exclusively to health care professional liability insurance, all types of insurance have several key elements in common. They all have as their primary purpose the protection of persons or entities with insurable legal interests in specific property or people. All types of insurance are characterized by the concepts of *risk pooling* and *risk transfer*. Risk pooling means that neither the innocent victims of misfortune, nor those who negligently or otherwise wrongfully cause injury to other persons or their property, bear the financial losses of their misfortunes personally. All of those who are jointly insured by an insurance company share in each payable loss through their payment of insurance premiums. The larger the pool of insured contributors, the greater the spread of risk of financial loss. Risk transfer means that the specific responsibility to pay for insured losses rests with insurance companies, rather than with individuals responsible for occasioning such losses.

Insurance law is largely a matter of state, rather than federal law.[1] State legislatures enact applicable statutes governing insurance activities conducted within their states. State administrative agencies establish applicable insurance rules and regulations and enforce compliance. Litigation over insurance matters is generally under the jurisdiction of state courts (absent diversity of citizenship or a relevant federal question).

The Insurer-Insured Relationship

The relationship between insured and insurer is a contractual one, with the policy representing the contractual legal instrument. The same rules that govern the formation, administration, and execution of business contracts in general also govern insurance policies.

The parties to the insurance contract are the insured, who is legally considered to be the offeror of an application for insurance. The insurer, or insurance company, as offeree, accepts the prospective insured's offer to purchase insurance and issues a policy. Intermediaries potentially involved in insurance contracts include brokers (representing insured persons) and underwriters and agents (representing insurance companies).

The mutual consideration in support of the validity of a health professional liability insurance policy includes the insured party's promise to pay (in the form of a lump-sum payment or periodic insurance premiums) and the insurer's promise to indemnify the insured against personal liability for covered losses. Indemnification means that the insurer "holds" the insured financially "harmless" by guaranteeing competent legal representation of the insured to defend the parties' mutual interests, up to the amount of insurance coverage, and by guaranteeing payment up to the maximum amount of insurance coverage in the event of settlement or an adverse judgment in court.

Health care professional liability insurance policies, reflecting state law requirements and public policy considerations, do not normally insure against liability for malicious intentional misconduct (such as malicious battery or sexual battery committed against patients). Nor do most such policies insure against liability for wanton reckless conduct, such as the conscious disregard of known contraindications to selected interventions in the course of treatment. These circumstances and other exclusions are stated in the exclusions section of an insurance policy.

Health care professional liability insurance policies do, however, normally insure against liability arising from non-malicious intentional treatment-related conduct generally, as long as such conduct does not involve a specific intent to cause harm to a patient. The inclusion of coverage for intentional conduct is critically important to rehabilitation professionals, including occupational, physical, respiratory, and speech-language therapists, nurses, physicians, and others, since their professional interventions necessarily involve the "laying on of hands."

Consider the following hypothetical example of a case in which coverage and indemnification for intentional treatment-related conduct by a health professional would be allowable under a typical professional liability insurance policy.

A board-certified orthopedic physical therapist evaluates a patient with a diagnosis of cervical facet syndrome. The family practice physician who referred the patient for physical therapy requested only that the physical therapist "evaluate and treat" the patient. The accompanying full cervical radiographic series taken just two days before physical therapy evaluation is negative. In the course of the physical therapy evaluation, the physical therapist reaches a diagnosis of a mild, chronic right-sided C6-7 facet subluxation. The therapist chooses to manipulate the patient's neck to resolve the patient's moderate local pain symptoms. As a result of manipulation, the patient's condition worsens. The patient's local pain begins to radiate to the right arm. Eventually, a C6-7 discectomy is required. The patient sues the physical therapist for professional negligence. The state physical therapy practice act is silent on whether physical therapists are privileged to carry out cervical orthopedic manipulation, as is the state's medical practice act.

Does the defendant-physical therapist's individual professional liability insurance policy protect him against personal liability in the event of an adverse judgment? Yes. Spinal manipulation is clearly within the customary scope of practice of orthopedic physical therapy, even if it is not specifically enumerated as an element of professional practice in the state practice act. The physical therapist did not violate the provisions of the referral order. The facts of the case, as stated, do not support the

227

contention that the physical therapist acted maliciously or recklessly. The defendant-physical therapist's professional liability insurer should both defend and indemnify the physical therapist against personal liability, to the maximum coverage limit of the policy. Remember, however, that once the insurer pays money to the plaintiff in settlement or judgment on the insured's behalf, the physical therapist's name must be reported for inclusion in the National Practitioner Data Bank.[2]

State insurance law may also prohibit indemnification of a health professional's liability for punitive damages, also on public policy grounds. Insurance entities normally may, however, insure for and indemnify against employers' vicarious liability for punitive damages levied against their employees who were acting within the scope of employment at the time of alleged wrongdoing, since no public policy is normally violated in such circumstances.

While an insurer's duty to indemnify an insured party against personal liability may be greatly affected by public policy considerations, its legal duty to defend its insured clients is governed largely by contract law (i.e., the private law of the parties). In most cases, an insurer has the contractual obligation to defend an insured client in a legal action against the client whenever there is a potential reasonable basis for indemnification of the insured by the insurer. (The customary practice is for an insurer to contract with outside legal counsel, who are civil trial experts, to represent its insured on behalf of the insurer.) In such cases, however, an insurer defends an insured party under an express reservation that indemnification is conditioned on a finding that permits indemnification under the insurance contract.

Both parties to an insurance contract are charged with the mutual implied duty of good faith. Consider the following hypothetical example.

An insured occupational therapist is sued by a patient for alleged professional negligence incident to post-stroke rehabilitation. In the course of managing the legal case, the defendant-occupational therapist has the affirmative duty to cooperate with the insurer, including, among other considerations:

- giving timely notice of the adverse patient event (i.e., P.C.E., or potentially compensable event)
- cooperating with appointed legal counsel representing the insured and insurer's mutual interests, especially in formulating a legitimate case strategy most favorable to the defense
- cooperating with legal counsel (for both sides) in pre-trial processes (including answering *interrogatories* and attending *depositions*
- appearing and testifying at trial, if the case proceeds to that point

The insurer also has affirmative good faith contractual duties. These include:

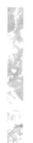

- using its best professional judgment and expending its best efforts to achieve a result most favorable for the insured

- working closely with the insured (and the insured party's personal legal counsel, if one or more is involved in the case) and keeping the insured apprised of developments in the case

- attempting to settle a claim or lawsuit within policy limits, so as to avoid exposing the insured to personal liability for amounts in excess of insurance coverage

State law may require that an insurer obtain an insured party's reasonable consent before settling a high-dollar claim. In a 1988 Missouri case, an insured health care professional was allowed to bring a breach of contract legal case against his professional liability insurer (and the law firm that the insurer hired to defend the case) for settling a case against the insured without the insured's consent, as was required under the policy.[3]

Because an attorney retained by an insurer to defend a health care professional in a malpractice case represents both the insured and the insurer, there is always the potential for a conflict of interest. The same potential for a conflict of interest exists when an employer's (vicarious) liability insurer co-represents the employer and a health care professional employee charged with negligence or wrongdoing, incident to employment. Attorneys in such circumstances are required by law to inform the insured of the nature of the dual representation, and obtain the insured party's informed consent to the relationship.

If an actual conflict of interest between the parties represented arises, then the attorney is legally and ethically obligated to sever representation of the health care professional and advise the health care professional to retain substitute legal counsel. The attorney severing the attorney-client relationship with the health care professional is then precluded from revealing to anyone (except substitute counsel) prejudicial confidential communications made to him or her by the health care professional-client.

Because of the potential for a conflict of interest in health care malpractice litigation, health care professionals should consider retaining personal legal counsel to assist them in defense of their personal interests if and when they are claimed against or sued. The exercise of this option has several advantages and disadvantages.

Personal legal counsel exclusively represents the legal interests of the health care professional-client, not those of an employer or insurance company. Hence, there is no potential conflict of interest, and personal counsel may be in a better position to recommend a course of action most favorable to the health care professional. Health care professionals may feel more at ease with such co-representation, especially if they have long-standing relationships with their personal legal counsel. The resultant diminution in the health care professional's stress level should work to everyone's advantage on the defense team, as the defendant will probably be a more effective witness in deposition and at trial.

There are two principal disadvantages to employing personal legal counsel to assist in health care malpractice defense cases in which insurance counsel is involved. First, the cost to retain personal counsel is potentially great. Second, the provider's personal and insurance counsel may not agree on case strategies and disposition. If such a disagreement is irreconcilable, then the provider's insurer may attempt to withdraw from representation, alleging failure on the part of the insured to cooperate with the insurer.

Occurrence vs. Claims-Made Professional Liability Insurance

During the 1970s, there was a substantial increase in the number and severity of health care malpractice claims and lawsuits. As a result, a health care professional liability insurance crisis ensued, leading first to decreased availability, and later to decreased affordability, of professional liability insurance. By the mid-1980s, health care professional liability insurers turned to writing claims-made, rather than occurrence coverage, professional liability insurance policies.[4]

Occurrence coverage means that a health care professional is indemnified for covered adverse incidents which occurred while the professional was insured by the insurer, irrespective of when a claim is filed. It does not matter, under occurrence coverage, whether the health professional is still insured by the insurer at the time the claim is filed.

Before the advent of the insurance affordability crisis of the 1980s, occurrence coverage for health care professional liability insurance was the industry standard. However, as the numbers of health care malpractice claims and lawsuits rose precipitously during the 1970s and 1980s, the "tail" period for liability and indemnity exposure grew very long. Health care malpractice claims and legal judgments can take years to come to fruition, leading to significant uncertainty both for health professionals and their professional liability insurers.

As a result, most health care professional liability insurers began to write exclusively claims-made policies, reflecting their fear of uncertainty under the health care and global litigation crises. Under *claims-made* health care professional liability policies, claims brought against insurers for covered adverse incidents must be made while the health professional is still insured by the insurer in order to be payable under the policy.

In order to minimize personal liability exposure incident to health care practice, health care professionals who are insured under claims-made policies must purchase an endorsement to their professional liability insurance policies called "tail coverage." The purchase of tail coverage, in essence, converts a claims-made professional liability insurance policy into an occurrence policy.

A sometimes costly alternative to tail coverage is "prior acts" coverage, also referred to as "nose coverage." Prior acts coverage consists of an endorsement to a new professional liability insurance policy offered by a new insurer for yet-to-be-claimed adverse incidents that may have occurred while the insured was covered under a previous policy. Prior acts coverage is not only more expensive than tail coverage; it is a less certain option for insured professionals and may be fraught with additional limitations and exclusions.[5]

The relative advantages of claims-made health care professional liability insurance policies are (1) their cost is lower than for occurrence-coverage policies, and (2) liability limits can be modified from year to year. The relative advantage of an occurrence-coverage policy is its longer-term (i.e., "tail") protection.[6]

Managed care poses particular professional liability insurance-related threats to the personal financial security of health care professionals. Because of the uncertainty of employment or affiliation in managed care environments, a health care professional must be sure to purchase tail coverage when the provider moves from one managed care relationship to another. In addition, all providers are cautioned to consult both with their legal advisors and agents for their professional liability insurance companies before signing managed care contracts under which they promise to "hold harmless" the managed organizations for provider conduct. A providers' primary health care malpractice insurance coverage may not indemnify the insured provider under such circumstances.

The Need for Professional Liability Insurance

Who needs professional liability insurance? Almost everyone does. Every health care professional involved in clinical practice, with the exception of those professionals who are federal employees (or state employees, under similar circumstances), need the protection of professional liability insurance coverage. Federal health care professionals enjoy worldwide protection from personal monetary liability for official acts incident to their federal duties under the Federal Employees Liability Reform and Tort Compensation Act of 1988.[7]

Until March 1991, it was not certain that federal employees were totally immune from personal liability for alleged health care malpractice. In 1987, a military service member and his wife filed a federal diversity health care malpractice lawsuit in the U.S. District Court for the Central District of California against a military physician. The lawsuit alleged medical malpractice incident to the delivery of their child at an Army hospital in Italy. The U.S. Court of Appeals for the Ninth Circuit ruled that the lawsuit could proceed against the military physician as a private defendant, because, in the opinion of the court, he did not have personal immunity from suit for malpractice actions arising outside of the territorial limits of the United States. The U.S. Supreme Court reversed the ruling in a 1991 decision, in which the Court ruled that the Federal Employees Liability Reform and Tort Compensation Act of 1988 provides an absolute shield of personal immunity (worldwide) for federal employees acting within the scope of their employment.[8] In this case, the plaintiffs were left without a legal remedy, because the federal government (which otherwise would have been substituted for the military physician as the defendant in the case) has not waived its sovereign immunity, under the Federal Tort Claims Act,[9] for incidents that occur abroad.

Hint *The Federal Employees Liability Reform and Tort Compensation Act of 1988 provides an absolute shield of personal immunity for federal employees acting within the scope of their employment, meaning that federal employees do not need professional liability insurance coverage for their official duties.*

Experts disagree over whether health care professionals should carry individual professional liability insurance, or should be content to rely on the coverage in liability policies carried by their employers.[10] In support of not purchasing individual professional liability insurance, it has been argued that knowledge on the part of a health care malpractice plaintiff of the very existence of individual professional liability insurance makes it more likely that the patient will sue. However, the peace of mind associated with the security that individual professional liability insurance coverage provides more than offsets this consideration. In addition, an individual providers' insurance legal counsel can contribute significantly in defense of a health care malpractice legal case and may actually decrease the likelihood of a finding of liability (with all of its adverse consequences to the defendant-provider).

Chapter Summary

Insurance coverage is one of the most effective ways to minimize personal liability risk. The insurance policy is similar in all respects to other business contracts, under which both the insured and the insurer voluntarily assume legal duties toward one another. The insured assumes the legal duties of promptly notifying the insurer in the event of a potentially compensable event, cooperating with insurance counsel in the adjudication of a claim or lawsuit, and paying for coverage in a timely manner, as provided by the agreement. The insurer acts as a *fiduciary*, or one in a special position of trust, toward the insured.

As a result of the litigation crisis of the 1970s and 1980s, the availability and affordability of health care professional liability insurance were jeopardized. Insurers began, in the 1980s, to issue claims-made vs. occurrence-coverage health care professional liability insurance policies in an attempt to minimize their potential liability exposure. Managed care initiatives have highlighted the need for providers to have seamless insurance coverage for potential liability incident to health care delivery.

Everyone needs professional liability insurance (except federal health care professionals, while acting exclusively within the scope of their federal duties). Everyone who needs insurance probably needs individual coverage, in addition to any coverage that employers or managed care organizations may carry on behalf of providers.

Cases and Questions

1. *A*, a physical therapist in private practice, is charged with commission of sexual battery on patient *B* during a therapeutic massage treatment. A civil malpractice lawsuit ensues, in which the jury awards a judgment in favor of *B*, with punitive damages. Is *A*'s professional liability insurer obligated to indemnify *A*?

2. *C*, a military occupational therapist, works part-time at a civilian rehabilitation center treating pediatric patients. Does *C* need to purchase professional liability insurance?

Suggested Answers to Cases and Questions

1. No. State insurance law normally prohibits indemnification of insured persons for willful misconduct. Even if not disallowed under state law, a judge would probably decline to enforce execution of a contract that violates public policy, as this one seemingly would.

2. Yes. The Federal Employees Liability Reform and Tort Compensation Act of 1988 only provides for personal immunity for federal employees while they are acting within the scope of their federal employment. Here, the military occupational therapist is acting in a private capacity and is subject to the same personal liability exposure as any of her civilian professional colleagues. (As a side note, military providers should ensure that all of their official duties are referenced on their federal job descriptions, so that there is no question of immunity under the Federal Employees Liability Reform and Tort Compensation Act of 1988 in the event of an adverse patient or client incident.)

References

1. With the McCarran-Ferguson Act of 1945, 15 United States Code Sections 1012–1014, Congress affirmed that the insurance industry is primarily the business of the states, creating a general legislative exemption for state insurance activities from application of federal antitrust law.
2. Individual health care professionals who personally pay money to plaintiffs in settlement of malpractice claims are not required to self-report to the National Practitioner Data Bank. Spaeth, D. "ADA Wins Appeal of Data Bank Suit." *ADA News*, 1993; 24(16):1, 9–10.
3. "Court Rules Physician May Sue Lawyer for Malpractice Settlement." *PT Bulletin*, September 14, 1988, p. 5.
4. Johnson, K.B., Hatlie, M.J., Johnson, I.D. *The Guide to Medical Professional Liability Insurance*. Chicago, IL: American Medical Association, 1991, pp. 13–14.
5. "Occurrence vs. Claims-Made Medical Professional Liability Insurance Policies: Fundamental Differences in the Concept of Coverage." *Journal of the American Medical Association*, 1991; 266:1570–1572.
6. Kelley, K. "In Practice: Occurrence vs. Claims-Made Policies." *PT: The Magazine of Physical Therapy*, 1994; 2(7):17.

7. The Federal Employees Liability Reform and Tort Compensation Act of 1988, 28 United States Code Section 2679(b)(1).

8. *United States* v. *(Marcus S.) Smith*, 499 U.S. 160 (1991).

9. The Federal Tort Claims Act, 28 United States Code Section 2671 *et seq*.

10. Aiken, T.D. *Legal, Ethical, and Political Issues in Nursing*. Philadelphia, PA: Davis Company, 1994, pp. 166–170.

Suggested Readings

1. Aiken, T.D. *Legal, Ethical, and Political Issues in Nursing*. Philadelphia, PA: Davis Company, 1994.

2. Ashcroft, C.E. "Your Professional Liability Policy." *Clinical Management*, 1991; 11(5):16–18.

3. Dobbyn, J.F. *Insurance Law in a Nutshell*. St. Paul, MN: West Publishing Company, 1981.

4. Johnson, K.B., Hatlie, M.J., Johnson, I.D. *The Guide to Medical Professional Liability Insurance*. Chicago, IL: American Medical Association, 1991.

5. Kelley, K. "In Practice: Occurrence vs. Claims-Made Policies." *PT: The Magazine of Physical Therapy*, 1994; 2(7):17.

6. "Occurrence vs. Claims-Made Medical Professional Liability Insurance Policies: Fundamental Differences in the Concept of Coverage." *Journal of the American Medical Association*. 1991; 266:1570–1572.

7. Scott, R.W. *Health Care Malpractice: A Primer on Legal Issues for Professionals*. Thorofare, NJ: Slack, Inc., 1990, pp. 127–130.

8. The McCarran-Ferguson Act of 1945, 15 United States Code Sections 1012–1014.

9. The Federal Employees Liability Reform and Tort Compensation Act of 1988, 28 United States Code Section 2679(b)(1).

10. The Federal Tort Claims Act, 28 United States Code Section 2671 *et seq*.

Chapter 10

Business Law

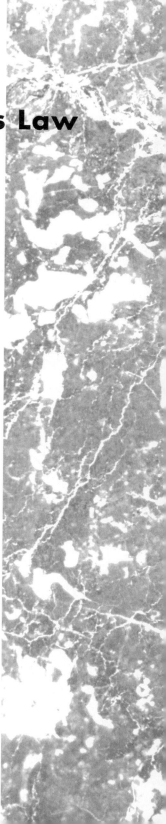

T his chapter introduces basic business law concepts, beginning with a discussion of administrative law and the important role of federal and state administrative agencies in overseeing health care business operations. Other concepts discussed include antitrust law; attorney-client relations (including deposition preparation and practice); business tort litigation; forms of business organizations (sole proprietorships, partnerships, corporations, and hybrid forms); managed care, nursing home, and reimbursement issues; and professional advertising. Specialized topics discussed include Good Samaritan statutes, the Patient Self-Determination Act, and the Safe Medical Devices Act.

Administrative Law

Administrative law encompasses all of the legal principles governing the activities and procedures of federal, state, and local governmental agencies, boards, commissions, and other similar entities. The influence of the hundreds of administrative agencies over business and professional affairs in the United States has become so pervasive over the past half-century that administrative agencies have come to be referred to as the "fourth branch" of government. Professor Kenneth Culp Davis, the preeminent administrative law scholar, has noted that people in business and other professionals have greater interface with state and federal administrative agencies than with any other branch of government at all levels of interaction.[1] In fact, businesspeople, including health care professionals and administrators, have continuous interaction with administrative agencies on issues such as licensure, reimbursement, taxation, and workplace safety, among a myriad of others.

Administrative agencies have grown in number and risen in prominence since World War II for several reasons. First and foremost, the complexity of modern-day society and the business environment has led generally to a perceived need for greater governmental assistance, oversight, and intervention in business and professional affairs. From environmental regulation and health care administration to labor relations and professional licensure, governmental administrative agencies at all levels have become ever more involved in rule-making and regulation of business activities. In addition to becoming more complex, society also has become less averse to governmental regulation of business in the twentieth century (although there currently is an equivocal counter-swing of the pendulum of public opinion in this regard). The doctrine of *laissez faire* was replaced by an attitude of trust in the ability and integrity of government to protect the public from unethical and incompetent businesspeople.

Administrative agencies, especially at the federal level, possess attributes of all three traditional branches of government. Under a valid constitutional delegation of legislative authority (often under very vague guidelines), administrative agencies make rules (a legislative function); investigate matters under their jurisdiction pursuant to broad discretionary powers (an executive function); and enforce their rules through adjudication and the award of sanctions against violators (a judicial function).

To survive legal scrutiny, the activities of administrative agencies must fall within the constitutionally permissible delegation of federal or state legislative authority. In addition to carrying out activities pursuant to a valid delegation of legislative authority, administrative agency activities also must afford *procedural due process* (notice; opportunity to be heard) to those under their jurisdiction.

When the meanings of statutes are not altogether clear, the rules and decisions of administrative agencies must be found by the courts to be reasonable interpretations of such statutes. Administrative rules and decisions must be reasonable and reasoned, not arbitrary or capricious. Courts typically defer to the proper exercise of administrative agency authority.[2]

Three important federal statutes warrant mentioning in this section. The Administrative Procedure Act of 1946 (APA)[3] provides a statutory framework for most decision making by federal administrative agencies. The Freedom of Information Act of 1966 (FOIA)[4] requires federal governmental agencies to expeditiously make public documents available to requesters, absent statutory exemptions to their release. The Privacy Act of 1974[5] requires federal agencies to inform individuals about the purposes and uses of information collected about them. Like FOIA, the Privacy Act contains a number of exceptions authorizing release of personal information about individuals to federal agencies and to entities outside the federal government without their consent. State governments commonly have similar statutory schemes for administrative procedure, release of public records, and protection of privacy.

Antitrust Law

Antitrust law, consisting of statutes, case law, and administrative regulations and rulings, has as its primary purpose the promotion of competition among private sector businesses that benefits the general public. The three federal statutes that provide the framework for federal antitrust regulation are the Sherman Act of 1890,[6] the Clayton Act of 1914,[7] and the Federal Trade Commission Act of 1914.[8] States also enact antitrust laws, but the federal courts have exclusive jurisdiction over federal antitrust law.

The Sherman Act has two sections. Section One prohibits business agreements or arrangements that unreasonably interfere with interstate commerce (restraint of trade). Certain types of business practices are so blatantly anticompetitive that they are always considered to be illegal, such as agreements to fix prices and group boycotts of competitors (per se violations). The legality of other types of agreements are analyzed on a case-by-case basis under the "rule of reason." Section Two prohibits the willful acquisition or maintenance of monopoly power in a given market or the attempt to achieve such control. Willful monopolization of a market or industry is done with the intent to adversely affect competition.

The Clayton Act prohibits specific anticompetitive business practices, including unjustified price discrimination by sellers and unreasonable mergers and acquisitions, among other practices. The Federal Trade Commission Act created the Federal Trade Commission (FTC), an administrative agency which, along with the Department of Justice, administers federal antitrust law. The Department of Justice can bring either criminal or civil legal actions against alleged violators of the Sherman Act. Private parties personally injured by such violations can sue civilly, and if successful, recover triple (*treble*) damages and the cost of their attorney fees.

Certain entities enjoy statutory or judicial exemptions from the enforcement of federal antitrust laws. Those of particular interest to health care professionals include:

- state governments and their political subdivisions, as well as private parties who are acting (with active state supervision) under clear statutory authority ("state action doctrine")[9]
- activities of industries highly regulated by federal agencies, including transportation, communications, and banking
- the insurance industry
- labor unions
- cooperative research activities involving small businesses
- concerted political action by private businesspeople to affect or create law (the Noerr-Pennington doctrine)[10]

The health care field is not exempt from compliance with antitrust laws, although health care was largely ignored, for purposes of antitrust enforcement, by government agencies and the courts until very recently.[11] That changed in 1975 when the U.S. Supreme Court, in *Goldfarb* v. *Virginia State Bar*,[12] disallowed a "learned professions" exemption for health care and other professional services.

Since 1975, there have been a number of prominent applications of federal antitrust laws to health care service delivery. In 1988, in *Patrick* v. *Burget*,[13] the U.S. Supreme Court held that private medical staff privileging actions that are not actively supervised by state governmental agencies do not enjoy "state action" immunity from antitrust scrutiny. In 1990, the U.S. Supreme Court, in *Wilk* v. *American Medical Association*,[14] denied review of the Seventh Circuit Court of Appeals' decision that the American Medical Association had carried out an illegal boycott of the chiropractic profession in violation of Section One of the Sherman Act. In 1993, the

Department of Justice and the Federal Trade Commission jointly issued antitrust guidelines for health care professionals and entities, designed to create safe zones within which individuals and entities could escape potential civil and criminal liability involving hospital mergers, hospital and physician joint ventures, purchasing arrangements, and dissemination of health-related information to the public.[15] Recent managed-care-related developments are bound to raise antitrust questions, such as the prospective merger between Aetna Life & Casualty Company and U.S. Healthcare, Inc.,[16] which would create the largest medical benefits company in the United States.

Advertising Professional Services

When it comes to advertising professional health care services, the traditional adage of *caveat emptor* ("let the buyer beware") is tempered by legal and ethical considerations favoring patient rights. Until the late 1970s, health professional ethics codes and that of the legal profession proscribed professional advertising.

Advertising in any form by health care and legal professionals was formerly considered inappropriate for a number of reasons. It was argued that advertising of health care and legal services had an adverse effect on professionalism, was misleading, and engendered undesirable economic consequences, including increased overhead cost passed on to consumers and creation of a substantial entry barrier to more junior professional colleagues attempting to enter or penetrate a market. In 1977, these arguments were systematically addressed and refuted by the U.S. Supreme Court in *Bates and Van O'Steen* v. *State Bar of Arizona*,[17] the landmark legal case involving professional advertising.

In *Bates*, the U.S. Supreme Court held that the advertising of professional services fell within the rubric of First Amendment free speech rights. Specifically, the Court declared that truthful advertising about the availability and cost of professional service delivery serves an important societal interest—to ensure that consumers make informed decisions about professional services based on readily available, complete, and reliable information.

Because professional advertising is a form of "commercial speech," it does not enjoy the broadest constitutional protection otherwise afforded to political or literary speech under the First Amendment. Government entities are free to regulate professional advertising to prevent the dissemination of misleading, deceptive, or false advertising, and advertisements for illegal activities (such as regulated health services rendered by unauthorized providers). As with other forms of protected speech, states may impose reasonable restrictions on the time, place, and manner of professional advertising.

Forms of health care professional advertising that might be prohibited as misleading, deceptive or false could include advertisements that compare the relative quality of services offered among competitors ("comparative competitor claims"). In addition to being subject to constitutionally permissible state regulation, such advertisements might expose the advertising professional to common-law business tort liability (discussed below).

238

Subsequent to *Bates*, many health disciplines revised their ethics codes to reflect the change in legal status of professional advertising. For example, Sections 6.2 B and C of the American Physical Therapy Association's *Guide for Professional Conduct*[18] read:

> B. Physical therapists may advertise their services to the public.
> C. Physical therapists shall not use, or participate in the use of, any form of communication containing a false, plagiarized, fraudulent, misleading, deceptive, unfair, or sensational statement or claim.

Principle 5C of the *Occupational Therapy Code of Ethics*[19] does not address professional advertising directly, but reads in pertinent part:

> Occupational therapy personnel shall refrain from using or participating in the use of any form of communication that contains false, fraudulent, deceptive, or unfair statements or claims.

The advertising of professional services requires a balance between legal and ethical considerations and the right of professionals to free speech. Such a balance is not always easy to maintain.

Attorney-Health Care Professional Client Relations

How, When, and Where to Seek Legal Advice

In the potentially litigious business environment in which they work, health care professionals need to have available legal counsel for confidential advice. Providers need to consult with their attorneys, not only when a potentially compensable event such as patient injury arises, but also for everyday business and personal affairs.

Every health care professional—whether self-employed or employed by another person or entity—should individually form a professional relationship with an attorney of choice. In no other professional relationship is a client able to openly discuss business and personal matters and know that, with few exceptions, the information conveyed to the advisor will be held in strict confidence. Such is the nature of the attorney-client relationship.[20] Rule 1.6 of the Model Rules of Professional Conduct reads:

Confidentiality of Information

> (a) A lawyer shall not reveal information relating to representation of a client unless the client consents after consultation, except for disclosures that are impliedly authorized in order to carry out the representation, and except as stated in paragraph (b).

(b) A lawyer may reveal such information to the extent the lawyer reasonably believes necessary:

(1) to prevent the client from committing a criminal act that the lawyer believes is likely to result in imminent death or substantial bodily harm; or

(2) to establish a claim or defense on behalf of the lawyer in a controversy between the lawyer and the client, to establish a defense to a criminal charge or civil claim against the lawyer based upon conduct in which the client was involved, or to respond to allegations in any proceeding concerning the lawyer's representation of the client.

How does one locate an attorney? The best ways to find an attorney are through word-of-mouth recommendations of professional colleagues[21] and through communication with bar association lawyer referral services. Bar associations usually offer lawyer referral services at no fee or at a very low fee for the initial consultation, and refer only to highly reputable attorneys who are specialists in areas of client interest. One of the least effective ways to choose an attorney is to randomly select one from listings in a telephone directory.

An attorney representing a health care professional optimally should be intimately familiar with the legal issues pertinent to the client's discipline. To the extent that an attorney is not familiar with a health professional client's discipline, it is the responsibility of the client to educate the attorney about the discipline and pertinent issues affecting the client. At all times, the client should be in control of the attorney-client relationship.[22]

Attorneys have frequently been the subject of humor and ridicule in recent times.[23,24] To a certain degree, the levity is harmless and the public's angst understandable. However, in their defense, attorneys have probably the most extensive history of *pro bono publico* (free of charge or reduced-fee) service to socioeconomically disadvantaged clients of any professionals.[25] In the best light, attorneys are champions for their clients and defenders of justice and order. In the least favorable light, attorneys are personifications of societal problems that are exacerbated all the more with their presence. The public ridicule of attorneys has had horrific destructive and violent consequences, including the murders of eight people who were lawyers, paralegals, or visitors in a law office in San Francisco on July 1, 1993, hyperbolically dubbed "the ultimate in lawyer bashing."[26]

Hint *Every health care professional should form a professional relationship with an attorney of personal choice.*

Pretrial Depositions: The Make or Break Point in Malpractice Litigation

Depositions are pre-trial procedures in which parties and (fact and expert) witnesses are questioned by attorneys and give answers under oath concerning issues which are or may be pertinent to pending litigation. Everything said in a deposition is recorded and transcribed by a court reporter, and the transcript is reduced to written form for introduction at trial.

Health care professionals undergoing deposition must take them seriously. The adage, "A witness in deposition today may be a defendant tomorrow" is one that health professional *deponents* should always remember.

No witness should undergo deposition without being prepared for the process by his or her attorney. Deposition preparation of a deponent by an attorney has been called "the most important trip to the woodshed."[27] The following are some important tips for prospective non-expert deponents:

- Always remember that a deposition is serious business. Dress in business attire for your deposition. Do not make jokes with your attorney, the opposing attorney, or anyone else in the process.

- Keep in mind that a major purpose for a deposition is to find out or "discover" important information favorable to a party in litigation. The deposition process is sometimes referred to as a "fishing expedition."

- Do not bring any items with you to a deposition that are not demanded of you by opposing counsel in a *subpoena duces tecum*.

- Irrespective of how nice or friendly the opposing attorney appears, he or she is not a friend of the deponent. Treat opposing counsel with caution and respect.

- Wait for a question to be completely stated before answering. Consider pausing to think before answering. (Pauses before answering should not be reflected in a deposition transcript, unless they are also indicated in the record for the attorneys and others who speak during the deposition.)

- Do not argue with opposing counsel.

- Do not use statements such as, "Do I have to answer that?" and "Can we go off the record?"

- If you do not understand a question, ask for it to be repeated. If you do not know an answer, state that you do not know the answer. Do not guess!

- Do not volunteer information. As a deponent, carefully limit your answers to respond only to the precise questions asked, and do so in as few words as possible.

- If your attorney objects on the record to a question, stop speaking immediately and do not resume until the objection is resolved by the attorneys.

- Do not let opposing counsel put words in your mouth by summarizing what you have testified to. Carefully correct improper characterizations of your testimony.

- Freely admit, if asked, that you have been prepared for your deposition by your attorney.

- If, at any time, you need to take a break to use the restroom or get a drink of water, state that you need a break. Do not let opposing counsel question you for hours on end without taking a reasonable number of breaks. (A tired deponent becomes careless and shows anger with opposing counsel more easily than one who is refreshed. A jury may consider an agitated and argumentative deponent to be an untruthful person.)

- Exercise your rights to review and correct your deposition after it is transcribed. Carefully review, correct, and sign it with assistance of counsel.

Consider the following hypothetical deposition scenarios and their attendant problems:

1. *T* is an occupational therapist being sued by *P*, a patient, for professional negligence for injury incident to a functional capacity assessment. *T*'s deposition is being taken by *P*'s attorney in the attorney's law office. *T*, who is eight-and-a-half months pregnant, is represented at the deposition by her attorney. The deposition begins at 8:30 AM. After one morning restroom break, a 30-minute lunch break, and one afternoon restroom break, *T* is visibly physically and emotionally exhausted. She begins to argue with, and make sarcastic remarks to, *P*'s attorney during questioning. What should *T*'s attorney do? *T*'s attorney should, considering the fact that *T* is eight-and-a-half months pregnant, demand that the session be suspended until the next day and state the reason for the demand on the record, and further inquire of the opposing counsel on the record about the projected length of the residual portion of *T*'s deposition. (*P*'s attorney may be deliberately trying to wear *T* down physiologically and emotionally so that *T*'s testimony will favor *P*'s case. Unless the deposition is videotaped, a jury will not know that *T* was pregnant while being deposed.)

2. *W* is a PhD and physical therapist-academician and an expert witness for *X*, an occupational therapist in a malpractice case being brought against *X* by *Y*, a former patient. The principal allegation against *X* is that *X* negligently mobilized *Y*'s traumatized finger post-operatively, allegedly causing a surgically-repaired tendon to rupture. *W* is properly *qualified* by *X*'s attorney to testify in the case based on her credentials and her special expertise in hand rehabilitation. Near the close of *W*'s deposition, *Q*, *Y*'s attorney who is questioning *W*, attempts to summarize *W*'s testimony incorrectly. What should *W* do? *W* should immediately state that the summarization of her testimony by *Q* is inaccurate, then correctly summarize her testimony on the record. (Be careful. The opposing counsel will be listening for *W* to make any inconsistent statements under pressure that can later be attacked.)

Health care administrators and facility clinic and risk managers should consider implementing ongoing inservice education programs on legal issues targeted to specific disciplines or interdisciplinary groups of professionals. Discussions about, and even simulations of, depositions (under attorney guidance) should be included in such programs. Education about legal issues may enhance professionals' sense of confidence in their practices and reduce stress[28] and costly defensive health care practice.

Hint *Health care professionals undergoing deposition must take the process seriously because "a witness in deposition today may be named as a defendant in the case tomorrow."*

Business Torts

Business torts are wrongs committed against the legitimate proprietary business interests of individuals, partnerships, or corporations. There are many variations of actionable business torts from state to state. Three that have the potential to arise frequently in health care settings are discussed in this section. They are tortious interference with a contractual relationship, interference with a prospective business relationship, and business disparagement.

Tortious or *wrongful interference with a contractual relationship* involves wrongful conduct on the part of a person or business entity to intentionally induce another person or business to breach an existing contract. An example of wrongful interference with an existing contract would be the situation in which one managed health care organization wrongfully caused a physical therapist-employee, who is under contract with a competitor, to breach the contract and come to work for the tortfeasor. Keep in mind that, absent the existence of a valid, enforceable contract (normally including contracts terminable at the will of the parties), the tort of wrongful interference with a contractual relationship is not normally actionable. Absent predatory, malicious conduct by a party, competition by rivals for employees or other business interests constitutes legitimate business practice.

Wrongful interference with a prospective business relationship occurs when one party intentionally and wrongfully acts to interfere with a pending business relationship. Such a situation would include wrongfully inducing a party in contract negotiations with another party to break off negotiations. In one legal case, a court ruled that the faxing of a civil lawsuit to one party (an invalid means of service of legal process), which caused a party who was negotiating a contract with the party receiving the fax to demand greater collateral, constituted actionable interference with a prospective business relationship.[29]

Business disparagement involves the wrongful communication of false information about a businessperson or entity which causes injury to the victim's business reputation or interests. The tort of disparagement is also commonly known, in its various forms, as injurious falsehood, slander of quality or of title, and trade libel.

Forms of Business Organizations

When one or more people create a business, they can form one of several legal forms of business organization. The forms of business organization, with various hybrids, include sole proprietorship, partnership, corporation, and limited liability company.

In a *sole proprietorship*—the simplest form for a business—an individual business owner personally makes all decisions and receives all of the profits generated by the business. In this scenario, the owner/entrepreneur is truly a one-person show. There is maximal flexibility in this form of business organization and minimal legal constraints on the formation and operation of the business. Business income and deductions are reported on the owner's individual tax returns.

The principal disadvantage of a sole proprietorship is that the owner personally bears the entire financial risk of loss, ranging from business losses to liability incident to claims and lawsuits. (Of course, the owner can and should transfer liability risks through the purchase of insurance.) Other relative disadvantages of the sole proprietorship include potential difficulty in attracting funds and discontinuity of operations in the event of serious illness or the death of the proprietor.

A *general partnership* is a contractual agreement between two or more people or other legal entities to establish and operate a business for profit. The partnership contractual agreement may be either express (oral or written) or implied. Like the sole proprietorship, partnership law is based in common, rather than statutory law.

Absent other agreement, partners manage the business equally and share in, and pay taxes individually, on their proportional share of profits. (The partnership itself reports income, but does not pay income tax.) Each partner is the agent for the other partner(s), and all partners are joint and severally liable for partnership business debts and tort liability.

The principle advantages of the general partnership are the sharing of business expenses and the availability of multiple sources of input for business decision making. The main disadvantage is the unlimited personal liability of each partner for partnership activities.

The *limited partnership* is a statutorily-created form of business, which consists of at least one general partner and one or more limited partners. It is a business arrangement under which the limited partners do not manage the operational affairs of a business, but share in its profits. The personal liability of limited partners is normally limited to the amount of their investment in the business.

Most jurisdictions do not allow professionals to form generic limited partnerships.[30] Other forms of limited partnerships may be available for health professionals in some states. For example, Texas law[31] permits the formation of a registered *limited liability partnership*, in which individual partners enjoy some protection from liability for other partners' or agents' tortious conduct.

A *joint venture* is very much like a general partnership, with two important differences. A joint venture is formed for a specific, limited purpose, and the members of the venture have only limited agency authority to bind their fellow members.

A *corporation* is a form of business organization that is recognized as a legal person apart from its owners (shareholders) with most of the rights and duties of natural persons. Corporations are governed by statutory law, which varies from state to state. All states have relatively strict statutory requirements associated with the formation and administration of corporations that do not apply to proprietorships and partnerships.

The personal liability of corporate shareholders for the debts of the corporation is normally limited to the amount of their investment in the business, unless a court "pierces the corporate veil" to reach additional assets of shareholders when they have ignored corporate statutory formalities or have failed to adequately capitalize the business.[32] Piercing of the corporate veil is only rarely done by courts.

In addition to limited shareholder liability, another advantage of the corporate form of business is perpetual existence. A corporation, unlike a proprietorship or partnership, does not cease to exist upon the death of its owner(s). A major disadvantage to incorporating is double taxation upon the net profits of a corporation and upon its shareholders for disbursed dividends.[33]

Many states require licensed professionals to incorporate under special professional corporation statutes. Under the Texas Professional Corporation Act,[34] for example, certain health care professionals licensed by the state may incorporate under the statute and be shielded from personal liability (beyond their proportional share of the assets of the corporation) for the conduct of other corporate owners. Of course, being in a corporation does not shield a professional from liability for his or her own conduct.

Professional corporations may operate for profit, or be nonprofit entities, in which case they do not issue stock. In some states, physicians form distinct professional associations[35] which share characteristics with *professional corporations*.

The *limited liability company*,[36] a relatively recent hybrid form of business organization, is becoming increasingly popular. The limited liability company shares characteristics of professional corporations and partnerships. Like a corporation, its owners have the benefit of limited personal liability for contract and tort actions against the company. Like a partnership, company income is passed through to the owners for unitary taxation at the individual level.

The decision of which form of business organization to adopt is a complicated one. Health professional entrepreneurs are urged to consult proactively with legal counsel for advice regarding such a decision.[37]

Good Samaritan Laws

The *American College Dictionary* defines *Good Samaritan* as "a person who is compassionate and helpful to one in distress," citing a Biblical passage, Luke 10:30–37, as authority. A more jurisprudential definition is found in *Black's Law Dictionary*, in which *Good Samaritan* is defined as one who aids another person in imminent or serious peril. Under law, a Good Samaritan rendering to another may be granted immunity from civil liability for negligence incident to such assistance.

Under the laws of the United States (unlike those of many other nations), unless there is some preexisting duty to come to another's aid, no one is obligated to help another person in peril.[38] One may have a moral duty to do so—especially where the rescuer faces no personal danger—but not a legal duty. Clinical health care professionals, of course, have a pre-existing duty to patients under their care and must come to their aid in emergencies to the extent of their professional competence.

Good Samaritan Statutes

After World War II, state legislatures became concerned that physicians and other competent rescuers would refrain from assisting strangers in emergency situations out of fear of liability exposure. As a result, first California (in 1959) and then every other state and the District of Columbia enacted Good Samaritan statutes to shield physicians and others from liability for emergency medical treatment, as long as specific statutory requirements were met.

There are about 118 statutes nationwide granting Good Samaritan immunity to various rescuers under a variety of circumstances.[39] Certain common guidelines pervade these Good Samaritan statutes, including:

- the requirement that an emergency exist for statutory protections to apply
- identification of who is protected from liability under the statute
- delineation of the degree of culpability that causes a rescuer to lose statutory immunity from liability
- determination of whether the statute applies to emergency aid rendered within a medical facility
- determination of whether a statutorily-protected rescuer must act without the expectation of compensation

Physicians are protected by Good Samaritan statutes in all 50 states and the District of Columbia. In at least 37 other states, anyone who renders emergency aid to accident victims is also protected. Many states expressly protect specific classes of persons who may render emergency care to others. For example, two states—Michigan and New York—expressly grant Good Samaritan immunity to physical therapists.[40]

Emergency and Good Faith

The two requirements most commonly observed in Good Samaritan statutes are that a bona fide emergency exist and that the rescuer act in good faith in administering assistance. Few statutes, however, clearly define "emergency" or "good faith," and there is very little case law addressing these points.

Most statutes also require that protected aid be rendered at or near the scene of an accident or emergency. Some allow for immunity even when aid in provided in hospital or other health care facility setting, so long as the Good Samaritan does not have a professional-patient relationship with the victim.

Culpability and Gratuitous Aid

Two other parameters of Good Samaritan statutes concern (1) the effect of gross negligence or more culpable conduct on the part of a person rendering emergency aid, and (2) the requirement that a rescuer offer assistance without expectation of compensation. The overwhelming majority of Good Samaritan statutes deny immunity when a rescuer acts in a grossly negligent, reckless, or malicious way and causes injury to an accident victim. A majority of statutes require gratuitous assistance for protection; however, almost half of the statutes do not disallow reasonable compensation for services rendered. The legislative intent behind the statutes that disallow compensation for emergency services presumably is to foster altruistic behavior on the part of would-be rescuers. The legislative intent behind the statutes that are silent on the issue of compensation may be to prevent unjust enrichment by accident victims who receive valuable services.

The Need for Reform and Professional Education

The lack of uniformity among the states regarding Good Samaritan immunity from liability[41] creates significant confusion and may dissuade competent health care professionals and others from rendering emergency aid to victims, a consequence clearly contrary to the intent of these statutes. A legislative solution to this dilemma is to create a uniform Good Samaritan statute that could be adopted nationwide, similar to uniform laws and guidance currently in effect governing commercial transactions and partnership and probate matters. Any uniform law should provide for immunity from liability for simple negligence for any rescuer who acts reasonably within the scope of his or her competency.

All health care professionals, support personnel, clinical managers, and facility administrators should become knowledgeable about their particular state laws providing Good Samaritan immunity before they find themselves in situations in which they are required to render emergency aid to patients or others. Periodic presentations by facility attorneys or legal consultants concerning Good Samaritan laws makes an excellent addition to any health care facility in-service education program.

Intellectual Property

Intellectual property refers to writings, computer software, depictions, inventions, symbols, and other intangible creations of the mind. Federal law protects the legitimate rights of creators of such contributions. The federal courts have exclusive jurisdiction over patent, trademark, and copyright matters.

A *patent* is an exclusive grant to an original inventor (or inventors jointly) to make, sell, and use an invention for a period of years. Currently, the U.S. Patent and Trademark Office (PTO) grants utility patents on new and useful processes, machines, and compositions of matter for a period of 20 years. An inventor must file a patent application with PTO within one year after public use of an invention or be statutorily barred from obtaining a patent for the invention.[42] Absent a contractual agreement otherwise, an employee personally owns the patent rights to inventions made by the employee during the course of employment.

A *trademark* is a distinctive symbol, word, or group of letters representing a particular product. A *service mark* is a distinctive symbol, word, or group of letters representing a professional service. The grant of an exclusive trademark or service mark to a businessperson serves to protect the proprietary and quality interests of the owner of these distinctive product and service representations. Trademarks and service marks should be registered with PTO in order to ensure universal protection; they are renewable indefinitely as long as they remain distinctive and are used by the owner.

A *copyright* protects an author's expression of a creative idea. That expression can be in the form of a writing, painting, computer program, or some other tangible means of expression. The owner of a copyright is legally entitled to exclusive rights in a work for the life of the author plus 50 years. A corporation that owns a copyright is granted exclusive rights in a work for 75 years.

Registration of a creative work with the U.S. Copyright Office is not a prerequisite to statutory copyright protection. Any original creative work in a tangible form is protected upon its creation. It is not even required that creators of copyrighted works affix the copyright symbol, ©, to their works, in order to enjoy statutory protection. Registration of a copyright, however, provides *prima facie* evidence of the validity of the copyright and facilitates enforcement of the copyright holder's rights against unlawful infringement.

Unlike with patents, copyright ownership for a work created by an employee in the scope of employment resides in an employer, absent agreement otherwise. The copyright to a "work for hire," written by a contractor for another person, is owned by the party commissioning the creation of the work. The "fair use" doctrine entitles use or reproduction of copyrighted materials without the permission of copyright owners for limited purposes enumerated in the Copyright Act,[43] including:

criticism, comment, news reporting, teaching (including multiple copies for classroom use), scholarship, [and] research.[44]

Information in the public domain, including government documents, are not subject to copyright protection. Recitations of publicly-known facts are also not protected; however, unique compilations or presentations of existing facts may enjoy copyright protection.

Legal Research Made Easy (or at Least Easier)

Health care professionals, clinical managers, and health care administrators should know (or learn) how to conduct basic legal research in order to aid them in meeting their legal responsibilities. The basic types of law that can easily be accessed are case decisions, statutes, and administrative rules and regulations.

Case law can most easily be retrieved through computerized legal databases. The two main legal computer services are LEXIS[45] and Westlaw.[46] These systems contain separate databases for each state court system and for the federal courts. They also permit mega-searches of federal or state systems for information. Legal cases can be retrieved by using case names or by topic areas using search words such as "physical and occupational therapy malpractice."

Because of restricted access and the relatively high cost for non-attorneys to use computerized legal databases, lay researchers may wish to access legal cases in textual legal case reporters, which are generally available to the public at law school, bar association, and large public libraries. Honing in on specific cases can easily be accomplished by using topic indices collocated with the textual case reporters.

A case citation (reference) contains, in addition to the names of the parties, a numerical designator indicating the reference volume in which the case is found, the reference series for the case, the initial page number for the case, and the date or year in which the case was decided. For example, the official citation for *Barragn v. Workers' Compensation Appeals Board and Hartford Accident and Indemnity Company*, a case addressing worker's compensation coverage for an injured physical therapy student extern, is: 240 Cal. Rptr. 811 (Cal. App. 1987), indicating that the case is found in the 240th volume of the California Reporter series, beginning at page 811. The parenthetical information reveals that the case was decided by a California state appellate-level court.

Legal researchers typically "brief" or summarize judicial cases in four sections: pertinent facts, legal issues, the court's holding (decision), and the rationale for the court's holding. Lay researchers may wish to begin their review of legal cases by carefully reading the case summaries that commonly precede the complete legal opinions.

Federal statutory law is found, in 50 broad subject areas, in the 50-title *United States Code* (U.S.C.) series. For example, Title 29 , entitled "Labor," includes all labor-related topics, including the Labor Management Relations Act of 1947, found at 29 U.S.C. Section 173. Rules and regulations of federal administrative agencies are found in the *Code of Federal Regulations* (C.F.R.), which, like the United States Code, consists of 50 titles.

Many other legal search instruments are also available to researchers, including the computerized *Index to Legal Periodicals*, law dictionaries and encyclopedias, and law reviews (consisting of scholarly essays on selected legal topics and case and statutory analyses). Friendly in-person assistance can usually be obtained at law libraries from reference and research librarians and their assistants.

Managed Care Issues

The advent of managed health care delivery in the 1980s, and its exponential growth during the 1990s, has resulted in both problems and promise for health care professionals. *Managed care* is an amorphous concept that has been defined in different ways by various authorities.[47,48,49] Everyone agrees, however, that managed care has the following characteristics:

- *integration* of the financing and delivery of health care services
- *cost containment* as its paramount concern

The managed care model that best typifies the integration of financing and delivery of services is the health maintenance organization, or HMO. Subscribers (patients) contract to receive all of their health care services from a pre-established, restricted set of providers under one of four models (staff, group, network, or independent practice association). Except for emergency care, subscribers are not normally insured for care received outside of the HMO. The other primary managed care organizational types include:

- Preferred provider organizations (PPOs), under which subscribers choose their caregivers from a list of network providers, who contract with payors to provide health care services at deeply discounted rates. Subscribers are not prohibited from electing care outside of the PPO network, but personally bear an increased proportion of cost when they choose to receive care from non-network providers.

- Exclusive provider organizations (EPOs), which are similar to PPOs, except that the cost for care rendered outside the EPO network is borne exclusively by subscribers.

- Point of service (POS) plans, which share characteristics of HMOs and PPOs. POS plans are often referred to as "open-ended HMOs."

- Other managed care organization types include physician organizations (POs), owned, managed, and staffed by physicians; physician-hospital organizations (PHOs), jointly owned and operated by physicians and hospitals [the subject of recent antitrust litigation[50]]; and management service organizations (MSOs), providing management, contracting, and administrative services to payors.[51]

Managed care has created profound challenges for professionals in all health care disciplines and for specialists within specific disciplines. Rehabilitation health care professionals, for example, find themselves being asked to assume ever-increasing responsibilities in multiple roles as multiskilled clinicians,[52] supervisors of increasing numbers and types of support and "extender" personnel, administrators, educators, researchers, and consultants.[53] Managed care forces a refocusing of health care delivery from optimizing quality of care in general to optimizing quality within the constraints of reimbursement. Strict utilization review and the constant threat of denial of reimbursement for services[54] has resulted in more careful documentation standards and a quest to expeditiously validate services based on beneficial outcomes.[55] Outcome studies have, in turn, generated growing numbers of clinical practice guidelines.[56]

Patients are not the only participants in managed care delivery systems who may be denied access to services. Unless states have in effect *any willing provider laws* (under which all qualified providers who are willing to participate must be included in provider networks), managed care organizations may contract exclusively with select health care providers and groups for service delivery and exclude all others from participation.[57] Rehabilitation professionals must be aware of pitfalls associated with managed care contracting, particularly those agreements structured under the *capitation* model, under which providers must provide all covered services to all subscribers for a periodic fixed fee per subscriber.[58]

The potential for malpractice liability exposure may be increased with managed care.[59] Theories of liability for managed care organizations include, among others, negligent care delivery, breach of contract, fraud, and vicarious liability for providers' conduct.[60] Over 400 legislative bills restricting managed care initiatives have been proposed so far in 1996; 33 states already have some form of restrictive managed care laws in place.[61]

The Pew Health Professions Commission recently reported that, although there will be a surplus of up to 150,000 physicians and 300,000 nurses by the year 2000, the demand for health care providers from other selected disciplines will increase.[62] The Office of Employment Projections of the Bureau of Labor Statistics predicts the following growth figures for physical and occupational therapists and assistants from 1994 to 2005: physical therapist assistants, 83 percent; certified occupational therapy assistants, 82 percent; physical therapists, 80 percent; and occupational therapists, 72 percent.[63]

Managed care is the private sector analog to public-sector health care reform initiatives. Although wholesale federal health care reform has been temporarily tabled (largely because of political considerations), some federal governmental initiatives have been enacted, such as Stark I and II, which restrict the ability of physicians to refer patients to facilities in which they have an ownership interest, including facilities providing occupational and physical therapy services, durable medical equipment, orthotic and prosthetic devices, clinical laboratory and diagnostic radiology services, and home health services, among other services.[64]

Nursing Home Issues

Health care malpractice civil cases and criminal prosecutions involving providers in long-term care settings are both increasing in number. Common allegations against long-term care providers and facilities include a pattern of substandard care and/or neglect of residents and intentional misconduct, including intentional infliction of emotional distress incident to verbal abuse, improper restraint, and battery.[65]

The Health Care Financing Administration (HCFA) surveys long-term care facilities for Medicare and Medicaid certification, based on compliance with more than 100 requirements delineated in the Nursing Home Reform Act, part of the Omnibus Budget Reconciliation Act of 1987 (OBRA).[66] OBRA greatly expanded the rights of long-term care residents and included the right to be free from improper physical restraint.[67]

OBRA prohibits the use of physical restraints on long-term care residents, except as adjuncts to treatment for specific medical conditions. Restraints include not only traditional arm and leg cuffs and lap belts, but also bedding materials such as sheets, when they are used to limit a patient's free movement. Whenever physical restraints are to be used, providers must justify their use through clear documentation in a patient's treatment records, including clinical justification and a statement that less restrictive alternatives to physical restraint have been tried and found to be inadequate.[68] Since OBRA's implementation, the former widespread use of physical restraints in long-term care facilities has plummeted as much as 90 percent, from 41 to 4 percent of residents, according to one study.[69]

Patient Self-Determination Act

The Patient Self-Determination Act of 1990 (PSDA)[70] is a federal statute that codifies patients' right to control treatment-related decisions, both routine and extraordinary.[71] The PSDA obligates hospitals, HMOs, long-term care facilities, home health agencies, hospices, and other health care organizations receiving Medicare and Medicaid funds to its provisions.

A fundamental purpose of the PSDA is to educate patients about their rights to formulate *advance directives*. Advance directives are legal instruments which memorialize a patient's desires concerning life-sustaining measures to be undertaken in the event of the patient's incapacitation, which a patient executes while still legally competent. Common varieties of advance directives include living wills and durable powers of attorney for health care decisions.

A *living will* is a legal document, signed by a patient, which states the patient's wishes concerning life-sustaining measures to be undertaken in the event of the patient's subsequent incompetence. Statutory "natural death acts" are forms of living wills in effect in many states. Most states require that a patient be both legally incompetent and terminally ill in order for a living will to become operative. Some states allow a living will to become operative when a patient is in a "persistive vegetative state." A *durable power of attorney for health care decisions*, a special power of attorney, is a legal document signed by a patient, which delegates health care decision making to an agent of the patient's choice. The power becomes operative upon the patient's legal incompetence to make such decisions for him- or herself. The patient normally may designate anyone—a spouse, relative, friend, attorney, or other trusted person—as the surrogate health care decision maker.

The principle premise underlying the PSDA is respect for a patient's inherent right to self-determination and control over treatment decision making. A health care provider must, according to this premise, disclose to a patient sufficient information about a proposed course of treatment—i.e., the nature of the recommended intervention; its material risks, if any; reasonable alternatives to the proposed intervention; and expected benefits of treatment—to empower the patient to analyze the options and make an informed choice about whether to undergo or reject treatment.

The PSDA does not create any new substantive patient rights. Instead, it imposes affirmative procedural obligations on health care providers and facilities to whom the law applies. Among other requirements, the PSDA requires providers and facilities to:

- provide written information to patients concerning their rights under state law to give informed consent to, or refusal of, treatment and to make advance directives

- provide patients with copies of institutional policies concerning informed patient decision making and advance directives

- document in patient records whether or not patients have executed advance directives concerning treatment[72]

Reimbursement Issues

Reimbursement for professional service delivery is of paramount importance for health care providers and organizations. Reimbursement principles are ever-changing, especially in light of the political environment and the evolving managed care model of health care delivery/financing. Under managed care, payors are especially concerned with "value," i.e., maximizing optimal quality services at the lowest possible cost.[73] The basic aspects of managed care have already been addressed in an earlier section of this chapter. An important point to reiterate regarding reimbursement under a *capitation* managed care model, under which providers must provide all covered services to all subscribers for a periodic fixed fee per subscriber, is that providers must ensure, to the maximal degree of certainty possible, that their projected revenues will exceed projected costs so that the enterprise generates a profit. The capitation model of managed health care delivery transfers financial risk from payors to providers, making health care providers into insurers of services.[74]

Health care delivery is perhaps the most regulated commercial business in the United States. Federal health programs, including Medicare and Medicaid are the responsibility of the Department of Health and Human Services (HHS). The Health Care Financing Administration (HCFA) is the agency within HHS directly responsible for administering these health care programs.

Medicare, the largest payor of health care services in the United States, reimburses health providers and institutions more than $150 billion annually, a figure that is increasing at 10.5 percent per year.[75] Medicare's two components, Part A (covering institutional care and some home health services) and Part B (covering outpatient care, durable medical equipment (DME), physical therapists in independent practice (PTIP) services, and some home health services), operate under different rules. Part A health insurance coverage (with a moderate deductible) is automatic for persons who have paid into the Part A Trust Fund for ten or more years and who are either age 65 or permanently disabled, while Part B provides elective coverage for Part A-eligible beneficiaries for a modest monthly premium and a substantial copayment for covered services. More than ten percent of Medicare's 37 million beneficiaries are covered by federally-approved HMO managed care plans.[76] Managed care Medicare users typically pay no deductible for hospitalization and only a nominal copayment for outpatient services.

Medicare covers rehabilitative services that are reasonable and necessary and that constitute affirmative treatment vs. maintenance services. Medicare pays providers and institutions in one of several ways: under a prospective payment system (PPS) based on pre-established diagnostic-related groups (DRGs) for acute care hospitalizations; through a cost-related reimbursement system for outpatient care; and by using a fee schedule for outpatient physician and incidental services and PTIP. (Physicians are reimbursed according to a physician fee schedule, based on the resource-based relative value scale (RBRVS). PTIP are limited to $900 per year per eligible patient.)

Billing Medicare for services provided to beneficiaries may be accomplished either under the Current Procedural Terminology (CPT) or HCFA's Common Procedure Coding (HCPCS Level II) Systems. Reimbursement claims are processed by functional intermediaries and private carrier organizations that contract with HCFA for these roles.

Denial of Medicare claims is best avoided by carefully documenting services in such a way as to justify reimbursement. Documenting rehabilitation treatment goals in terms of concise, objective, functional outcomes; demonstrating incremental patient improvement; and employing nomenclature which complements the billing classification are important considerations. Appeals of Medicare claims denials proceed through progressively more complex steps through administrative bodies and ultimately to the courts with progressively increasing minimal amounts in controversy (similar to diversity jurisdiction, discussed in Chapter 1) for successive steps.

The Office of the Inspector General (OIG) of HHS bears primary responsibility for ensuring compliance by providers with statutory and administrative Medicare mandates. A finding of Medicare "program-related misconduct" (e.g., the filing of fraudulent claims for reimbursement[77]) can lead to mandatory exclusion from participation in federally funded health programs administratively and to criminal prosecution for fraud by the Criminal Division of the Department of Justice. Not only providers are subject to criminal prosecution for fraud, but also contracting entities that process claims. In the first case of its kind, Blue Shield of California, a Medicare claims administrator, recently agreed to plead guilty to three criminal counts of conspiracy and obstructing federal Medicare audits incident to the activities of six of its employees.[78]

This section has provided only a sketchy overview of basic reimbursement issues and is focused almost exclusively on Medicare, the largest payor for health services in the United States. For additional information on reimbursement issues, readers are strongly urged to review a superb text by Rasmussen, B., entitled *Reimbursement and Fiscal Management in Rehabilitation*. Alexandria, VA: American Physical Therapy Association, 1995.

Safe Medical Devices Act

The Safe Medical Devices Act of 1990 (SMDA),[79] administered by the Food and Drug Administration (FDA), requires health care facilities to report incidents involving serious patient injury, illness, or death resulting from defective medical equipment. Under the SMDA, a designee of the facility (typically the facility risk manager) must submit a report directly to the FDA within ten working days whenever a death occurs and to the product manufacturer (or directly to the FDA, if the name of the product manufacturer is not known) for cases involving injury or illness.

Such reports enjoy limited qualified immunity from use against the facility in civil litigation, unless the facility intentionally makes a false report.[80] In addition to generating an agency report under the SMDA, the clinical manager for the area in which patient injury from equipment occurred should turn off and sequester the allegedly defective equipment; generate an internal incident report concerning the event; and ensure that documentation of the patient's post-injury evaluation and care are retained by medical records personnel as potential litigation documents.

Chapter Summary

A key component of a proactive liability risk management program in business is regularly-recurring education of professional, support, and administrative personnel of the basic principles of, and developments in, business law. Business law is extremely complex, and in near-constant flux, requiring that continuing legal education in this area be given by attorneys, rather than non-attorneys.

The arm of government that health care business entrepreneurs interact with most often is the administrative branch, consisting of federal and state administrative agencies like the EEOC, HCFA, IRS, and OSHA, to name just a few. Every health care professional contemplating the formation of a business should consult proactively with an attorney of choice for early and ongoing advice.

Cases and Questions

1. A physical therapist who has treated a patient for post-operative spinal rehabilitation exercises is being deposed as a fact witness in the patient's medical malpractice case against the patient's orthopedic surgeon. The patient's attorney asks the physical therapist to describe the lumbar intervertebral disc. The witness explains, at length, how the lumbar intervertebral disc is like a jelly doughnut. The patient's attorney impeaches (challenges the credibility of) the witness by saying, "You

don't really mean to say that the lumbar intervertebral disc in human beings is similar to a jelly doughnut, do you?" After that exchange, the patient's attorney asks the witness to concede that a particular orthopedic physical therapy text is generally recognized as an authoritative work. The witness concedes that the text is authoritative. The patient's attorney then proceeds to impeach the witness using remote passages from the text which recite propositions with which the witness does not agree. How should the witness have approached these two trick questions?

2. A patient undergoing work conditioning activities in occupational therapy allegedly sustains a minor musculoskeletal arm injury from a piece of medical equipment. What legal reporting responsibilities, if any, does the occupational therapy service have?

Suggested Answers to Cases and Questions

1. First and foremost, this witness should have been thoroughly prepared for deposition by an attorney, because a fact witness today may be named as a malpractice defendant tomorrow. The witness should not have attempted to describe in detail the anatomy and physiology of the lumbar intervertebral disc in the deposition, unless the witness is an anatomist or physiologist. Instead, the witness should have declined to give a detailed description of the disc, based on the fact that such a description is beyond the scope of the witness's professional competence. Similarly, the question asking the witness to declare a text authoritative was designed to enable the patient's attorney to impeach the witness, using remote textual passages. This witness should have stated that, while the text in question may be a legitimate reference text, without further review, the witness is unwilling to casually declare it to be authoritative. (By "authoritative," the witness concedes that the work is accurate from cover to cover.)

2. The occupational therapist or assistant overseeing the patient's treatment should generate an internal incident report concerning the adverse patient incident. The facility employee who witnessed the alleged incident, if any, should write the narrative part of the report. The report should include information about the post-injury evaluation, care of the patient, and detailed identification of the equipment involved. The incident report, once reviewed by the clinic chief, must be forwarded to the facility risk manager for review and retention. There is no legal requirement in this case to make a report to the equipment's manufacturer or to the FDA under the Safe Medical Devices Act, since neither serious injury/illness nor death occurred. (It might be prudent, however, to notify the equipment manufacturer of the incident, but not to release a copy of the internal incident report.)

References

1. Davis, K.C., Pierce, R.J., Jr. *Administrative Law Treatise*, 3rd ed. Boston, MA: Little, Brown and Company Publishing, Vol. I, 1994, pp. 6–7.

2. *Chevron, USA, Inc., v. Natural Resources Defense Council*, 467 U.S. 837 (1984).

3. The Administrative Procedure Act of 1946, 5 United States Code Sections 551–559, 701–706.

4. The Freedom of Information Act, 5 United States Code Section 552.

5. The Privacy Act, 5 United States Code Section 552a.

6. The Sherman Act of 1890, 15 United States Code Sections 1–3.

7. The Clayton Act of 1914, 15 United States Code Sections 15a, 19.

8. The Federal Trade Commission Act of 1914, 15 United States Code Section 41 *et seq.*

9. Marx, D., Jr., Laing, M.A. "The State Action Doctrine: Can It Be Applied to a Private Hospital's Acquisition of a Public Hospital?" *The Health Lawyer*, 1995; 8(3):1, 3–5.

10. *Eastern Railroad Presidents Conference* v. *Noerr Motor Freight*, 365 U.S. 127 (1961); *United Mine Workers of America* v. *Penning*, 381 U.S. 657 (1965).

11. Furrow, B.R., Johnson, S.H., Jost, T.S., Schwartz, R.L. *Health Law: Cases, Materials and Problems*, 2nd ed. St. Paul, MN: West Publishing Company, 1991, p. 785.

12. *Goldfarb* v. *Virginia State Bar*, 421 U.S. 773 (1975).

13. *Patrick* v. *Burget*, 486 U.S. 94 (1988).

14. *Wilk* v. *American Medical Association*, 895 F.2d 352, cert. denied, 498 U.S. 982 (1990).

15. Freed, C. "Antitrust Reform for Physicians Network Joint Ventures." *San Antonio Medical Gazette*, October 13–19, 1995, pp. 6, 23.

16. Smolowe, J. "A Healthy Merger?" *Time*, April 15, 1996, pp. 77–78.

17. *Bates and Van O'Steen* v. *State Bar of Arizona*, 433 U.S. 350 (1977).

18. *Guide for Professional Conduct.* Alexandria, VA: American Physical Therapy Association, Judicial Committee, Sections 6.2B, C, 1996.

19. *Occupational Therapy Code of Ethics.* Bethesda, MD: American Occupational Therapy Association, Commission on Standards and Ethics, Principle 5C, 1994.

20. Rule 1.6. *Annotated Model Rules of Professional Conduct*, 2nd ed. Chicago, IL: American Bar Association, 1992.

21. Ginsburg, W.H. "How to Evaluate a Lawyer." *Physician's Management*, December 1991, pp. 90–99.

22. Overman, S. "How to Work With Your Lawyer." *HR Magazine*, July 1992, pp. 41–45.

23. Behrman, S. *The Lawyer Joke Book*. New York: Dorset Press, 1991.

24. "Readers Love Lawyer Jokes." *California Bar Journal*, January 1994, p. 10.

25. Geyelin, M. "ABA Is Asking Lawyers to Boost Help for the Poor." *Wall Street Journal*, April 30, 1993, p. B2.

26. "Anger Against Lawyers Left Many Dead." *National Law Journal*, December 27, 1993–January 3, 1994, p. S5.

27. McElaney, J.W. "Preparing Witnesses for Depositions." *Journal of the American Bar Association*, June 1992, pp. 84–86.

28. Bamonte, A.M. "Program Builds Staff Confidence, Eases Stress of Lawsuits." *Hospital Risk Management*, January 1993, pp. 9–11.

29. McMorris, F.A. "Judge Permits Claim That a Fax Could Interfere With Contract." *Wall Street Journal*, December 20, 1995, p. B8.

30. Novis, J.H., Friedman, M.J. "Taxes and the Independent Contractor: Part 2." *PT: Magazine of Physical Therapy*, 1993; 1(5):63–65.

31. Texas Uniform Partnership Act (Registered Limited Liability Partnership), Texas Rev. Civ. Stat. Ann. art. 6132b.

32. Huckstep, A., Wilson, J.C., Carmody, R.P. *Corporate Law for the Healthcare Provider: Organization, Operation, Merger and Bankruptcy*. Washington, DC: National Health Lawyers Association Focus Series Publication, 1993, p. 26.

33. Yagoda, B.J., Klingenberg, E. "The Taxman Cometh." *Journal of the American Bar Association*, November 1991, pp. 78–81.

34. Texas Professional Corporation Act, Texas Rev. Civ. Stat. Ann. art. 1528e.

35. Texas Professional Association Act, Texas Rev. Civ. Stat. Ann. art. 1528f.

36. *Corporate Law for the Healthcare Provider*, note 32, 5.

37. Schutzer, A.I. "Does Incorporation Still Make Sense?" *Medical Economics*, May 20, 1991, pp. 157–160.

38. One exception is Vermont, whose Stat. Ann. 12, Section 519 requires citizens to render aid to others in grave harm when it can safely be done. Klein, C.A. "Good Samaritan Acts, Part I." *Nurse Practitioner*, March 1984, pp. 66–67.

39. Mason, R. "Good Samaritan Laws, Legal Disarray: An Update." *Mercer Law Review*, 1987; 38:1339–1375.

40. Scott, R.W. "Good Samaritan Immunity." *Clinical Management*, 1991; 11(4):11–12.

41. Helminski, F. "Ghosts From Samaria: Good Samaritan Laws in the Hospital." *Mayo Clinic Proceedings*, 1993; 68:400–401.

42. 35 United States Code Section 102(b).

43. The Copyright Act, 17 United States Code Section 101 *et seq.*

44. *Ibid.*, Section 107.

45. Mead Data Central, 9393 Springboro Pike, Dayton, OH 45401.

46. West Publishing Company, 50 W. Kellogg Blvd., St. Paul, MN 55164.

47. Morris, A. "Through the Looking Glass: Managed Care and Healthcare Reform." *Synergy*, February 1994, pp. 5, 11.

48. Schunk, C. "Understanding Managed Care: A Glossary of Terminology." *GeriNotes*, 1995; 3(1):20–21.

49. Werning, S.C. "A Primer on Managed Care." *Healthcare Trends & Transitions*, 1993; 5(1):10–13, 26–28, 46.

50. Enders, R.T.J. "PHO Contracting Under the Microscope." *Inside Health Law*, 1996; 1(1):9–11.

51. Olsen, G.G. "The Coming Wave: PSNs, PHOs, and PCCOs." *Rehab Management*, October/November 1995, pp. 101–102.

52. Arthur, P.R. "The Restructuring of America's Hospitals: Acute Orthopedic Services." *PT: Magazine of Physical Therapy*, 1994; 2(7):35–45.

53. Richardson, J.K. "The Challenging Roles Facing PTs." *Healthcare Trends & Transitions*, 1993; 5(1):34–35.

54. Framroze, A. "Reimbursement Update." *Rehab Management*, August/September 1994, pp. 24–28.

55. Monahan, B. "Managing Under Managed Care." *PT: Magazine of Physical Therapy*, 1993; 1(7):34–40.

56. Hadorn, D.C., McCormick, K., Diokno, A. "An Annotated Algorithm Approach to Clinical Practice Guidelines." *Journal of the American Medical Association*, 1992; 267:3311–3314.

57. Jirank, A.L., Baker, S.D. "Any Willing Provider Laws: Regulating the Health Care Provider's Contractual Relationship with the Insurance Company." *Health Lawyer*, 1994; 7(4):1, 3–6.

58. Weil, D.A., Diamond, J.T. "Managed Care Contract Provision Requiring Attention." *Health Lawyer*, 1995; 8(5):3–9.

59. Applebaum, P.S. "Legal Liability and Managed Care." *American Psychologist*, 1993; 48(3):251–257.

60. Poland, S.C. "Medical Malpractice Actions Against HMOs in the 1990s." *Exchange Plus Quarterly*, February 1996, pp. 2–4.

61. "HMO Backlash Spurs Wave of Restrictive Litigation." *San Antonio Express News*, March 15, 1996, p. 10B.

62. *Critical Challenges: Revitalizing the Health Professions for the Twenty-First Century: Third Report of the Pew Health Professions Commission*. San Francisco, CA: UCSF Center for the Health Professions, 1995, pp. 36, 42, 48.

63. *Therapy Student Journal*, Spring 1996, pp. 1–6.

64. Wachler, A.B., Kopson, M.S., Avery, P.A. "Stark I Final Regulations: Implications for Health Care Providers and Suppliers." *Health Lawyer*, August 1995 (Special Edition), pp. 1–14.

65. Kelly, B.L., Harkins, M.J. "The Devil You Don't Know: Litigation and Enforcement Trends in Long-Term Care." *Health Lawyer*, 1995; 8(3): 6–9.

66. Omnibus Budget Reconciliation Act of 1987, Public Law 100-203, 101 Stat. 1330, 42 United States Code Sections 1395i-3 and 1396r *et seq*.

67. Murphy, J., Breske, S. "Nursing Homes: Continue to Restrain Restraints." *Advance for Physical Therapists*, February 26, 1996, pp. 8, 24.

68. Scott, R.W. *Legal Aspects of Documenting Patient Care*. Gaithersburg, MD: Aspen Publishers, Inc., 1994, p. 190.

69. Murphy & Breske, note 67, at 8.

70. The Patient Self-Determination Act of 1990, 42 United States Code Sections 1395cc and 1396a.

71. Scott, R.W. "Guaranteeing Patient Rights: It's the Law." *Advance for Directors in Rehab*, September/October 1992, pp. 43–44.

72. Patient Self-Determination Act, Section 1395cc(f).

73. Framroze, note 54, at 24.

74. Rasmussen, B. *Reimbursement and Fiscal Management in Rehabilitation*. Alexandria, VA: American Physical Therapy Association, 1995, p. 120.

75. Anders, G., McGinley, L. "Managed Eldercare: HMOs Are Signing Up New Class of Member: The Group in Medicare." *Wall Street Journal*, April 27, 1995, pp. A1, A5.

76. Jeffrey, N.A. "Sign of the Times: Medicare Users Turn to HMOs." *Wall Street Journal*, October 20, 1995, pp. C1, C18.

77. Scott, note 68, at 201.

78. Rundle, R.L. "Medicare Fraud Case Draws Guilty Plea." *Wall Street Journal*, April 29, 1996, p. B2.

79. The Safe Medical Devices Act of 190, 21 United States Code Sections 301note, 321, 360d, 360hh *et seq.*

80. "The Safe Medical Devices Act: Does It Increase Hospital Liability?" *Hospital Risk Management*, May 1991, pp. 55–58.

Suggested Readings

1. Anders, G., McGinley, L. "Managed Eldercare: HMOs Are Signing Up New Class of Member: The Group in Medicare." *Wall Street Journal*, April 27, 1995, pp. A1, A5.

2. Applebaum, P.S. "Legal Liability and Managed Care." *American Psychologist*, 1993; 48(3):251–257.

3. Arthur, P.R. "The Restructuring of America's Hospitals: Acute Orthopedic Services." *PT: Magazine of Physical Therapy*, 1994; 2(7):35–45.

4. Bamonte, A.M. "Program Builds Staff Confidence, Eases Stress of Lawsuits." *Hospital Risk Management*, January 1993, pp. 9–11.

5. *Critical Challenges: Revitalizing the Health Professions for the Twenty-First Century: Third Report of the Pew Health Professions Commission*. San Francisco, CA: UCSF Center for the Health Professions, 1995.

6. Davis, K.C., Pierce, R.J., Jr. *Administrative Law Treatise*, 3rd ed. Boston, MA: Little, Brown and Company Publishing, 1994.

7. Driskell, C. "Ethics: Advertising Your Services." *Clinical Management*, 1992: 12(2):16–17.

8. Enders, R.T.J. "PHO Contracting Under the Microscope." *Inside Health Law*, 1996; 1(1):9–11.

9. Framroze, A. "Reimbursement Update." *Rehab Management*, August/September 1994, pp. 24–28.

10. Freed, C. "Antitrust Reform for Physicians Network Joint Ventures." *San Antonio Medical Gazette*, October 13–19, 1995, pp. 6, 23.

11. Furrow, B.R., Johnson, S.H., Jost, T.S., Schwartz, R.L. *Health Law: Cases, Materials and Problems*, 2nd ed. St. Paul, MN: West Publishing Company, 1991.

12. Ginsburg, W.H. "How to Evaluate a Lawyer." *Physician's Management*, December 1991, pp. 90–99.

13. *Guide for Professional Conduct*. Alexandria, VA: American Physical Therapy Association, 1996.

14. Hadorn, D.C., McCormick, K., Diokno, A. "An Annotated Algorithm Approach to Clinical Practice Guidelines." *Journal of the American Medical Association*, 1992; 267:3311–3314.

15. Helminski, F. "Ghosts From Samaria: Good Samaritan Laws in the Hospital." *Mayo Clinic Proceedings*, 1993; 68:400–401.

16. "HMO Backlash Spurs Wave of Restrictive Litigation." *San Antonio Express News*, March 15, 1996, p. 10B.

17. Huckstep, A., Wilson, J.C., Carmody, R.P. *Corporate Law for the Healthcare Provider: Organization, Operation, Merger and Bankruptcy*. Washington, DC: National Health Lawyers Association Focus Series Publication, 1993.

18. *Integrated Delivery Systems in a Changing Health Care Environment: New Legal Challenges*. American Bar Association, Forum on Health Law, Monograph 1, 1994.

19. Jeffrey, N.A. "Sign of the Times: Medicare Users Turn to HMOs." *Wall Street Journal*, October 20, 1995, pp. C1, C18.

20. Jirank, A.L., Baker, S.D. "Any Willing Provider Laws: Regulating the Health Care Provider's Contractual Relationship with the Insurance Company." *Health Lawyer*, 1994; 7(4):1, 3–6.

21. Kelly, B.L., Harkins, M.J. "The Devil You Don't Know: Litigation and Enforcement Trends in Long-Term Care." *Health Lawyer*, 1995; 8(3): 6–9.

22. Klein, C.A. "Good Samaritan Acts, Part I." *Nurse Practitioner*. March 1984, pp. 66–67.

23. Klein, C.A. "Good Samaritan Acts, Part II." *Nurse Practitioner*, April 1984, pp. 56–58.

24. La Puma, J., Orentlicher, D., Moss, R.J. "Advance Directives on Admission: Clinical Implications and Analysis of the Patient Self-Determination Act of 1990." *Journal of the American Medical Association*, 1991; 266:402–405.

25. Lewis, C.B. "Think Like a Lawyer: Tips for PTs Who Testify in Court." *PT Today*, February 12, 1996.

26. Marx, D., Jr., Laing, M.A. "The State Action Doctrine: Can It Be Applied to a Private Hospital's Acquisition of a Public Hospital?" *The Health Lawyer*, 1995; 8(3):1, 3–5.

27. Mason, R. "Good Samaritan Laws, Legal Disarray: An Update." *Mercer Law Review*, 1987; 38:1339–1375.

28. McElaney, J.W. "Preparing Witnesses for Depositions." *Journal of the American Bar Association*, June 1992, pp. 84–86.

29. Monahan, B. "Managing Under Managed Care." *PT: Magazine of Physical Therapy*, 1993; 1(7):34–40.

30. Morris, A. "Through the Looking Glass: Managed Care and Healthcare Reform." *Synergy*, February 1994, pp. 5, 11.

31. Murphy, J. "Can I Get a Witness? Tips on Testifying—And How to Avoid It." *Advance for Physical Therapists*, March 11, 1996, pp. 5, 30.

32. Murphy, J., Breske, S. "Nursing Homes: Continue to Restrain Restraints." Advance for Physical Therapists, February 26, 1996, pp. 8, 24.

33. Novis, J.H., Friedman, M.J. "Taxes and the Independent Contractor: Part 2." *PT: Magazine of Physical Therapy*, 1993; 1(5):63–65.

34. *Occupational Therapy Code of Ethics*. Bethesda, MD: American Occupational Therapy Association, Commission on Standards and Ethics, 1994.

35. Olsen, G.G. "The Coming Wave: PSNs, PHOs, and PCCOs." *Rehab Management*, October/November 1995, pp. 101–102.

36. Omnibus Budget Reconciliation Act of 1987, Public Law 100-203, 101 Stat. 1330, 42 United States Code Sections 1395i-3 and 1396r *et seq.*

37. Overman, S. "How to Work With Your Lawyer." *HR Magazine*, July 1992, pp.

41-45.

38. Patient Self-Determination Act of 1990, 42 United States Code Sections 1395cc and 1396a.

39. Poland, S.C. "Medical Malpractice Actions Against HMOs in the 1990s." *Exchange Plus Quarterly*, February 1996, pp. 2–4.

40. Rasmussen, B. *Reimbursement and Fiscal Management in Rehabilitation*. Alexandria, VA: American Physical Therapy Association, 1995.

41. Richardson, J.K. "The Challenging Roles Facing PTs." *Healthcare Trends & Transitions*, 1993; 5(1):34–35.

42. Rundle, R.L. "Medicare Fraud Case Draws Guilty Plea." *Wall Street Journal*, April 29, 1996, p. B2.

43. Safe Medical Devices Act of 1990, 21 United States Code Sections 301note, 321, 360d, 360hh *et seq*.

44. Schunk, C. "Understanding Managed Care: A Glossary of Terminology." *GeriNotes*, 1995; 3(1):20–21.

45. Schutzer, A.I. "Does Incorporation Still Make Sense?" *Medical Economics*, May 20, 1991, pp. 157–160.

46. Scott, R.W. "Good Samaritan Immunity." *Clinical Management*, 1991; 11(4):11–12.

47. Scott, R.W. "Guaranteeing Patient Rights: It's the Law." *Advance for Directors in Rehab*, September/October 1992, pp. 43–44.

48. Scott, R.W. *Legal Aspects of Documenting Patient Care*. Gaithersburg, MD: Aspen Publishers, Inc. 1994.

49. Smolowe, J. "A Healthy Merger?" *Time*, April 15, 1996, pp. 77–78.

50. "The Safe Medical Devices Act: Does It Increase Hospital Liability?" *Hospital Risk Management*, May 1991, pp. 55–58.

51. Van Lieshout, B. "'Restraint' Not a Bad Thing (When Used Properly)." *Advance for Physical Therapists*, December 4, 1995, pp. 24–25.

52. Wachler, A.B., Kopson, M.S., Avery, P.A. "Stark I Final Regulations: Implications for Health Care Providers and Suppliers." *Health Lawyer*, August 1995 (Special Edition), pp. 1–14.

53. Weil, D.A., Diamond, J.T. "Managed Care Contract Provision Requiring Attention." *Health Lawyer*, 1995; 8(5):3–9.

54. Werning, S.C. "A Primer on Managed Care." *Healthcare Trends & Transitions*, 1993; 5(1):10–13, 26–28, 46.

55. Williams, M.A. "The Safe Medical Devices Act." *Southern Hospitals*, March/April 1992, pp. 16–17.

56. Yagoda, B.J., Klingenberg, E. "The Taxman Cometh." *Journal of the American Bar Association*, November 1991, pp. 78–81.

Chapter 11

Health Care Ethics

This chapter briefly introduces the topics of professional ethics and frameworks for ethical decision making by health care professionals. The provisions of the codes of ethics of the American Physical Therapy Association and the American Occupational Therapy Association are studied and contrasted. The administrative procedures for disciplinary action of the two health professions are examined, as are those of the National Board for Certification in Occupational Therapy. Disciplinary actions taken by voluntary, private associations are compared to those "state actions" undertaken by public regulatory agencies.

A Framework for Ethical Decision Making

Health care decision making, whether in educational, clinical, research, school, home, or other settings, requires careful compliance with professional and institutional ethical standards. As with legal requirements, ignorance of ethical responsibilities is no excuse for non-compliance.

Hint *Ignorance of ethical responsibilities is no excuse for noncompliance.*

There are several recognized frameworks for ethical decision making for health care professionals.[1,2,3] Ethical decision-making models governing patient care are based on the foundational ethical principles of beneficence, nonmaleficence, autonomy, and justice, and are reflective of the professional duties of competency, confidentiality, fidelity, and truth. Conducting oneself in conformity with these principles and duties is seemingly more difficult under the current health care delivery model of managed care, which presents significant potential conflicts of interest.

Most analytical ethical decision-making models have common core elements:

- identification of a problem having ethical implications
- identification of relevant facts, assumptions, and unknowns associated with the problem
- delineation and analysis of courses of action to resolve the problem

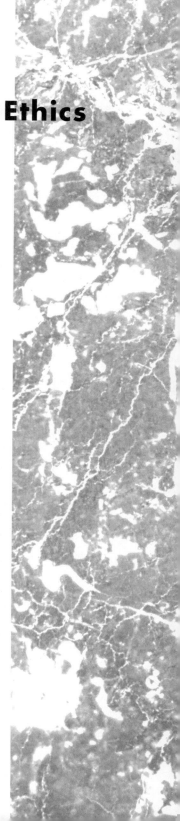

- selection of an option based on an appropriate ethics approach and ethical guidelines and in conformity with any governing ethical and legal directives

Ethical principles may be grounded in religion, in other duty-based moral theory (such as Immanuel Kant's deontological approach),[4] or in other philosophical theory (such as John Stuart Mill 's outcome-oriented utilitarianism).[5] Health care professions, through their professional associations, formalize fundamental ethical principles governing the official conduct of members of the profession into codes of ethics.

Today, law and ethics have largely been blended into common standards of professional conduct. Very often, professional conduct that constitutes a breach of ethics also constitutes a violation of law, and vice versa. For example, commission of nonconsensual sexual battery upon a patient is universally accepted as a breach of professional ethics, as well as a violation of civil and criminal law.

Professional conduct may, however, be a violation of ethical standards, but not a violation of the law. Consider the following hypothetical example:

An employment contract between a health care professional and a managed care organization contains in it a provision which prohibits the health care professional from discussing treatment options with patients that are not offered by the managed care organization. (Such a contractual provision is commonly referred to as a "gag clause."[6]) While compliance by the health care professional with the gag clause might be upheld by a court as a legally acceptable course of action, such conduct might still constitute an actionable breach of professional ethics. Under traditional ethical standards governing patient informed consent to treatment, a competent patient must be informed by a clinical health care professional of *all* reasonable alternatives to a proposed intervention, irrespective of whether or not a managed care entity elects to offer them as a matter of its business judgment. The health care professional in this case might face adverse administrative or association action for a breach of professional ethics, in spite of the legality of the contract.

Educational Settings

In professional education settings, academicians, clinical faculty, and students all have ethical responsibilities. The same fundamental duties of competency, confidentiality, fidelity, and truth that apply to professional-patient relationships also apply to relationships between students and faculty. Many of these ethical duties are codified into case law and statutes, making them legal duties as well. For example, the legal duty of confidentiality of student records incumbent upon academicians is governed by the Family Educational Rights and Privacy Act of 1974 (the "Buckley Amendment").[7]

Students, as well as faculty, have fundamental ethical duties governing their conduct. For example, relative to truth, students have the ethical duties not to cheat on examinations and not to plagiarize the work product of others. Health professional students also have the ethical duty not to intentionally defraud prospective employers by signing pre-employment contracts solely to receive current financial incentives.

Sanctions for violations of ethical duties in professional education exist along a progressive continuum, just as they do along the disciplinary continuum in employment settings. Students who violate ethical obligations may face a failing grade or suspension or expulsion from their programs for serious breaches of ethics. Faculty who breach ethical standards may incur the loss of a chance for tenure or the loss of employment for serious breaches of their ethical responsibilities.

Faculty and student ethical responsibilities are commonly spelled out with varying degrees of clarity in faculty and student handbooks, respectively. While standards may appear vague, sanctions for violations of standards cannot be vague, because of the due process considerations of notice and substantive fairness which are prerequisites to adverse action.

Clinical Settings

It is perhaps easiest to understand the meanings of the foundational ethical principles of beneficence, nonmaleficence, autonomy, and justice[8] when they are applied to health care clinical scenarios. Health professions identify themselves as being altruistic and, specifically, patient welfare-focused. The profession of occupational therapy in particular characterizes its core values around seven fundamental concepts: altruism, equality, freedom (autonomy), justice, dignity, truth, and prudence.[9] Whether express or implied, all health professions espouse similar values and attitudes.

Beneficence means that a health care professional's conduct relative to a particular patient will be carried out in accordance with that patient's best interests. *Nonmaleficence* means that health care professionals will not intentionally cause harm to patients under their care. *Autonomy* recognizes the inherent human right of self-determination in every competent patient. *Justice* reflects the desire to achieve fundamental fairness in health care delivery, at individual, group, societal, and global levels.

As will be seen below, the provisions of the American Physical Therapy Association's ethical *Guide for Professional Conduct*[10] (applicable to member-physical therapists) and *Guide for Conduct of the Affiliate Member*[11] (applicable to physical therapist assistants) are largely focused specifically on professional-patient relations, although the provisions of the guides apply to all physical therapy professionals—clinicians, academicians, researchers, and others. (Section 4.3 of the *Guide for Professional Conduct* is a comprehensive provision addressing the ethical conduct of researchers.[12]) The principles of the *Occupational Therapy Code of Ethics*[13] (applicable to all occupational therapy personnel) are more global in their jurisdiction of providers and focus on "recipients of services."

The developing paradigm of managed health care delivery brings with it a number of potential ethical dilemmas for health care professionals, who face ever more sharply divided loyalty issues involving their employers and patients. A recent backlash of legislative initiatives has begun at the state and federal levels and is designed to curb managed care practices that restrict patient access to and funding of health care.[14]

Assistance to health care professionals facing ethical dilemmas is provided in health care institutions by institutional ethics committees. These multidisciplinary committees may have several roles, including policy making, education, and provision of consultation services.

Research Settings

Ethical issues in research settings center largely on two issues: the protection of human research subjects and the integrity of research processes.[15] The history of the protection of human subjects—including discussion of subject informed consent procedures—has already been discussed in detail in Chapter 4. Federal (Department of Health and Human Services) regulations governing the use of human subjects in research[16] are derived, in part, from domestic law and custom and, in part, from customary international law and multinational human rights treaties. Responsibility for the protection of human research subjects rests with institutional review boards, which are multidisciplinary committees that establish research protocol guidelines; review and approve research proposals for their institutions that involve human research subjects; and enforce compliance with federal, state, and institutional requirements.

The integrity of research scientists is of paramount concern to the research community for obvious reasons. From the funding of research projects to public trust, research, especially involving human subjects, must have the respect of the scientific community, government, and the public-at-large.

Researchers, just like health care clinicians, academicians, and students, have ethical responsibilities. Scientists have the same core values that all others within a profession do[17] and are bound by the same professional codes of ethics governing their respective disciplines.

Researchers are ethically bound to protect the well-being of research subjects and to ensure that they are provided with detailed disclosure of information regarding the research, so that they give informed consent to participate. They must also maintain appropriate confidentiality of the personal identities of research subjects. Researchers must avoid conflicts of interest that might bias their research findings. They are similarly obliged to avoid distorting or misrepresenting results. They must appropriately credit others for their source materials and contributions to research projects.[18]

Professional Association Codes of Ethics

Every health care professional discipline association has in place a code of ethics governing the official conduct of its members. This section examines the ethics codes for the professions of physical and occupational therapy. Readers are invited to research other health professional codes of ethics of interest, and conduct a comparative analysis of those codes and the ethics codes governing the physical and occupational therapy professions.

Standards

Codes of ethics may contain two general types of provisions: directive and nondirective. Directive provisions address required conduct. Nondirective provisions are of two types, addressing permissive and recommended conduct. Directive provisions normally contain the action verbs *shall*, *will*, *may not*, *shall not*, or *will not*. Nondirective provisions addressing permissive conduct may contain the action verb *may*, while nondirective provisions addressing recommended conduct typically contain the action verbs *should* or *should not*. Examples of directive and nondirective ethics provisions from the American Physical Therapy Association's *Guide for Professional Conduct* are:

> *Directive*: Physical therapists *shall* recognize that each individual is different from all other individuals and shall respect and be responsive to those differences.[19]

> *Nondirective (permissive conduct)*: Physical therapists *may* enter into agreements with organizations to provide physical therapy services if such agreements do not violate the ethical principles of the Association.[20]

> *Nondirective (recommended conduct)*: Physical therapists *should* render pro bono publico (reduced or no fee) services to patients lacking the ability to pay for services, as each physical therapist 's practice permits.[21]

The provisions in the *Occupational Therapy Code of Ethics*[22] are not differentiated into directive and nondirective components. All of the ethical principles in the *Occupational Therapy Code of Ethics* are directive, and all contain the action verb *shall*. For example, Principle 2A states that:

> Occupational therapy personnel *shall* collaborate with service recipients or their surrogate(s) in determining goals and priorities throughout the intervention process.

The American Physical Therapy Association's *Code of Ethics* and implementing *Guide for Professional Conduct* contain directive and nondirective ethical provisions regulating the official conduct of member-physical therapists. The framework of the *Guide for Professional Conduct* is as follows:

Principle 1 (Respect for Rights and Dignity)
   1.1 Attitudes
   1.2 Confidentiality
   1.3 Patient Relations
   1.4 Informed Consent

Principle 2 (Compliance with Laws and Regulations)
   2.1 Professional Practice

Principle 3 (Responsibility, Professional Autonomy)
   3.1 Responsibility
   3.2 Delegation

3.3 Provision of Services

3.4 Referral Relationships

3.5 Practice Arrangements

Principle 4 (Standards: Maintenance, Promotion)

4.1 Continuing Education

4.2 Review and Self-Assessment

4.3 Research

4.4 Education

Principle 5 (Renumeration)

5.1 Fiscally Sound Renumeration

5.2 Business Practices/Fee Arrangements

5.3 Endorsement of Equipment or Services

5.4 Gifts

Principle 6 (Professional Information Dissemination)

6.1 Information About the Profession

6.2 Information About Services

Principle 7 (Professional Responsibility)

7.1 Consumer Protection

7.2 Disclosure of Potential Conflicts of Interest

Principle 8 (Public Health)

8.1 Pro Bono Service

The American Physical Therapy Association's *Standards of Ethical Conduct for the Physical Therapist Assistant* and implementing *Guide for Conduct of the Affiliate Member* contains directive and nondirective ethical provisions regulating the official conduct of member-physical therapist assistants. The framework of the *Guide for Conduct of the Affiliate Member* is as follows:

Standard 1 (Performance of Services Under Supervision)

1.1 Supervisory Relationships

1.2 Performance of Services

Standard 2 (Respect for Rights and Dignity)

2.1 Attitudes

2.2 Requests for Release of Information

2.3 Protection of Privacy

2.4 Patient Relations

Standard 3 (Standards: Maintenance, Promotion)

3.1 Information About Services

3.2 Organizational Equipment

3.3 Endorsement of Equipment

3.4 Financial Considerations

3.5 Exploitation of Patients

268

Standard 4 (Compliance with Law)
    4.1 Supervisory Relationships
    4.2 Representation
Standard 5 (Exercise of Judgment)
    5.1 Patient Treatment
    5.2 Patient Safety
    5.3 Qualifications
    5.4 Discontinuance of Treatment Programs
    5.5 Continuing Education
Standard 6 (Professional Responsibility)
    6.1 Consumer Protection

All but four of the standards and their sections in the *Guide for Conduct of the Affiliate Member* are directive in nature. Those four nondirective provisions are all of the permissive type.

The American Occupational Therapy Association's *Occupational Therapy Code of Ethics* is binding on all occupational therapy personnel who are members of the professional association. Its framework is as follows:

Principle 1 (Beneficence)
    A. Equitable provision of services
    B. Professional relationships
    C. Avoidance of harm to recipients of services
    D. Reasonableness of fees[23]

Principle 2 (Respect for Rights of Service Recipients)
    A. Continuous collaboration on goals and priorities
    B. Patient informed consent
    C. Research subject informed consent
    D. Right to refuse services or participation
    E. Confidentiality

Principle 3 (Competence)
    A. Credentials
    B. Standards of practice
    C. Professional development
    D. Accurate and current information
    E. Appropriate delegation
    F. Appropriate supervision
    G. Referral, consultation

Principle 4 (Compliance with Laws and Policies)
    A. Personal compliance
    B. Communication of legal and administrative duties
    C. Compliance by those under supervision

       D. Accurate documentation and communication

Principle 5 (Accuracy in Information About Services)
       A. Personal representation
       B. Actual and potential conflicts of interests
       C. False, deceptive, unfair communications

Principle 6 (Professional Relations)
       A. Confidentiality
       B. Representation of qualifications
       C. Reporting of breaches of ethics

Enforcement of Ethics Codes: Disciplinary Processes

Health professional ethical standards are enforced by professional associations, credentialing bodies, and state licensure or regulatory administrative agencies. The jurisdictional models and procedural processes for physical and occupational therapy are presented in this section. Readers are invited to research the ethical jurisdiction and complaint processes for their respective professions, and compare them to those in place for physical and occupational therapy.

Participants and Processes

Physical therapy The American Physical Therapy Association has ethical jurisdiction over the more than 60,000 physical therapists and physical therapist assistants who are members of the association.[24] A written complaint of unethical conduct on the part of member-physical therapists or physical therapist assistants is the starting point for initiation of investigation and disciplinary action, pursuant to the Procedural Document on Disciplinary Action of the American Physical Therapy Association.[25]

A complaint can be made by anyone having knowledge (firsthand or otherwise) of a suspected ethical violation by an association member. The signed, written complaint is forwarded to the state chapter president, who (1) forwards an informational copy of the complaint to the judicial committee, and (2) makes an initial determination as to whether the complaint is actionable or not. Acknowledgment of receipt of the complaint must be forwarded to the *complainant* by the chapter president within 15 days of receipt. Along with acknowledgment, the chapter president advises the complainant that the *respondent* may have the right to learn the complainant's identity.

If a complaint is non-actionable because an allegation does not involve a violation of the Code of Ethics or Standards of Ethical Conduct, or, if in the judgment of the chapter president, the allegation does not warrant action, the complaint is dismissed by the chapter president. If the complaint is actionable, the respondent-member is notified of the charge(s) and of the specific provisions of the Code or Standards allegedly violated.

A chapter president may initiate action on his or her own (without a written complaint), based on public information. Proof of commission of a crime related to a member's professional status, or of a felony, or of revocation of licensure, is *prima facie* (presumptive) evidence of an actionable ethics violation and triggers interim suspension of membership until judicial committee action at its next regularly scheduled semiannual meeting.

In all other actionable cases, the chapter president forwards the case file to the chapter ethics committee (CEC) for processing. The CEC either summarily dismisses charges, based on available evidence, or appoints an investigator, who conducts a comprehensive, unbiased investigation of the charges against the respondent, compiles an investigative file, and makes findings of fact (but not conclusions or recommendations).

If the CEC determines that charges against a respondent are unsubstantiated, then the CEC may summarily dismiss the complaint, under which option the respondent does not have the right to learn of the name of the complainant. Otherwise, the respondent is notified of his or her right to a copy of the investigative file and to a hearing of the charges.

With or without a hearing, the CEC makes specific conclusions and recommendations on charges against a respondent, which must be either dismissal of the charges or disciplinary action by the judicial committee. Judicial committee disciplinary actions include written reprimands, membership probation (from six months to two years in length), membership suspension (of one year or longer), and expulsion from the association.

Once properly notified of the CEC recommendations, a respondent has the right to request a hearing before the judicial committee at its next semiannual meeting in Alexandria, Virginia. At this hearing, as at the state level, the respondent may be accompanied by an attorney, who serves as a silent advisor to the respondent during the proceedings.

With or without another hearing, the judicial committee takes action on a complaint, as follows. The judicial committee may adopt the disciplinary recommendation(s) of the CEC, dismiss charges or award a less severe disciplinary sanction, or *remand* the case to the CEC for further action.

After appropriate notification, a respondent has the right to appeal the judicial committee's decision to the Board of Directors within 30 days. The board of directors may affirm the decision of the judicial committee, dismiss charges or impose a less severe disciplinary sanction, or remand the case to the judicial committee for further action. Once final, publication of disciplinary action takes place in the association's publications of general circulation. Published information is limited to the name of the respondent, the disciplinary action taken, and the effective date of the action. Beyond this summary information, the details of disciplinary proceedings are confidential, and further information about proceedings is not normally disseminated without a court order.

Occupational therapy

American occupational therapy association   The American Occupational Therapy Association has ethical jurisdiction over the more than 48,000 occupational therapists and certified occupational therapy assistants who are members of the association.[26] The procedures for receiving, evaluating, and adjudicating ethical complaints against members of the American Occupational Therapy Association are analogous to those employed by the American Physical Therapy Association, with a few important differences.[27]

A complaint of an ethical violation against a member of the association may be filed by anyone having knowledge of a suspected ethical violation by an association member. A signed, written complaint is filed with the Standards and Ethics Commission (SEC), for which an appointed investigation committee conducts a preliminary investigation to determine whether there is substantial evidence of an ethical violation. The investigation committee is empowered to make findings and recommendations concerning suspected ethical violations. If such evidence is found to exist, the SEC may issue a formal charge, which it forwards to the president of the Association, who then appoints a judicial counsel to adjudicate the charge.

The ad hoc judicial counsel, comprised of three members of the Association, presides at a hearing on charges against a member and is represented by legal counsel. A respondent may also be represented at such a hearing by legal counsel.

A finding that a member has committed an ethical violation may result in the award of one of the following disciplinary sanctions: censure, membership suspension, or expulsion from the Association. A respondent is notified in a certified writing of the judicial counsel's decision by the president of the Association.

A respondent may file a timely written appeal of a disciplinary action to the executive director of the Association. Such an appeal is heard by a three-member panel, comprised of the vice-president, secretary, and treasurer of the association. An appeals hearing may or may not take place, at the discretion of the appeals panel. The decision of the appeals panel is final.

National board for certification in occupational therapy

The National Board for Certification in Occupational Therapy (NBCOT), formerly known as the American Occupational Therapy Certification Board, is the national nongovernmental agency responsible for certification and recertification of occupational therapists and certified occupational therapy assistants.[28] It has jurisdiction to investigate complaints and take disciplinary action against all NBCOT-certified (and eligible) occupational therapists and certified occupational therapy assistants. In addition to adjudicating ethical complaints, NBCOT investigates and takes action on complaints alleging incompetence and impairment on the part of certified occupational therapy professionals. Its *Procedures for Disciplinary Action*[29] spells out procedures that are similar to those employed by the American Occupational and Physical Therapy Associations.

The spectrum of disciplinary sanctions that can be awarded by the NBCOT includes, in order of progressive severity:

- formal written reprimand
- public censure

- compulsory community service
- compulsory participation in remediation programs
- suspension of certification to practice for a definite term
- ineligibility for certification, either for a definite term, or indefinitely
- revocation of certification

Unlike the American Occupational and Physical Therapy Associations, NBCOT may also issue advisory opinions on matters under its jurisdiction, similar to procedures utilized by the American Bar Association, which governs the ethical conduct of member attorneys.

Actions by State Regulatory Agencies

In addition to adverse action by professional associations and certification entities, disciplinary action for ethical violations against health care professionals can be undertaken by state regulatory and licensure agencies. These entities are public bodies, so that all of the federal and state constitutional safeguards and procedures that apply to state actions generally also apply to their actions.

Health professional regulatory entities have jurisdiction over professionals privileged to practice in the state and those who practice without proper credentials. They operate pursuant to the state "police power" to make and enforce standards for public health and safety.[30]

Administrative procedures for adjudicating disciplinary complaints alleging ethics violations (of practice acts or professional codes) are similar to those utilized by private associations and boards, except that, as public entities, state regulatory bodies must pay strict attention to procedural and substantive due process requirements (as discussed below). Disciplinary sanctions that may be awarded by public regulatory entities include, among other possible adverse actions, public censure and suspension and revocation of licensure or practice privileges.

Public censure means dissemination of offenses and disciplinary sanctions to the general public. As with news about other public figures, the public has the constitutional "right to know" about disciplinary actions taken by states against licensed or otherwise regulated health care professionals. Recent examples of public censure of health professionals by state regulatory agencies include license suspension or revocation for corporal punishment of a spouse in one case and for prostitution in another,[31] and announcement of impending licensure suspension authority for nonpayment of child support by licensees.[32]

Private associations and boards adjudicating disciplinary actions against health care professionals may or may not communicate formally with state regulatory entities about their activities. The policies of the American Occupational Therapy Association and NBCOT are to communicate information about disciplinary actions taken against occupational therapy professionals to state regulatory entities via the Disciplinary Action Information Exchange Network.[33] The official policy of the American Physical Therapy Association is to not routinely communicate specific information about its disciplinary proceedings to state regulatory entities, without a statute, regulation, or court order requiring such communication.[34] Of course, the proceedings of state regulatory entities are available to private associations and individuals, because they are public records.

Due Process and Judicial Oversight

In adverse administrative disciplinary actions by state regulatory agencies against health professionals, the federal constitutional due process clause of the Fourteenth Amendment requires that the government afford procedural and substantive due process to respondents. State constitutions, statutes, and case law may afford additional protections to respondents.

Procedural due process means adequate notice of an adverse action and a reasonable opportunity to be heard. In the case of adverse professional licensure actions, a reasonable opportunity to be heard is synonymous with the right to a hearing. *Substantive due process* means that a disciplinary procedure must be fundamentally fair, especially in light of the fact that a health professional respondent faces potential loss of a constitutionally-recognized property interest in the earned privilege of professional practice.

For disciplinary actions taken by voluntary, private (nongovernmental) associations and boards, constitutional due process considerations do not strictly apply. Instead, the internal affairs of voluntary private associations are governed by their charters, constitutions, and bylaws. The private association analog of due process is that such associations must follow their own rules and procedures when administering discipline.

Courts always have oversight jurisdiction over state administrative agencies and their decisions, and the activities of voluntary, private associations. Courts are reluctant to reverse the decisions of administrative bodies, however, for several reasons. These include deference to the reasonable decisions of administrative entities and considerations of time management. Reasons justifying reversal of administrative decisions for public agencies include the denial of due process and instances in which decisions are characterized as arbitrary, capricious, or the result of bias. Reasons for reversal of decisions of voluntary private associations include, among others, fraud, malice, bias, the prejudicial failure to follow association rules and procedures, and instances in which decisions contravene law or public policy.

Chapter Summary

Ethics involves doing what is "right" under the circumstances. Health care professionals are governed by professional codes of ethics which are developed and enforced by professional associations. Frameworks for ethical decision making by professionals include the following elements: identification of a problem having ethical implications; identification of relevant facts, assumptions, and unknowns about the problem; delineation and analysis of reasonable courses of action; and selection of an option, based on an appropriate ethics approach and ethical guidelines, and in conformity with any governing ethical and legal directives.

Ethics apply in all professional settings, including, but not limited to, the clinical, school, and research settings. Professional association codes of ethics and state licensure laws and regulations govern the official conduct of professionals within a specific discipline.

The American Physical Therapy Association, the American Occupational Therapy Association, and the National Board for Certification in Occupational Therapy all have detailed administrative procedures for receiving, investigating, and adjudicating complaints of ethical misconduct lodged against members and credentialed providers, respectively. Similar administrative procedures apply to disciplinary actions taken by state regulatory entities against health care professionals, with the additional consideration that disciplinary actions by public agencies meet constitutional due process requirements.

The most important consideration that health care professionals should remember is that ignorance of one's ethical responsibilities, just like ignorance of the law, is not a valid excuse for noncompliance.

Cases and Questions

1. As an individual or group exercise, identify as many practices as possible, under managed health care, that may create ethical dilemmas. How might individual health care professionals or groups of professionals focus attention on and help to resolve such dilemmas?

2. As an individual or group exercise, examine your discipline's code of ethics. Is it comprehensive in scope? If not, what provisions are missing?

Suggested Answers to Cases and Questions

1. Managed care may adversely affect health care professionals and patients in several ways. For patients, freedom of choice is limited, as may be the right to be informed of all reasonable options to a proposed treatment in informed consent processes (autonomy). It may also be unjust and unsafe for non-health professionals to make triaging decisions concerning provision of care (justice, nonmaleficence). The denial of the most effective treatment or intervention, based on a cost-benefit analysis, may work adversely to a patient's best interests (beneficence). For providers, dual loyalties to patients and managed care organizations may create irreconcilable conflicts of interest, especially where the provider's compensation is based on a minimization of financial outlays by the organization (beneficence, nonmaleficence, justice). Compliance with a gag order limiting information disclosure during informed consent processes is evidence that a provider places a contractual business relationship above the exercise of independent judgment and respect for patient autonomy.

2. A code of ethics governing a health care discipline should:

- be grounded in the fundamental ethical principles of beneficence, nonmaleficence, autonomy, and justice
- address the conduct of all personnel within the discipline
- address conduct in all settings, including, but not limited to, clinical practice, research, education, and home
- include directive (mandatory compliance) and nondirective (requested compliance) guidance

Acknowledgment

I wish to publicly thank and recognize Mr. Paul Ellsworth, MPH, OTR, FAOTA, Associate Professor, Department of Occupational Therapy, University of Texas Health Science Center, San Antonio, Texas, for his review of this chapter and sage comments before it was submitted for final publication.

References

1. Anderson, G.R., Glesnes-Anderson, V.A. *Health Care Ethics: A Guide for Decision Makers*. Gaithersburg, MD: Aspen Publishers, Inc., 1987, pp. 7–8.
2. Kyler-Hutchinson, P. *Everyday Ethics: Common Concerns in Occupational Therapy*. Rockville, MD: American Occupational Therapy Association, 1995, pp. 14–21.
3. Purtilo, R. *Ethical Dimensions in the Health Professions*, 2nd ed. Philadelphia, PA: W.B. Saunders Company, 1993, pp. 49–57.
4. Mappes, T.A., Zembaty, J.S. *Biomedical Ethics*, 3rd ed. New York: McGraw-Hill, Inc., 1991, pp. 16–21.
5. *Ibid.* at 29–30.
6. "HMO Backlash Spurs Wave of Restrictive Legislation." *San Antonio Express-News*, March 15, 1996, p. 10B.
7. The Family Educational Rights and Privacy Act of 1974, 20 United States Code Section 1232 *et seq.*
8. Beauchamp, T.L., Childress, J.F. *Principles of Biomedical Ethics*, 4th ed. New York: Oxford Press, 1994, pp. 120–394.
9. "Core Values and Attitudes of Occupational Therapy Practice." *American Journal of Occupational Therapy*, 1993; 47(12):1085–1086.
10. *Guide for Professional Conduct*. Alexandria, VA: American Physical Therapy Association, Judicial Committee, 1996.
11. *Guide for Conduct of the Affiliate Member*. Alexandria, VA: American Physical Therapy Association, Judicial Committee, 1996.
12. Section 4.3, Research, reads:

    A. Physical therapists shall support research activities that contribute knowledge for improved patient care.
    B. Physical therapists engaged in research shall ensure:

1. the consent of subjects;
2. confidentiality of the data on individual subjects and the personal identities of the subjects;
3. well-being of all subjects in compliance with facility regulations and the laws of the jurisdiction in which the research is conducted;
4. the absence of fraud and plagiarism;
5. full disclosure of support received;
6. appropriate acknowledgment of individuals making a contribution to the research; and
7. that animal subjects used in research are treated humanely and in compliance with facility regulations and laws of the jurisdiction in which the research experimentation is conducted.

C. Physical therapists shall report to appropriate authorities any acts in the conduct or presentation of research that appear unethical or illegal.

13. *Occupational Therapy Code of Ethics*. Rockville, MD: American Occupational Therapy Association, 1994.

14. "HMO Backlash Spurs Wave of Restrictive Legislation." *San Antonio Express-News*, March 15, 1996, p. 10B.

15. Portney, L.G., Watkins, M.P. *Foundations of Clinical Research: Applications to Practice*. Norwalk, CT: Appleton & Lange, Publishing, 1993, pp. 27–31.

16. *Title 45 Code of Federal Regulations, Part 46: Protection of Human Subjects*. Washington, DC: Department of Health and Human Services, 1983.

17. *On Being a Scientist: Responsible Conduct in Research*, 2nd ed. Washington, DC: National Academy Press, 1995, pp. 6–8.

18. *Ibid*. 8–18.

19. *Guide for Professional Conduct*. Alexandria, VA: American Physical Therapy Association, Judicial Committee, Section 1.1, 1996.

20. *Ibid*. Section 5.2C.

21. *Ibid*. Section 8.1

22. *Occupational Therapy Code of Ethics*. Rockville, MD: American Occupational Therapy Association, 1994.

23. Principle 1D of the *Occupational Therapy Code of Ethics*, like Section 8.1 of the American Physical Therapy Association's *Guide for Professional Conduct*, addresses the provision of services for socioeconomically disadvantaged patients. It reads:

    Occupational therapy personnel shall strive to ensure that fees are fair, reasonable, and commensurate with the service performed and *are set with due regard for the service recipient's ability to pay* [emphasis added].

    Note that, unlike the physical therapy ethical provision on pro bono service, the occupational therapy standard is directive in tenor.

24. *Commonalities and Differences Between the Professions of Physical Therapy and Occupational Therapy: An American Physical Therapy Association White Paper*. Alexandria, VA: American Physical Therapy Association, 1995, p. 32.

25. *Procedural Document on Disciplinary Action of the American Physical Therapy Association*. Alexandria, VA: Judicial Committee, American Physical Therapy Association, 1996, as amended.

26. *Commonalities and Differences Between the Professions of Physical Therapy and Occupational Therapy: An American Physical Therapy Association White Paper*. Alexandria, VA: American Physical Therapy Association, 1995, p. 34.

27. *Enforcement Procedure for Occupational Therapy Code of Ethics*. Bethesda, MD: American Occupational Therapy Association, 1988, as amended.

28. *Occupational Therapy Board Announces New Certification Renewal Program, Changes Name*. Press Release, Gaithersburg, MD: National Board for Certification in Occupational Therapy, April 4, 1996.

29. *Procedures for Disciplinary Action*. Gaithersburg, MD: National Board for Certification in Occupational Therapy, 1989.

30. In states where unlicensed practitioners fall outside of the jurisdiction of regulatory agencies, standards and disciplinary action are taken by the Office of the State Attorney General. For more on this topic, see "Disciplinary Procedures & Unlicensed Practitioners." *Federation of State Boards of Physical Therapy Newsletter*, 1996; 11(1):2.

31. *Medical Boards of California Action Report*, January 1995, p. 13.

32. "License Suspension for Non-Payment of Child Support." *Communique: Texas Board of Physical Therapy Examiners*, Fall 1995, p. 1.

33. Kyler-Hutchinson, P. *Everyday Ethics: Common Concerns in Occupational Therapy*. Rockville, MD: American Occupational Therapy Association, 1995, p. 31.

34. Bennett, J.J. Memorandum. October 11, 1995, p. 3.

Suggested Readings

1. Anderson, G.R., Glesnes-Anderson, V.A. *Health Care Ethics: A Guide for Decision Makers*. Gaithersburg, MD: Aspen Publishers, Inc., 1987.

2. Beauchamp, T.L., Childress, J.F. *Principles of Biomedical Ethics*, 4th ed. New York: Oxford Press, 1994.

3. *Commonalities and Differences Between the Professions of Physical Therapy and Occupational Therapy: An American Physical Therapy Association White Paper*. Alexandria, VA: American Physical Therapy Association, 1995.

4. "Core Values and Attitudes of Occupational Therapy Practice." *American Journal of Occupational Therapy*, 1993; 47(12):1085–1086.

5. "Disciplinary Procedures & Unlicensed Practitioners." *Federation of State Boards of Physical Therapy Newsletter*, 1996; 11(1):2.

6. *Enforcement Procedure for Occupational Therapy Code of Ethics*. Bethesda, MD: American Occupational Therapy Association, 1988, as amended.

7. *Guide for Conduct of the Affiliate Member*. Alexandria, VA: Judicial Committee, American Physical Therapy Association, 1996.

8. *Guide for Professional Conduct*. Alexandria, VA: Judicial Committee, American Physical Therapy Association, 1996.

9. "HMO Backlash Spurs Wave of Restrictive Legislation." *San Antonio Express-News*, March 15, 1996, p. 10B.

10. Jonsen, A.R., Siegler, M., Winslade, W.J. *Clinical Ethics: A Practical Approach to Ethical Decisions in Clinical Medicine*, 3rd ed. New York: McGraw-Hill, Inc., 1992.

11. Kyler-Hutchinson, P. *Everyday Ethics: Common Concerns in Occupational Therapy*. Rockville, MD: American Occupational Therapy Association, 1995.

12. Mappes, T.A., Zembaty, J.S. *Biomedical Ethics*, 3rd ed. New York: McGraw-Hill, Inc., 1991.

13. Monagle, J.F., Thomasma, D.C. *Health Care Ethics: Critical Issues*. Gaithersburg, MD: Aspen Publishers, Inc., 1994.

14. *Occupational Therapy Code of Ethics*. Rockville, MD: American Occupational Therapy Association, 1994.

15. *On Being a Scientist: Responsible Conduct in Research*, 2nd ed. Washington, DC: National Academy Press, 1995.

16. Portney, L.G., Watkins, M.P. *Foundations of Clinical Research: Applications to Practice*. Norwalk, CT: Appleton & Lange, Publishing, 1993.

17. *Procedural Document on Disciplinary Action of the American Physical Therapy Association*. Alexandria, VA: Judicial Committee, American Physical Therapy Association, 1996.

18. *Procedures for Disciplinary Action*. Gaithersburg, MD: National Board for Certification in Occupational Therapy, 1989.

19. Purtilo, R. *Ethical Dimensions in the Health Professions*, 2nd ed. Philadelphia, PA: W.B. Saunders Company, 1993.

20. The Family Educational Rights and Privacy Act of 1974, 20 United States Code Section 1232 *et seq.*

21. *Title 45 Code of Federal Regulations, Part 46: Protection of Human Subjects*. Washington, DC: Department of Health and Human Services, 1983.

Future Directions

The organization and processes for delivery of health care services are in a state of great flux. Fundamental changes in health care delivery affect providers, professions, organizations, governmental entities, and, most importantly, patients. While health care service delivery is a business, it is more than merely another commercial enterprise. Health care professionals stand in a fiduciary relationship with their patients, in a direct and important way unlike any other professionals, except perhaps attorneys vis-a-vis their clients. For that reason, it is awkward, if not inappropriate, to label health care an "industry."

Under managed care, characterized by a strong, new emphasis on the dollar value of health professional services, the inherent ethical dilemma surrounding the conflict of interest between provider and health care organizational self-interest and interest in the welfare of patients is made more pronounced. The preeminent duty owed by a health professional is always to the patient. The legal system will continue to zealously protect patient rights, because the law has not changed to a significant degree to accommodate the business of managed care.

Many good things have come from managed health care delivery thus far. Cost-containment, seriously undertaken at all levels, will prevent bankruptcy of the health care delivery system. The opening up of the traditional practices and interventions of health professionals to public and scientific scrutiny is likewise beneficial, and will hopefully lead to validation of (and routine reimbursement for) the most efficacious procedures. Similarly, the formalization of acceptable practice parameters in the form of guidelines and (where appropriate) protocols will clarify the meaning of the standard of care and lead to a diminution in health care malpractice litigation.

There is evidence that managed care, as a business concept, has reached the limit of its usefulness in multiple areas; for example, in establishing the appropriate length of patient hospitalizations (Anders, *Wall Street Journal*, May 2, 1996, p. B8). As the United States and the world evolve from a dollar-focused system of managed care to a patient-welfare-focused system of managed health over the next several years and decades, the process of fine-tuning the massive, beautiful, and critically important health care delivery system will be complete.

Table of Cases Cited

Table of Statutes, Regulations, Treaties, and Declarations Cited

Glossary of Terms

Abandonment: improper unilateral termination by a treating health care provider of a professional-patient relationship.

Actual causation: a situation in which, but for a defendant's conduct, a plaintiff would not have sustained injury.

Actus reus: (Latin for "criminal act"); one of two essential components of a crime.

Administrative law: all of the legal principles governing the activities and procedures of federal, state, and local governmental agencies, boards, commissions, and similar entities.

Advance directives: legal instruments memorializing personal choices concerning the drafter's authorization for life-sustaining interventions in the event of that individual's subsequent incompetence.

Affidavit: sworn statement.

Answer: a defendant's initial responsive pleading, in which the defendant responds to the charges in the plaintiff's complaint.

Antitrust law: laws whose primary purpose is to promote competition among businesses for the benefit of the public.

Apparent agency: a legal concept under which an employer may be held liable for a contractor's conduct, when the contractor is indistinguishable from an employee in the eyes of the public.

Appeal: mandatory or discretionary review of a criminal or civil case by an appellate judicial body.

As a matter of law: a binding legal conclusion by a judge in a case.

Assault: reasonable anticipation or fear by a person of an impending battery.

Assumption of the risk: a defense to a tort action, based on the argument that the plaintiff voluntarily accepted the risks of harm associated with a known dangerous activity.

Autonomy: a foundational ethical principle, which recognizes the right of self-determination in patients.

Battery: unjustified and unexcused harmful, offensive, or otherwise impermissible intentional contact by a tortfeasor with another person.

Beneficence: a foundational ethical principle, under which a health professional's conduct relative to a patient is carried out in accordance with the patient's best interests.

Beyond a reasonable doubt: criminal law standard of proof of a defendant's guilt, to a moral certainty.

Bilateral contract: two or more parties legally obligated to perform under contract.

Bona fide occupational qualification (BFOQ): a (rarely allowed) legal justification for employment discrimination based on gender, religion, or national origin.

Breach of contract: failure of a party to a contract to perform as promised.

Breach of warranty: failure of a commercial product to meet promised or reasonably expected performance standards.

Burglary: the unlawful breaking and entering onto another's property, with the specific intent to commit a felony crime on the victim's premises.

Business disparagement: verbal or other communication that harms a target person's business reputation in the community.

Business torts: wrongs committed against the legitimate proprietary interests of individuals, partnerships, or corporations.

Capacity: legal ability of prospective parties to enter into enforceable contracts; in criminal proceedings, the ability of a defendant to understand charges and assist in the defense of the case.

Case in chief: a party's substantive case presentation, intended to meet all legal burdens of proof and persuasion.

Caveat emptor: "Let the buyer beware," used to imply that parties to business contracts personally bear the full risks of their contractual undertakings.

Civil law: the law governing private legal actions initiated by one or more private plaintiffs against one or more private defendants.

Claims-made professional liability insurance: requires liability clams to be made while a health care professional is still insured by an insurer in order to be payable under the policy.

Clear and convincing evidence: an intermediate-tier standard of proof in a legal case, equating to "much more probable than not."

Clinical affiliation agreement: contract between an academic institution and a clinical site for health student intern placement.

Code of Federal Regulations: 50 bound volumes containing federal administrative agency rules and regulations.

283

Collateral estoppel: prohibition against relitigating an issue that has already been adjudicated.

Collateral source rule: a legal rule under which a jury in a tort case is prevented from learning of a plaintiff's collateral sources of recovery for injuries, such as personal insurance.

Collective bargaining: (organized) labor-management negotiations over compensation, benefits, and conditions of employment.

Commercial speech: business speech protected under the First Amendment, but to a lesser degree than literary or political speech.

Common law: judge-made case law.

Comparative fault: the process of apportioning culpability between a plaintiff and defendant in a civil case, with a proportional reduction in monetary damages according to the percentage of fault attributed to the plaintiff.

Compensatory damages: monetary damages designed to make a tort victim "whole."

Complainant: a person initiating adverse administrative or professional association action against a member-health care professional.

Complaint: a plaintiff's initial pleading, detailing allegations of wrongdoing or other conduct that justify a legal remedy.

Condition precedent: a precondition to an obligation to perform under a contract.

Condition subsequent: a contingent event terminating a future performance obligation under contract.

Conditions concurrent: simultaneous performance conditions under contract.

Consequential damages: contractual monetary damages awarded to an aggrieved party for indirect financial losses.

Consideration: the process of mutual bargaining between contractual parties, evidenced by legal benefit or detriment to the parties.

Contract: bargained-for promises between parties, enforceable as legal obligations.

Contributory negligence: conduct by a plaintiff which falls below a standard mandated by law for self-protection against unreasonable harm.

Copyright: federal statutory protection of an author's expression of a creative idea from infringement by others.

Corporate liability: primary health care organization liability for negligent hiring, oversight, or retention of professional personnel.

Corporation: form of business organization recognized as a legal entity apart from its owners (shareholders) who have only limited liability for the obligations of the corporation.

Counteroffer: a new offer made by an offeree after rejecting a contractual offer.

Covenant not to compete: a provision in an employment contract restricting an employee's right to compete with the employer after termination of employment.

Crime: conduct which violates a recognized duty owed to society as a whole, for which society will demand satisfaction in the form of punishment.

Criminal negligence: gross negligence or recklessness punishable as a criminal offense.

Damages: money awarded to a plaintiff in a tort case designed to make the plaintiff whole.

Defamation: false communication of purported fact about a person that harms the victim's positive personal reputation in the eyes of a significant number of other people in the victim's community.

Defamation per quod: a communication which, although not defamatory on its face, becomes defamatory when coupled with an extrinsic fact.

Defamation per se: a clearly defamatory communication that is actionable without proof of damages.

Defendant: a party against whom litigation is initiated.

Deponent: a party or witness undergoing a deposition.

Deposition: pre-trial civil litigation discovery procedure consisting of sworn testimony of parties and witnesses.

Development: as a human resource management concept, the furtherance of knowledge or skill under education or training.

Dicta: judicial remarks not directly related to a court's decision in a case.

Directive professional ethical principles: those provisions in a code of ethics demanding compliance by members of the profession.

Disability: a physical or mental impairment that substantially limits one or more major life activities.

Discovery: the pre-trial processes of gathering evidence and formulating a case strategy and trial tactics.

Disparate impact: neutral employment practices that have a particular adverse impact on protected classes of workers.

Disparate treatment: intentional employment discrimination against protected classes of workers.

Diversity of citizenship: a basis for federal jurisdiction, when all plaintiffs are citizens of different states than are all defendants.

Do not resuscitate (DNR) orders: medical orders precluding the automatic initiation of cardiopulmonary resuscitation efforts for a patient in cardiorespiratory distress.

Due process: a federal constitutional protection, requiring government to treat people with fairness and to afford them notice and opportunity to be heard on governmental actions affecting them.

Durable power of attorney for health care decisions: a legal instrument giving a surrogate decision maker the right to make health care decisions for a legally incompetent principal.

Education: acquisition of general or specific knowledge, with or without specific learning goals.

Emergency doctrine: an exception to the requirement to obtain patient informed consent, applicable when a patient presents with a life-threatening emergency and is unable to communicate his or her wishes regarding treatment due to incapacitation. Absent knowledge of contrary patient desires, it is presumed that life-saving medical intervention is desired.

Employment at will: the common law doctrine that permits an employee or employer to unilaterally terminate the employment relationship without adverse legal consequences.

Equal protection: a federal constitutional protection, requiring government to treat similarly-situated people in a similar manner.

Ethics: principles governing the official conduct of professional or institutional group members; doing what is "right" under the circumstances.

Exculpatory release: an attempt, by one party, to limit that party's tort liability by contract.

Execution: full performance of contractual obligations by one or more parties to an agreement.

Expectancy damages: contractual damages for breach of contract that give the aggrieved party the full benefit of the contractual bargain.

Expert witness: one who is qualified based on in-depth knowledge about a material issue in a trial and familiarity with the applicable standard of care in the jurisdiction.

Extenuation and mitigation: factors offered by a criminal defendant in the sentencing phase of trial, or by a respondent in an adverse administrative proceeding, to lessen the severity of sanctions awarded.

Fair use doctrine: a provision of copyright law permitting the use or reproduction of copyrighted works for limited purposes.

False imprisonment: an intentional tort involving the unlawful restriction of a person's free movement.

Felony: a major crime, punishable by imprisonment for greater than one year or by death.

Fiduciary: one in a special position of trust vis-a-vis another person, such as the duty owed by a health care professional or attorney to a patient or client.

Four-fifths rule: evidence of possible employment discrimination based on demonstrated job selection rates for protected classes of job applicants less than 80 percent of that of the group with the highest selection rate.

Fraud: the intentional false representation (or concealment) of a material fact, designed to deceive another person, which causes that person to act (or not act) in some manner, to the victim's legal detriment.

General damages: the portion of a monetary judgment paid to a successful tort plaintiff for pain and suffering and the loss of enjoyment of life.

General partnership: contractual agreement between two or more parties to operate a business for profit, each having equal control over and bearing full liability for its operation.

Good Samaritan immunity: statutory immunity from liability for simple negligence incident to rendering emergency aid to an accident victim.

Guilt: culpability in a criminal case.

Health care malpractice: liability of health care providers for patient injury, caused by professional negligence, breach of a contractual promise, intentional conduct, dangerously defective treatment products, or abnormally dangerous treatment activities.

Health maintenance organization (HMO): managed care organization type characterized by integration of financing and delivery of health services to member subscribers.

Hearsay: out-of-court statements offered as evidence in legal proceedings for the truth of the matter asserted in them (i.e., "second-hand" speech).

Hold harmless: contractual promise in which one party agrees to indemnify another against financial risk of loss.

Homicide: the killing of one human being by another.

Hostile work environment: a type of legally-actionable sexual harassment case in which sexual harassment unreasonably interferes with either the target victim's or another person's work performance.

Human resource management: the comprehensive workplace management of the complex needs and wants of an organization's human (labor) resources.

Immunity: nonliability: sovereign- (governmental), charitable- (applicable to a religious or other non-profit entity).

Impeachment: legal challenge of a witness by opposing counsel.

Impossibility of performance: a legal defense to performance under a contract, which discharges contractual obligations by operation of law.

Incidental damages: contractual monetary damages directly incurred incident to performance by the aggrieved party.

Incident report: memorialization of facts surrounding an adverse event, such as patient injury, designed to

285

(1) alert management to safety concerns, and (2) create a legal record.

Independent contractor: a person who works independently of detailed control by an employer and for whose conduct the employer is not normally vicariously liable.

Infancy: minority; legal incapacity to contract or commit a crime.

Informed consent: the right of a patient or research subject to make a knowing, intelligent, voluntary, and unequivocal decision to accept or reject treatment or participation in an activity based on disclosure of the nature of the intervention, its material risks of harm, reasonable alternatives, and expected benefits.

Injunction: an equitable order by a court to a defendant to refrain from undertaking or continuing some offensive activity.

Insanity: a complete defense to criminal guilt, based on a lack of capacity on the part of a defendant to (depending on the jurisdiction) appreciate wrongful conduct, conform conduct to legal requirements, or distinguish right from wrong.

Institutional ethics committee: a multidisciplinary committee in a health care organization that advises physicians, other health professionals, patients, and their significant others on the ethical propriety of health care-related activities.

Institutional review board: a multidisciplinary committee of scientists (including at least one attorney or ethicist) which reviews research protocols involving human subjects for subject safety and informed consent.

Insurance: transfer of risk of financial loss incident to liability from a tortfeasor to a third party.

Intellectual property: writings, computer software, depictions, inventions, symbols, and other intangible creations of the mind.

Intentional infliction of emotional distress: an intentional tort involving extreme, outrageous conduct by a defendant that results in severe emotional distress to a plaintiff.

Intentional torts: intentional wrongs committed against individuals or property.

Interrogatories: formal written questions posed by opponents to parties in civil litigation.

Invasion of privacy: an intentional tort involving either (1) unreasonable intrusion upon a plaintiff's solitude, (2) false light publicity about a plaintiff, (3) misappropriation of a plaintiff's name or likeness, or (4) the public disclosure of private facts about a plaintiff.

Joint venture: business endeavor formed for a specific, limited purpose, whose members have only limited agency (authority) to bind their fellow members.

Judge-alone trial: legal case in which the trial judge acts as fact-finder in place of a jury.

Jurisdiction: the power of a court to adjudicate a legal case.

Justice: as a foundational health care ethical principle, the desire to achieve fundamental fairness in health care delivery, at individual, group, societal, and global levels.

Larceny: the unlawful taking of another's property with the intent to permanently deprive the true owner of its use.

Last clear chance: a contributory negligence concept in which the defendant has the last reasonable opportunity to prevent injuring the plaintiff, but fails to do so.

Liability: culpability in a civil proceeding.

Libel: a defamatory communication transmitted by means other than oral, including written, film, video-and audiotape, and computer transmissions.

Limited liability company: hybrid form of business organization resembling a professional corporation and a partnership.

Limited partnership: business partnership consisting of at least one general partner and one or more limited partners.

Living will: a legal document stating a person's wishes concerning life-sustaining measures to be undertaken in the event of that person's subsequent incompetence.

Loss of consortium: monetary damages paid to the spouse or child of a successful tort plaintiff for the value of lost services, society, and companionship.

Managed care: the integration of financing and delivery of health care services, with primary emphasis on value (optimal quality within cost constraints).

Manslaughter: unlawful homicide without either a specific intent to kill the victim or a reckless disregard for human life.

Mens rea: (Latin for "wrongful state of mind"); one of two essential components of a crime.

Misdemeanor: a crime of relatively minor importance, generally punishable by incarceration for less than one year and/or a fine of less than $1,000.

Moral turpitude: intentional criminal conduct that violates public standards of moral decency.

Murder: the unlawful killing of a person with malice aforethought (premeditation) or reckless disregard for human life.

Mutuality of assent: mutual agreement of parties to a bilateral contract to be legally bound to performance under the agreement, evidenced by mutual consideration.

Negligence: conduct by a person who owes another a legal duty, which falls below a standard established by law for the protection of others against unreasonable risk of harm.

Negligent hiring: primary employer liability for injury to others caused by the employer's failure to take reasonable steps to ascertain that a job applicant poses a danger to others.

Negligent homicide: a crime involving the death of a person by another's grossly negligent conduct.

Nondirective professional ethical principles: those provisions in a code of ethics recommending compliance by members of the profession or permitting specified official conduct.

Nonmaleficence: foundational ethical principle meaning "do no harm."

Occurrence professional liability insurance: indemnifies an insured party for covered adverse incidents which occur while the professional is insured by the insurer, irrespective of when a claim is presented.

Offeree (promisee): a party to whom a contractual offer is made.

Offeror (promisor): a party making an offer to be legally bound to perform under contract.

Ordinary reasonable person standard: legal standard requiring a fact-finder (judge or jury) to put him- or herself into the shoes of an ethereal person of ordinary care and diligence.

Parol evidence rule: a rule of interpretation regarding contracts that disallows evidence of prior or contemporaneous understandings between the parties not made part of the written agreement.

Past recollection recorded: an exception to the hearsay rule allowing introduction of documentation of past events with conditions.

Patent: exclusive grant by the federal government to an original inventor to make, sell, and use an invention for a period of years.

Percipient witness: a fact witness; one who perceives information concerning material issues in litigation.

Per se violations: clearly defined violations of antitrust law, such as price fixing and group boycotts of competitors.

Plaintiff: a party initiating litigation.

Plea bargaining: the formulation of an express contract between the state and a criminal defendant concerning charges, sentencing limitations, and other conditions.

Pleadings: litigation documents.

Police power: the federal constitutional power of states to make and enforce standards for public health and safety.

Preferred provider organization (PPO): managed care organization type characterized by networks of providers providing health services to subscribers at deeply discounted rates.

Premises liability: liability of owners/occupiers of land for injuries incurred by patrons or others coming onto their land.

Preponderance of evidence: civil law and administrative standard of proof by the greater weight of evidence.

Present recollection refreshed: witness recall of past events, induced by words, objects, or other means.

Prima facie evidence: evidence sufficient on its face to establish a disputed fact.

Primary liability: legal responsibility for one's own conduct.

Privacy, constitutional right to: the only implied federal constitutional right; the right to be free of unreasonable governmental intrusion on personal freedom.

Privilege: freedom not to disclose (or allow another to disclose) confidential communications; freedom from liability for defamation.

Probable cause: substantial, objective, credible evidence that a particular suspect committed a specific offense.

Procedural due process: adequate notice to a respondent of an adverse governmental or other official action and a reasonable opportunity to be heard on the matter.

Professional negligence: treatment-related negligence (substandard care).

Progressive discipline: disciplinary action taken against an employee along a continuum of possible actions, ranging at one extreme to no action, to discharge at the other.

Punitive damages: monetary damages designed to punish a tortfeasor and to deter similar future conduct.

Qualified individual with a disability: under the Americans with Disabilities Act, an employee or job applicant who is capable of performing essential job functions with or without reasonable accommodation.

Quasi-contract: (Latin for "analogous to a contract"); a situation in which a contractual-like obligation to perform is implied-in-law to prevent unjust enrichment to the party being obligated to perform.

Quid pro quo: a type of legally-actionable sexual harassment case in which a victim's response to sexual harassment forms the basis for employment-related decisions involving the victim or others.

Qui tam action: civil legal action initiated by a private citizen-informer for fraud.

Race-norming: scaling of raw scores on pre-employment tests for purposes of affirmative action.

Reasonable accommodation: under the Americans with Disabilities Act, any workplace change or adjustment that permits a qualified applicant or employee with a disability to perform the essential functions of a job.

Reliance damages: contractual damages for breach of contract that give the aggrieved party reasonable monetary damages to compensate for the other party's failure to perform.

Remand: the process of an appellate-level court returning a judicial case to a lower-level court for reconsideration.

Remedies: judicial resolutions in civil legal tort cases, to make victims "whole."

Remittitur: discretionary reduction by a judge of jury-awarded monetary damages in a civil legal case.

Reporting statutes: statutes requiring professionals to report certain findings about clients, such as suspected child, domestic, or elder abuse; trauma wounds; and communicable diseases.

Res ipsa loquitur: (Latin for "the thing speaks for itself"); reduction of a tort plaintiff's burden of proof under which a judge permits an inference or mandates a presumption of negligence, when the defendant's conduct makes it impossible for the plaintiff to prevail without such inference or presumption.

Res judicata: ("Latin for "the matter has been settled"); prohibition against relitigating a case that has already been adjudicated.

Respondeat superior: (Latin for "let the master answer"); vicarious liability.

Respondent: a member of a health care (or other) profession against whom a formal administrative or ethical complaint has been lodged.

Restitution damages: contractual damages for breach of contract that return the aggrieved party to the position he or she occupied before beginning performance under the contract (status quo ante).

Restrictive (employment contract) covenant: a contractual provision limiting a party's ability to act without restraint.

Reversible error: mistake by a trial-level judge justifying appellate reversal of the judge's decision in a case.

Risk management: business strategies and tactics designed to minimize organizational liability exposure.

Robbery: the unlawful, forcible taking of a victim's property from the person of the victim.

Sentencing principles: factors considered by a judge or jury in determining a criminal penalty, including retribution, isolation of an offender, specific and general deterrence, and rehabilitation.

Service mark: a distinctive symbol, word, or letter(s) representing a particular business service.

Sexual battery: any nonconsensual touching of a victim's (or perpetrator's) sexual or other body parts (or clothing) for the purpose of arousing or gratifying the sexual desires of either party or for the purpose of sexual abuse of the victim.

Sexual harassment: unwelcome sexual advances, request for sexual favors, and related verbal or physical conduct directed toward another person.

Slander: a defamatory communication transmitted orally or through signing.

Sole proprietorship: form of business organization in which an individual business owner personally controls the business and bears all liability incident to its operation.

Special damages: the portion of a monetary judgment paid to a successful tort plaintiff for specific out-of-pocket losses.

Specific performance: an equitable contract remedy compelling a party to perform as promised under contract.

Spoliation: intentional loss or destruction of documents relevant to litigation.

Stare decisis: (Latin for "the decision stands"); a legal principle requiring lower courts within a jurisdiction to abide by prior judicial pronouncements of higher-level courts within the jurisdiction, applicable to the same or similar facts (precedent).

State action: official governmental conduct triggering constitutional and other civil rights protections.

Statute of frauds: a law requiring certain classes of contracts to be in writing in order to be enforceable.

Statute of limitations: time period after injury during which an injured person must file a civil lawsuit or be forever barred (absent applicability of an exception) from later initiating legal action based on conduct allegedly causing the injury.

Statute of repose: under tort reform, an absolute time period for filing a specific class of legal action, such as a product liability lawsuit.

Statutory rape: consensual sexual relations with a legal minor, punishable as a crime (also called *carnal knowledge*).

Strict liability: liability for consequences of conduct without consideration of fault.

Subpoena duces tecum: a court order requiring a deponent to bring papers or other physical objects with him or her to a deposition or other proceeding.

Substandard care: care that fails to comply with legal and ethical standards; care that fails to meet at least minimally acceptable practice standards.

Substantive due process: the requirement that government treat people fairly when taking action that affects fundamental, important rights and liberties, such as employment and professional licensure.

Summary judgment: formal finding in a judicial proceeding that a case cannot or need not proceed to trial because of insufficient or defective evidence.

Surrogate decision maker: an agent appointed by a principal to make substituted decisions regarding health care and other significant interventions involving the principal.

Therapeutic privilege: an exception to the requirement to obtain patient informed consent, applicable when a physician reasonably believes that a particular patient is unable psychologically to process information concerning the patient's diagnosis or prognosis.

Tolling: suspension of the running of the statute of limitations.

Tort: a private civil wrong (other than breach of contract) that forms the basis for a claim or litigation.

Tortfeasor: wrongdoer.

Tort reform: legislative and judicial measures to prevent abuse of the tort legal system.

Trademark: a distinctive symbol, word, or letter(s) representing a particular product.

Training: the acquisition of job-specific or other activities-of-daily-living (ADL)-related proficiency skills.

Transferred intent: a situation in which a defendant intends to direct conduct toward one person, but unintentionally affects another person.

Treble damages: triple monetary damages available to victorious plaintiffs in antitrust litigation.

Undue hardship: under the Americans with Disabilities Act, employer excusal from reasonable accommodation of a qualified employee or job applicant disability based on excessive cost or disruption of the business.

Unilateral contract: a situation in which one party can consummate a binding contract only by completing some action (or omission) requested by another party.

United States Code: 50 bound volumes containing federal statutory law.

Vicarious liability: indirect legal and financial responsibility for the conduct of another person, such as an employer for an employee or a clinic volunteer.

Whistleblowing: the making of a good-faith report of a suspected violation of law to authorities.

Workers' compensation statutes: provide for income continuation and payment of related medical and rehabilitation expenses for covered employees injured on the job.

Work for hire: a literary work written under contract, the ownership rights of which reside with the entity commissioning the work.

Wrongful death: a tort action in which heirs recover the present economic value of reasonably anticipated future contributions of a decedent lost as a result of a defendant's tortious conduct.

Wrongful discharge: the unjustified termination of an employee.

Wrongful interference with a contractual relationship: wrongful conduct on the part of a person or business entity to intentionally induce another person or business to breach an existing contract.

PURPOSE

This *Guide for Professional Conduct* (Guide) is intended to serve physical therapists who are members of the American Physical Therapy Association (Association) in interpreting the *Code of Ethics* (Code) and matters of professional conduct. The Guide provides guidelines by which physical therapists may determine the propriety of their conduct. The Code and the Guide apply to all physical therapists who are Association members. These guidelines are subject to changes as the dynamics of the profession change and as new patterns of health care delivery are developed and accepted by the professional community and the public. This Guide is subject to monitoring and timely revision by the Judicial Committee of the Association.

INTERPRETING ETHICAL PRINCIPLES

The interpretations expressed in this Guide are not to be considered all inclusive of situations that could evolve under a specific principle of the Code, but reflect the opinions, decisions, and advice of the Judicial Committee. Although the statements of ethical principles apply universally, specific circumstances determine their appropriate application. Input related to current interpretations or to situations requiring interpretation is encouraged from Association members.

PRINCIPLE 1

Physical therapists respect the rights and dignity of all individuals.

1.1 Attitudes of Physical Therapists

   A. Physical therapists shall recognize that each individual is different from all other individuals and shall respect and be responsive to those differences.

   B. Physical therapists are to be guided at all times by concern for the physical, psychological, and socioeconomic welfare of those individuals entrusted to their care.

   C. Physical therapists shall not engage in conduct that constitutes harassment or abuse of, or discrimination against, colleagues, associates, or others.

1.2 Confidential Information

   A. Information relating to the physical therapist/patient relationship is confidential and may not be communicated to a third party not involved in that patient's care without the prior written consent of the patient, subject to applicable law.

   B. Information derived from component-sponsored peer review shall be held confidential by the reviewer unless written permission to release the information is obtained from the physical therapist who was reviewed.

   C. Information derived from the working relationships of physical therapists shall be held confidential by all parties.

   D. Information may be disclosed to appropriate authorities when it is necessary to protect the welfare of an individual or the community. Such disclosure shall be in accordance with applicable law.

1.3 Patient Relations

Physical therapists shall not engage in any sexual relationship or activity, whether consensual, or nonconsensual, with any patient while a physical therapist/patient relationship exists.

1.4 Informed Consent

Physical therapists shall obtain patient informed consent before treatment.

PRINCIPLE 2

Physical therapists comply with the laws and regulations governing the practice of physical therapy.

2.1 Professional Practice

Physical therapists shall provide consultation, evaluation, treatment, and preventive care, in accordance with the laws and regulations of the jurisdiction(s) in which they practice.

PRINCIPLE 3

Physical therapists accept responsibility for the exercise of sound judgment.

3.1 Acceptance of Responsibility

   A. Upon accepting an individual for provision of physical therapy services, physical therapists shall assume the responsibility for evaluating that individual; planning, implementing, and supervising the therapeutic program; reevaluating and changing that program; and maintaining adequate records of the case, including progress reports.

   B. When the individual's needs are beyond the scope of the physical therapist's expertise, or when additional services are indicated, the individual shall be so informed and assisted in identifying a qualified provider.

   C. Regardless of practice setting, physical therapists shall maintain the ability to make independent judgments.

   D. The physical therapist shall not provide physical therapy services to a patient while under the influence of a substance that impairs his or her ability to do so safely.

3.2 Delegation of Responsibility

   A. Physical therapists shall not delegate to a less-qualified person any activity which requires the unique skill, knowledge, and judgment of the physical therapist.

   B. The primary responsibility for physical therapy care rendered by supportive personnel rests with the supervising physical therapist. Adequate supervision requires, at a minimum, that a supervising physical therapist perform the following activities:

   1. Designate or establish channels of written and oral communication.

   2. Interpret available information concerning the individual under care.

   3. Provide initial evaluation.

   4. Develop plan of care, including short- and long-term goals.

   5. Select and delegate appropriate tasks of plan of care.

   6. Assess competence of supportive personnel to perform assigned tasks.

   7. Direct and supervise supportive personnel in delegated tasks.

   8. Identify and document precautions, special problems, contraindications, goals, anticipated progress, and plans for reevaluation.

   9. Reevaluate, adjust plan of care when necessary, perform final evaluation, and establish follow-up plan.

3.3 Provision of Services

A. Physical therapists shall recognize the individual's freedom of choice in selection of physical therapy services.

B. Physical therapists' professional practices and their adherence to ethical principles of the Association shall take preference over business practices. Provision of services for personal financial gain rather than for the need of the individual receiving the services is unethical.

C. When physical therapists judge that an individual will no longer benefit from their services, they shall so inform the individual receiving the services. Physical therapists shall avoid overutilization of their services.

D. In the event of elective termination of a physical therapist/patient relationship by the physical therapist, the therapist should take steps to transfer the care of the patient, as appropriate, to another provider.

3.4 Referral Relationships

In a referral situation in which the referring practitioner prescribes a treatment program, alteration of that program or extension of physical therapy services beyond that program should be undertaken in consultation with the referring practitioner.

3.5 Practice Arrangements

A. Participation in a business, partnership, corporation, or other entity does not exempt the physical therapist, whether employer, partner, or stockholder, either individually or collectively, from the obligation of promoting and maintaining the ethical principles of the Association.

B. Physical therapists shall advise their employer(s) of any employer practice which causes a physical therapist to be in conflict with the ethical principles of the Association. Physical therapist employees shall attempt to rectify aspects of their employment which are in conflict with the ethical principles of the Association.

PRINCIPLE 4

Physical therapists maintain and promote high standards for physical therapy practice, education, and research.

4.1 Continued Education

A. Physical therapists shall participate in educational activities which enhance their basic knowledge and provide new knowledge.

B. Whenever physical therapists provide continuing education, they shall ensure that course content, objectives, and responsibilities of the instructional faculty are accurately reflected in the promotion of the course.

4.2 Review and Self Assessment

A. Physical therapists shall provide for utilization review of their services.

B. Physical therapists shall demonstrate their commitment to quality assurance by peer review and self assessment.

4.3 Research

A. Physical therapists shall support research activities that contribute knowledge for improved patient care.

B. Physical therapists engaged in research shall ensure:

1. The consent of subjects.

2. Confidentiality of the data on individual subjects and the personal identities of the subjects.

3. The well-being of all subjects in compliance with facility regulations and laws of the jurisdiction in which the research is conducted.

4. The absence of fraud and plagiarism.

5. Full disclosure of support received.

6. Appropriate acknowledgment of individuals making a contribution to the research.

7. That animal subjects used in research are treated humanely and in compliance with facility regulations and laws of the jurisdiction in which the research experimentation is conducted.

C. Physical therapists shall report to appropriate authorities any acts in the conduct or presentation of research that appear to be unethical or illegal.

4.4 Education

A. Physical therapists shall support high-quality education in academic and clinical settings.

B. Physical therapists functioning in the educational role are responsible to the students, the academic institutions, and the clinical settings for promoting ethical conduct in educational activities. Whenever possible, the educator shall ensure:

1. The rights of students in the academic and clinical setting.

2. Appropriate confidentiality of personal information.

3. Professional conduct toward the student during the academic and clinical educational processes.

4. Assignment to clinical settings prepared to give the student a learning experience.

C. Clinical educators are responsible for reporting to the academic program student conduct which appears to be unethical or illegal.

PRINCIPLE 5

Physical therapists seek remuneration for their services that is deserved and reasonable.

5.1 Fiscally Sound Remuneration

A. Physical therapists shall never place their own financial interest above the welfare of individuals under their care.

B. Fees for physical therapy services should be reasonable for the service performed, considering the setting in which it is provided, practice costs in the geographic area, judgment of other organizations, and other relevant factors.

C. Physical therapists should attempt to ensure that providers, agencies, or other employers adopt physical therapy fee schedules that are reasonable and that encourage access to necessary services.

5.2 Business Practices/ Fee Arrangements

A. Physical therapists shall not:

1. Directly or indirectly request, receive, or participate in the dividing, transferring, assigning, or rebating of an unearned fee.

2. Profit by means of a credit or other valuable consideration, such as an unearned commission, discount, or gratuity in connection with furnishing of physical therapy services.

B. Unless laws impose restrictions to the contrary, physical therapists who provide physical therapy services in a business entity may pool fees and moneys received. Physical therapists may divide or apportion these fees and moneys in accordance with the business agreement.

C. Physical therapists may enter into agreements with organizations to provide physical therapy services if such agreements do not violate the ethical principles of the Association.

5.3 Endorsement of Equipment or Services

A. Physical therapists shall not use influence upon individuals under their care or their families for utilization of equipment or services based upon the direct or indirect financial interest of the physical therapist in such equipment or services. Realizing that these individuals will normally rely on the physical therapists' advice, their best interest must always be maintained as well as their right of free choice relating to the use of any equipment or service. Although it cannot be considered unethical for physical therapists to own or have a financial interest in equipment companies or services, they must act in accordance with law and make full disclosure of their interest whenever such companies or services become the source of equipment or services for individuals under their care.

B. Physical therapists may be remunerated for endorsement or advertisement of equipment or services to the lay public, physical therapists, or other health care professionals provided they disclose any financial interest in the production, sale, or distribution of said equipment or services.

C. In endorsing or advertising equipment or services, physical therapists shall use sound professional judgment and shall not give the appearance of Association endorsement.

5.4 Gifts and Other Considerations

A. Physical therapists shall not accept nor offer gifts or other considerations with obligatory conditions attached.

B. Physical therapists shall not accept nor offer gifts or other considerations that affect or give an objective appearance of affecting their professional judgment.

PRINCIPLE 6

Physical therapists provide accurate information to the consumer about the profession and about those services they provide.

6.1 Information About the Profession

Physical therapists shall endeavor to educate the public to an awareness of the physical therapy profession through such means as publication of articles and participation in seminars, lectures, and civic programs.

6.2 Information About Services

A. Information given to the public shall emphasize that individual problems cannot be treated without individualized evaluation and plans/programs of care.

B. Physical therapists may advertise their services to the public.

C. Physical therapists shall not use, or participate in the use of, any form of communication containing a false, plagiarized, fraudulent, misleading, deceptive, unfair, or sensational statement or claim.

D. A paid advertisement shall be identified as such unless it is apparent from the context that it is a paid advertisement.

PRINCIPLE 7

Physical therapists accept the responsibility to protect the public and the profession from unethical, incompetent, or illegal acts.

7.1 Consumer Protection

A. Physical therapists shall report any conduct which appears to be unethical, incompetent, or illegal.

B. Physical therapists may not participate in any arrangements in which patients are exploited due to the referring sources enhancing their personal incomes as a result of referring for, prescribing, or recommending physical therapy.

7.2 Disclosure

The physical therapist shall disclose to the patient if the referring practitioner derives compensation from the provision of physical therapy. The physical therapist shall ensure that the individual has freedom of choice in selecting a provider of physical therapy.

PRINCIPLE 8

Physical therapists participate in efforts to address the health needs of the public.

8.1 Pro Bono Service

Physical therapists should render pro bono publico (reduced or no fee) services to patients lacking the ability to pay for services, as each physical therapist's practice permits.

Issued by the Judicial Committee of the American
Physical Therapy Association
October 1981 Last Amended January 1996

Code of Ethics
of the
American Physical Therapy Association

Preamble

This *Code of Ethics* sets forth ethical principles for the physical therapy profession. Members of this profession are responsible for maintaining and promoting ethical practice. This *Code of Ethics*, adopted by the American Physical Therapy Association, shall be binding on physical therapists who are members of the Association.

Principle 1: Physical therapists respect the rights and dignity of all individuals.

Principle 2: Physical therapists comply with the laws and regulations governing the practice of physical therapy.

Principle 3: Physical therapists accept responsibility for the exercise of sound judgment.

Principle 4: Physical therapists maintain and promote high standards for physical therapy practice, education, and research.

Principle 5: Physical therapists seek remuneration for their services that is deserved and reasonable.

Principle 6: Physical therapists provide accurate information to the consumer about the profession and about those services they provide.

Principle 7: Physical therapists accept the responsibility to protect the public and the profession from unethical, incompetent, or illegal acts.

Principle 8: Physical therapists participate in efforts to address the health needs of the public.

Adopted by the House of Delegates, June 1981 Amended June 1987 and June 1991

PURPOSE

This *Guide for Conduct of the Affiliate Member* (Guide) is intended to serve physical therapist assistants who are affiliate members of the American Physical Therapy Association in the interpretation of the *Standards of Ethical Conduct for the Physical Therapist Assistant*, providing guidelines by which they may determine the propriety of their conduct. These guidelines are subject to change as new patterns of health care delivery are developed and accepted by the professional community and the public. This Guide is subject to monitoring and timely revision by the Judicial Committee of the Association.

INTERPRETING STANDARDS

The interpretations expressed in this Guide are not to be considered all inclusive of situations that could evolve under a specific standard of the *Standards of Ethical Conduct for the Physical Therapist Assistant*, but reflect the opinions, decisions, and advice of the Judicial Committee. Although the statements of ethical standards apply universally, specific circumstances determine their appropriate application. Input related to current interpretations or to situations requiring interpretation is encouraged from Association members.

STANDARD 1

Physical therapist assistants provide services under the supervision of a physical therapist.

1.1 Supervisory Relationships

Physical therapist assistants shall work under the supervision and direction of a physical therapist who is properly credentialed in the jurisdiction in which the physical therapist assistant works.

1.2 Performance of Service

A. Physical therapist assistants may not initiate or alter a treatment program without prior evaluation by and approval of the supervising physical therapist.

B. Physical therapist assistants may modify a specific treatment procedure in accordance with changes in patient status.

C. Physical therapist assistants may not interpret data beyond the scope of their physical therapist assistant education.

D. Physical therapist assistants may respond to inquiries regarding patient status to appropriate parties within the protocol established by a supervising physical therapist.

E. Physical therapist assistants shall refer inquiries regarding patient prognosis to a supervising physical therapist.

STANDARD 2

Physical therapist assistants respect the rights and dignity of all individuals.

2.1 Attitudes of Physical Therapist Assistants

A. Physical therapist assistants shall recognize that each individual is different from all other individuals and shall respect and be responsive to those differences.

B. Physical therapist assistants shall be guided at all times by concern for the dignity and welfare of those patients entrusted to their care.

C. Physical therapist assistants shall not engage in conduct that constitutes harassment or abuse of, or discrimination against, colleagues, associates, or others.

2.2 Request for Release of Information

Physical therapist assistants shall refer all requests for release of confidential information to the supervising physical therapist.

2.3 Protection of Privacy

Physical therapist assistants must treat as confidential all information relating to the personal conditions and affairs of the persons whom they serve.

2.4 Patient Relations

Physical therapist assistants shall not engage in any sexual relationship or activity, whether consensual or nonconsensual, with any patient while a physical therapist assistant/patient relationship exists.

STANDARD 3

Physical therapist assistants maintain and promote high standards in the provision of services, giving the welfare of patients their highest regard.

3.1 Information About Services

A. Physical therapist assistants may provide consumers with information regarding provision of services within the protocol established by a supervising physical therapist.

B. Physical therapist assistants may not use, or participate in the use of, any form of communication containing a false, fraudulent, misleading, deceptive, unfair, or sensational statement or claim.

3.2 Organizational Employment

Physical therapist assistants shall advise their employer(s) of any employer practice that causes them to be in conflict with the *Standards of Ethical Conduct for the Physical Therapist Assistant*.

3.3 Endorsement of Equipment

Physical therapist assistants may not endorse equipment or exercise influence on patients or families to purchase or lease equipment except as directed by a physical therapist acting in accord with the stipulation in paragraph 5.3.A. of the *Guide for Professional Conduct*.

3.4 Financial Considerations

Physical therapist assistants shall never place their own financial interest above the welfare of their patients.

3.5 Exploitation of Patients

Physical therapist assistants shall not participate in any arrangements in which patients are exploited. Such arrangements include situations in which referring sources enhance their personal incomes as a result of referring for, delegating, prescribing, or recommending physical therapy services.

STANDARD 4

Physical therapist assistants provide services within the limits of the law.

4.1 Supervisory Relationships

Physical therapist assistants shall comply with all aspects of law. Regardless of the content of any law, physical therapist assistants shall provide services only under the supervision and direction of a physical therapist who is properly credentialed in the jurisdiction in which the physical therapist assistant works.

4.2 Representation

Physical therapist assistants shall not hold themselves out as physical therapists.

STANDARD 5

Physical therapist assistants make those judgments that are commensurate with their qualifications as physical therapist assistants.

5.1 Patient Treatment

Physical therapist assistants shall report all untoward patient responses to a supervising physical therapist.

5.2 Patient Safety

A. Physical therapist assistants may refuse to carry out treatment procedures that they believe to be not in the best interest of the patient.

B. The physical therapist assistant shall not provide physical therapy services to a patient while under the influence of a substance that impairs his or her ability to do so safely.

5.3 Qualifications

Physical therapist assistants may not carry out any procedure that they are not qualified to provide.

5.4 Discontinuance of Treatment Program

Physical therapist assistants shall discontinue immediately any treatment procedures which in their judgment appear to be harmful to the patient.

5.5 Continued Education

Physical therapist assistants shall continue participation in various types of educational activities which enhance their skills and knowledge and provide new skills and knowledge.

STANDARD 6

Physical therapist assistants accept the responsibility to protect the public and the profession from unethical, incompetent, or illegal acts.

6.1 Consumer Protection

Physical therapist assistants shall report any conduct which appears to be unethical or illegal.

Issued by the Judicial Committee of the
American Physical Therapy Association
October 1981
Last Amended January 1996

American Physical Therapy Association
Standards of Ethical Conduct
for the Physical Therapist Assistant

Preamble

Physical therapist assistants are responsible for maintaining and promoting high standards of conduct. These *Standards of Ethical Conduct for the Physical Therapist Assistant* shall be binding on physical therapist assistants who are affiliate members of the Association.

Standard 1: Physical therapist assistants provide services under the supervision of a physical therapist.

Standard 2: Physical therapist assistants respect the rights and dignity of all individuals.

Standard 3: Physical therapist assistants maintain and promote high standards in the provision of services, giving the welfare of patients their highest regard.

Standard 4: Physical therapist assistants provide services within the limits of the law.

Standard 5: Physical therapist assistants make those judgments that are commensurate with their qualifications as physical therapist assistants.

Standard 6: Physical therapist assistants accept the responsibility to protect the public and the profession from unethical, incompetent, or illegal acts.

Adopted by the House of Delegates,
June 1982 Amended June 1991

The American Occupational Therapy Association's *Code of Ethics* is a public statement of the values and principles used in promoting and maintaining high standards of behavior in occupational therapy. The American Occupational Therapy Association and its members are committed to furthering people's ability to function within their total environment. To this end, occupational therapy personnel provide services for individuals in any stage of health and illness, to institutions, to other professionals and colleagues, to students, and to the general public.

The *Occupational Therapy Code of Ethics* is a set of principles that applies to occupational therapy personnel at all levels. The roles of practitioner (registered occupational therapist and certified occupational therapy assistant), educator, fieldwork educator, supervisor, administrator, consultant, fieldwork coordinator, faculty program director, researcher-scholar, entrepreneur, student, support staff member, and occupational therapy aide are assumed.

Any action that is in violation of the spirit and purpose of this Code shall be considered unethical. To ensure compliance with the Code, enforcement procedures are established and maintained by the Commission on Standards and Ethics. Acceptance of membership in the American Occupational Therapy Association commits members to adherence to the *Code of Ethics* and its enforcement procedures.

Principle 1

Occupational therapy personnel shall demonstrate a concern for the well-being of the recipients of their services. (beneficence)

A. Occupational therapy personnel shall provide services in an equitable manner for all individuals.

B. Occupational therapy personnel shall maintain relationships that do not exploit the recipient of services sexually, physically, emotionally, financially, socially or in any other manner. Occupational therapy personnel shall avoid those relationships or activities that interfere with professional judgment and objectivity.

C. Occupational therapy personnel shall take all reasonable precautions to avoid harm to the recipient of services or to his or her property.

D. Occupational therapy personnel shall strive to ensure that fees are fair, reasonable, and commensurate with the service performed and are set with due regard for the service recipient's ability to pay.

Principle 2

Occupational therapy personnel shall respect the rights of the recipients of their services. (autonomy, privacy, confidentiality)

A. Occupational therapy personnel shall collaborate with service recipients or their surrogate(s) in determining goals and priorities throughout the intervention process.

B. Occupational therapy personnel shall fully inform the service recipients of the nature, risks, and potential outcomes of any interventions.

C. Occupational therapy personnel shall obtain informed consent from subjects involved in research activities indicating they have been fully advised of the potential risks and outcomes.

D. Occupational therapy personnel shall respect the individual's right to refuse professional services or involvement in research or educational activities.

E. Occupational therapy personnel shall protect the confidential nature of information gained from educational, practice, research, and investigational activities.

Principle 3

Occupational therapy personnel shall achieve and continually maintain high standards of competence. (duties)

A. Occupational therapy practitioners shall hold the appropriate national and state credentials for providing services.

B. Occupational therapy personnel shall use procedures that conform to the Standards of Practice of the American Occupational Therapy Association.

C. Occupational therapy personnel shall take responsibility for maintaining competence by participating in professional development and educational activities.

D. Occupational therapy personnel shall perform their duties on **the basis of accurate and current information.**

E. Occupational therapy practitioners shall protect service recipients by ensuring that duties assumed by or assigned to other occupational therapy personnel are commensurate with their qualifications and experience.

F. Occupational therapy practitioners shall provide appropriate supervision to individuals for whom the practitioners have supervisory responsibility.

G. Occupational therapists shall refer recipients to other service providers or consult with other service providers when additional knowledge and expertise are required.

Principle 4

Occupational therapy personnel shall comply with laws and Association policies guiding the profession of occupational therapy. (justice)

A. Occupational therapy personnel shall understand and abide by applicable Association policies; local, state, and federal laws; and institutional rules.

B. Occupational therapy personnel shall inform employers, employees, and colleagues about those laws and Association policies that apply to the profession of occupational therapy.

C. Occupational therapy practitioners shall require those they supervise in occupational therapy related activities to adhere to the *Code of Ethics*.

D. Occupational therapy personnel shall accurately record and report all information related to professional activities.

Principle 5

Occupational therapy personnel shall provide accurate information about occupational therapy services. (veracity)

    A. Occupational therapy personnel shall accurately represent their qualifications, education, experience, training, and competence.

    B. Occupational therapy personnel shall disclose any affiliations that may pose a conflict of interest.

    C. Occupational therapy personnel shall refrain from using or participating in the use of any form of communication that contains false, fraudulent, deceptive, or unfair statements or claims.

Principle 6

Occupational therapy personnel shall treat colleagues and other professionals with fairness, discretion, and integrity. (fidelity, veracity)

    A. Occupational therapy personnel shall safeguard confidential information about colleagues and staff members.

    B. Occupational therapy personnel shall accurately represent the qualifications, views, contributions, and findings of colleagues.

    C. Occupational therapy personnel shall report any breaches of the *Code of Ethics* to the appropriate authority.

Prepared by the Commission on Standards and Ethics (SEC) (Ruth Hansen, PhD, OTR, FAOTA, Chairperson).
Approved by the Representative Assembly April 1977.
Revised 1979, 1988, 1994.
Adopted by the Representative Assembly July 1994.
This document replaces the 1988 Occupational Therapy Code of Ethics (American Journal of Occupational Therapy, 42, 795–796), which was rescinded by the 1994 Representative Assembly.

PREAMBLE

The physical therapy profession is committed to provide an optimum level of care and to strive for excellence in practice. The House of Delegates of the American Physical Therapy Association, as the responsible body representing this profession, attests to this commitment by adopting, publishing, disseminating, and promoting the application of the following *Standards of Practice for Physical Therapy*. These *Standards of Practice* are the profession's statement of conditions and performances which are essential for quality physical therapy. They provide a foundation for assessment of physical therapy practice.

ADMINISTRATION OF THE PHYSICAL THERAPY SERVICE

I. Purposes and Goals

A written statement of purposes and goals exists for the physical therapy service which reflects the needs of the individuals served, the physical therapy personnel, the facility, and the community.
Define scope and limitation of service.
Contain current description of purpose.
List objectives and goals of services provided.
Are appropriate for the population (community) served.
Provide a mechanism for annual review.

II. Organizational Plan

A written organizational plan exists for the physical therapy service.
Describes the interrelationships within the overall organization.
Provides for direction of service by a physical therapist.
Defines supervisory functions within the program/service.
Reflects current personnel functions.

III. Policies and Procedures

Written policies and procedures, which reflect the operation of the service, exist and are consistent with the purposes and goals of the physical therapy service.

Address pertinent information about the following:
- Clinical education
- Clinical research
- Criteria for access to, initiation, and termination of care
- Equipment maintenance
- Fire and disaster
- Infection control
- Job descriptions
- Medical emergencies
- Patient care policies and protocols
- Patient rights
- Personnel-related policies
- Position descriptions
- Quality assurance
- Record keeping
- Safety
- Staff orientation
- Supervisory relationships

Meet the requirements of external agencies and state law.
Meet the requirements of the overall organization.
Be reviewed on a regular basis.

IV. Administration

A physical therapist shall be responsible for the direction of the physical therapy service.

Assures that the service is consistent with established purposes and goals.
Assures that the service is provided in accordance with established policies and procedures.
Assures compliance with local, state, and federal requirements.
Complies with current APTA *Standards of Practice* and *Guide for Professional Conduct*.
Reviews and updates polices and procedures as appropriate.
Provides appropriate education, training, and review of physical therapy support personnel.

V. Staffing

The physical therapy personnel are qualified and sufficient in number to achieve the purposes and goals of the physical therapy service.

Meets legal requirements regarding licensure and/or certification of appropriate personnel.
Provides expertise appropriate to the case mix.
Provides adequate staff to patient ratio.
Provides adequate support staff to professional staff.

VI. Physical Setting

1. The physical setting is designed to provide a safe and effective environment that facilitates the achievement of the purposes and goals of the physical therapy service.

Meets all applicable legal requirements for health and safety.
Meets space needs appropriate for the number and type of patients served.

2. Equipment is safe and sufficient to achieve the purposes and goals of the physical therapy service.

Meets all applicable legal requirements for health and safety.
Meets equipment needs appropriate for the number and type of patients served.
Provides for routine safety inspection of equipment by a qualified individual.

VII. Fiscal Affairs

Fiscal planning and management of the physical therapy service are based upon sound accounting principles.

Include preparation and use of a budget.
Conform to legal requirements.
Are accurately recorded and reported.
Provide for optimum use of resources.
Include a plan for audit control.
Establish the basis for a fee schedule consistent with cost of service and within customary norms of fair and reasonable.

VIII. Quality Assurance

A written plan exists for the assessment of, and action to assure, the quality and appropriateness of the physical therapy service.

Provides for a current written plan for assessment of the service.
Provides evidence of ongoing review, evaluation of the service.
Resolves identified problems.
Is consistent with requirements of external agencies.

IX. Staff Development

A written plan exists which provides for appropriate ongoing development of staff.

Is reflected by evidence of ongoing education or attendance at continuing education activities.

PROVISION OF CARE

X. Informed Consent

The physical therapist obtains the patient's informed consent in accordance with jurisdictional law before initiating physical therapy.

XI. Initial Evaluation

The physical therapist performs and records an initial evaluation and interprets results to determine appropriate care for the individual.

> Is initiated prior to treatment.
> Is performed by the physical therapist in a timely manner.
> Is documented, dated, and signed by the physical therapist who performed the evaluation.
> Identifies physical therapy needs of the client.
> Includes pertinent information of the following:

- History
- Diagnosis
- Problem
- Complications and precautions
- Physical status
- Functional status
- Critical behavior/mentation
- Social/environmental needs

> Provides sufficient data to establish time-related goals.

> The physical therapist shall render care within the scope of the physical therapist's education and experience. Appropriate referral to other practitioners shall be made when necessary.

> The physical therapist utilizes objective measures to establish a baseline at the time of the initial evaluation.

> Is documented, dated, and signed by the physical therapist who performed the evaluation.

XII. Plan of Care

1. The physical therapist establishes and records a plan of care for the individual based on the results of the evaluation.

   Includes realistic goals and expected outcome.

   Is based on identified needs.

   Includes effective treatment, frequency, and duration.

   Recommends appropriate coordination of care with other professionals/services.

   Is documented, dated, and signed by the physical therapist who established the plan of care.

2. The physical therapist involves the individual/significant other in the planning, implementation, and revision of the treatment program.

3. The physical therapist plans for discharge of the individual, taking into consideration goal achievement, and provides for appropriate follow-up or referral.

XIII. Treatment

1. The physical therapist provides or delegates and supervises the physical therapy treatment consistent with the results of the evaluation and plan of care.

   Is under the ongoing personal care or supervision of the physical therapist.

   Reflects that delegated responsibilities are commensurate with the qualifications of the physical therapy personnel.

   Is altered in accordance with changes in individual status.

   Is provided at a level consistent with current physical therapy practice.

2. The physical therapist records, on an ongoing basis, treatment rendered, progress, and change in status relative to the plan of care.

XIV. Reevaluation

The physical therapist reevaluates the individual and modifies the plan of care as indicated.

> Is performed by the physical therapist in a timely manner.

> Reflects that the individual's progress is reassessed relative to initial evaluation and plan of care.

> Is documented, dated, and signed by the physical therapist who performed the evaluation.

EDUCATION

XV. Professional Development

The physical therapist is responsible for his/her individual professional development and continued competence in physical therapy.

XVI. Student

The physical therapist participates in the education of physical therapy students and other student health professionals.

RESEARCH

XVII.

The physical therapist utilizes research findings in practice and encourages or participates in research activities.

COMMUNITY RESPONSIBILITY

XVIII.

The physical therapist participates in community activities to promote community health.

LEGAL/ETHICAL

XIX. Legal

The physical therapist fulfills all the legal requirements of the jurisdictions regulating the practice of physical therapy.

XX. Ethical

The physical therapist practices according to the *Code of Ethics* of the American Physical Therapy Association.

American Physical Therapy Association
1111 North Fairfax Street, Alexandria, VA 22314-1488

Preface

These standards are intended as recommended guidelines to assist occupational therapy practitioners in the provision of occupational therapy services. These standards serve as a minimum standard for occupational therapy practice and are applicable to all individual populations and the programs in which these individuals are served.

These standards apply to those registered occupational therapists and certified occupational therapy assistants who are in compliance with regulation where it exists. The term *occupational therapy practitioner* refers to the registered occupational therapist and to the certified occupational therapy assistant, both of whom are in compliance with regulation where it exists.

The minimum educational requirements for the registered occupational therapist are described in the current *Essentials and Guidelines of an Accredited Educational Program for the Occupational Therapist* (American Occupational Therapy Association [AOTA], 1991a). The minimum educational requirements for the certified occupational therapy assistant are described in the current *Essentials and Guidelines of an Accredited Educational Program for the Occupational Therapy Assistant* (AOTA, 1991b).

Standard I: Professional Standing

1. An occupational therapy practitioner shall maintain a current license, registration, or certification as required by law.

2. An occupational therapy practitioner shall practice and manage occupational therapy programs in accordance with applicable federal and state laws and regulations.

3. An occupational therapy practitioner shall be familiar with and abide by AOTA's (1994) *Occupational Therapy Code of Ethics*.

4. An occupational therapy practitioner shall maintain and update professional knowledge, skills, and abilities through appropriate continuing education or in-service training or higher education. The nature and minimum amount of continuing education must be consistent with state law and regulation.

5. A certified occupational therapy assistant must receive supervision from a registered occupational therapist as defined by official AOTA documents. The nature and amount of supervision must be provided in accordance with state law and regulation.

6. An occupational therapy practitioner shall provide direct and indirect services in accordance with AOTA's standards and policies. The nature and scope of occupational therapy services provided must be in accordance with state law and regulation.

7. An occupational therapy practitioner shall maintain current knowledge of the legislative, political, social, and cultural issues that affect the profession.

Standard II: Referral

1. A registered occupational therapist shall accept referrals in accordance with AOTA's *Statement of Occupational Therapy Referral* (AOTA, 1994) and in compliance with appropriate laws.

2. A registered occupational therapist may accept referrals for assessment or assessment with intervention in performance areas, performance components, or performance contexts when individuals have or appear to have dysfunctions or potential for dysfunctions.

3. A registered occupational therapist, responding to requests for service, may accept cases within the parameters of the law.

4. A registered occupational therapist shall assume responsibility for determining the appropriateness of the scope, frequency, and duration of services within the parameters of the law.

5. A registered occupational therapist shall refer individuals to other appropriate resources when the therapist determines that the knowledge and expertise of other professionals is indicated.

6. An occupational therapy practitioner shall educate current and potential referral sources about the process of initiating occupational therapy referrals.

Standard III: Screening

1. A registered occupational therapist, in accordance with state and federal guidelines, shall conduct screening to determine whether intervention or further assessment is necessary and to identify dysfunctions in performance areas.

2. A registered occupational therapist shall screen independently or as a member of an interdisciplinary team. A certified occupational therapy assistant may contribute to the screening process under the supervision of a registered occupational therapist.

3. A registered occupational therapist shall select screening methods that are appropriate to the individual's age and developmental level; gender; education; cultural background; and socioeconomic, medical, and functional status. Screening methods may include, but are not limited to, interviews, structured observations, informal testing, and record reviews.

4. A registered occupational therapist shall communicate screening results and recommendations to appropriate individuals.

Standard IV: Assessment

1. A registered occupational therapist shall assess an individual's performance areas, performance components, and performance contexts. A registered occupational therapist conducts assessments individually or as part of a team of professionals, as appropriate to the practice settings and the purposes of the assessments. A certified occupational therapy assistant may contribute to the assessment process under the supervision of a registered occupational therapist.

2. An occupational therapy practitioner shall educate the individual, or the individual's family or legal guardian, as appropriate, about the purposes and procedures of the occupational therapy assessment.

3. A registered occupational therapist shall select assessments to determine the individual's functional abilities and problems as related to performance areas, performance components, and performance contexts.

4. Occupational therapy assessment methods shall be appropriate to the individual's age and developmental level; gender; education; socioeconomic, cultural, and ethnic background; medical status; and functional abilities. The assessment methods may include some combination of skilled observation, interview, record review, or the use of standardized or criterion-referenced tests. A certified occupational therapy assistant may contribute to the assessment process under the supervision of a registered occupational therapist.

5. An occupational therapy practitioner shall follow accepted protocols when standardized tests are used. Standardized tests are tests whose scores are based on accompanying normative data that may reflect age ranges, gender, ethnic groups, geographic regions, and socioeconomic status. If standardized tests are not available or appropriate, the results shall be expressed in descriptive reports, and standardized scales shall not be used.

6. A registered occupational therapist shall analyze and summarize collected evaluation data to indicate the individual's current functional status.

7. A registered occupational therapist shall document assessment results in the individual's records, noting the specific evaluation methods and tools used.

8. A registered occupational therapist shall complete and document results of occupational therapy assessments within the time frames established by practice settings, government agencies, accreditation programs, and third-party payers.

9. An occupational therapy practitioner shall communicate assessment results, within the boundaries of client confidentiality, to the appropriate persons.

10. A registered occupational therapist shall refer the individual to the appropriate services or request additional consultations if the results of the assessments indicate areas that require intervention by other professionals.

Standard V: Intervention Plan

1. A registered occupational therapist shall develop and document an intervention plan based on analysis of the occupational therapy assessment data and the individual's expected outcome after the intervention. A certified occupational therapy assistant may contribute to the intervention plan under the supervision of a registered occupational therapist.

2. The occupational therapy intervention plan shall be stated in goals that are clear, measurable, behavioral, functional, and appropriate to the individual's needs, personal goals, and expected outcome after intervention.

3. The occupational therapy intervention plan shall reflect the philosophical base of occupational therapy (AOTA, 1979) and be consistent with its established principles and concepts of theory and practice. The intervention planning processes shall include
   - (a) formulating a list of strengths and weaknesses
   - (b) estimating rehabilitation potential
   - (c) identifying measurable short-term and long-term goals
   - (d) collaborating with the individual, family members, other caregivers, professionals, and community resources
   - (e) selecting the media, methods, environment, and personnel needed to accomplish the intervention goals
   - (f) determining the frequency and duration of occupational therapy services
   - (g) identifying a plan for reevaluation
   - (h) discharge planning.

4. A registered occupational therapist shall prepare and document the intervention plan within the time frames and according to the standards established by the employing practice settings, government agencies, accreditation programs, and third-party payers. The certified occupational therapy assistant may contribute to the formation of the intervention plan under the supervision of the registered occupational therapist.

Standard VI: Intervention

1. An occupational therapy practitioner shall implement a program according to the developed intervention plan. The plan shall be appropriate to the individual's age and developmental level, gender, education, cultural and ethnic background, health status, functional ability, interests and personal goals, and service provision setting. The certified occupational therapy assistant shall implement the intervention under the supervision of a registered occupational therapist.

2. An occupational therapy practitioner shall implement the intervention plan through the use of specified purposeful activities or therapeutic methods to enhance occupational performance and achieve stated goals.

3. An occupational therapy practitioner shall be knowledgeable about relevant research in the practitioner's areas of practice. A registered occupational therapist shall interpret research findings as appropriate for application to the intervention process.

4. An occupational therapy practitioner shall educate the individual, the individual's family or legal guardian, non-certified occupational therapy personnel, and non-occupational therapy staff, as appropriate, in activities that support the established intervention plan. An occupational therapy practitioner shall communicate the risk and benefit of the intervention.

5. An occupational therapy practitioner shall maintain current information on community resources relevant to the practice area of the practitioner.

6. A registered occupational therapist shall periodically reassess and document the individual's levels of functioning and changes in levels of functioning in the performance areas, performance components, and performance contexts. A certified occupational therapy assistant may contribute to the reassessment process under the supervision of a registered occupational therapist.

7. A registered occupational therapist shall formulate and implement program modifications consistent with changes in the individual's response to the intervention. A certified occupational therapy assistant may contribute to program modifications under the supervision of a registered occupational therapist.

8. An occupational therapy practitioner shall document the occupational therapy services provided, including the frequency and duration of the services within the time frames and according to the standards established by the employing facility, government agencies, accreditation programs, and third-party payers.

Standard VII: Transition Services

1. The occupational therapy practitioner shall provide community-referenced services, as necessary, to identify occupational performance needs related to transition. Transition involves outcome-oriented actions which are coordinated to prepare or facilitate an individual for change, such as from one functional level to another, from one life stage to another, from one program to another, or from one environment to another.

2. The occupational therapy practitioner shall participate, when appropriate, in preparing a formal individualized transition plan based on the individual's needs and shall assist in the fulfillment of life roles (e.g., independent or community living, self-care, care for others, work, play, and leisure) through activities in such a plan.

3. The occupational therapy practitioner shall facilitate the transition process in cooperation with the individual and the multidisciplinary team or other community support systems (including family members), when appropriate. The registered occupational therapist shall initiate referrals to appropriate community agencies to provide needed services (e.g., direct service, consultation, monitoring).

4. The occupational therapy practitioner shall determine the effectiveness of transition programs and the extent to which individuals have achieved desired transition outcomes (e.g., degree to which the individual is integrated and successful in community living and work environments). This is done in conjunction with the individual and other team members, where appropriate.

Standard VIII: Discontinuation

1. A registered occupational therapist shall discontinue service when the individual has achieved predetermined goals or has achieved maximum benefit from occupational therapy services.

2. A registered occupational therapist, with input from a certified occupational therapy assistant where applicable, shall prepare and implement a discharge plan that is consistent with occupational therapy goals, individual goals, interdisciplinary team goals, family goals, and expected outcomes. The discharge plan shall address appropriate community resources for referral for psychosocial, cultural, and socioeconomic barriers and limitations that may need modification.

3. A registered occupational therapist shall document the changes between the initial and current states of functional ability and deficit in performance areas, performance components, and performance contexts. A certified occupational therapy assistant may contribute to the process under the supervision of a registered occupational therapist.

4. An occupational therapy practitioner shall allow sufficient time for the coordination and effective implementation of the discharge plan.

5. A registered occupational therapist shall document recommendations for follow-up or reevaluation when applicable.

Standard IX: Continuous Quality Improvement

1. An occupational therapy practitioner shall monitor and document the continuous quality improvement of practice, which may include outcomes of services, using predetermined practice criteria reflecting professional consensus, recent developments in research, and specific employing facility standards.

2. An occupational therapy practitioner shall monitor all aspects of individual occupational therapy services for effectiveness and timeliness. If actual care does not meet the prescribed standard, it must be justified by peer review or other appropriate means within the practice setting. Occupational therapy services shall be discontinued when no longer necessary.

3. A registered occupational therapist shall systematically assess the review process of patient care to determine the success or appropriateness of interventions. Certified occupational therapy assistants may contribute to the process in collaboration with the registered occupational therapist.

Standard X: Management

1. A registered occupational therapist shall provide the management necessary for efficient organization and provision of occupational therapy services.

2. A certified occupational therapy assistant, under the supervision of a registered occupational therapist, may perform the following management functions:

(a) education of members of other related professions and physicians about occupational therapy

(b) participation in (1) orientation, supervision, training, and evaluation of the performance of volunteers and other non-certified occupational therapy personnel, and (2) developing plans to remediate areas of skill deficit in the performance of job duties by volunteers and other non-certified occupational therapy personnel

(c) design and periodic review of all aspects of the occupational therapy program to determine its effectiveness, efficiency, and future directions

(d) systematic review of the quality of service provided, using criteria established by professional consensus and current research, as well as established standards for state regulation; accreditation; American Occupational Therapy Certification Board (AOTCB) certification; and related laws, policies, guidelines, and regulations

(e) incorporation of a fair and equitable system of admission, discharge, and charges for occupational therapy services

(f) participation in cross-disciplinary activities to ensure that the total needs of the individual are met

(g) provision of support (i.e., space, time, money as feasible) for clinical research or collaborative research when such projects have the approval of the appropriate governing bodies (e.g., institutional review board), and the results of which are deemed potentially beneficial to individuals of occupational therapy services now or in the future. A

References

American Occupational Therapy Association. (1979). The philosophical base of occupational therapy. *American Journal of Occupational Therapy, 33,* 785.

American Occupational Therapy Association. (1991a). Essentials and guidelines of an accredited educational program for the occupational therapist. *American Journal of Occupational Therapy, 45,* 1077–1084.

American Occupational Therapy Association. (1991b). Essentials and guidelines of an accredited educational program for the occupational therapy assistant. *American Journal of Occupational Therapy, 45,* 1085–1092.

American Occupational Therapy Association (1994). Occupational therapy code of ethics. *American Journal of Occupational Therapy, 48,* 1037–1038.

American Occupational Therapy Association (1994). Statement of occupational therapy referral. *American Journal of Occupational Therapy, 48,* 1034.

Prepared by the Commission on Practice (Jim Hinojosa, PhD, OTR, FAOTA, Chairperson).

Adopted by the Representative Assembly July 1994.

This document replaces the 1992 Standards of Practice for Occupational Therapy (American Journal of Occupational Therapy, 46, 1082–1085) and the 1987 Standards of Practice for Occupational Therapy in Schools (American Journal of Occupational Therapy, 41, 804–808), which were rescinded by the 1994 Representative Assembly.

INDEX